Infant and Early Childhood Mental Health

A Comprehensive
Developmental Approach to Assessment
and Intervention

Infant and Early Childhood Mental Health

A Comprehensive Developmental Approach to Assessment and Intervention

By

Stanley I. Greenspan, M.D.

Clinical Professor of Psychiatry and Pediatrics,
George Washington University Medical School,
Washington, DC

Serena Wieder, Ph.D.

Codirector,
Interdisciplinary Council for Developmental and
Learning Disorders,
Bethesda, Maryland

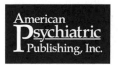

American Psychiatric Publishing, Inc.

Washington, DC
London, England

Copyright © 2006 American Psychiatric Publishing, Inc.
ALL RIGHTS RESERVED
Manufactured in the United States of America on acid-free paper
09   08   07   06   05   5   4   3   2   1
First Edition
Typeset in Italia Medium, AGaramond, and Frutiger 55 Roman.
American Psychiatric Publishing, Inc.
1000 Wilson Boulevard
Arlington, VA 22209–3901
www.appi.org
Library of Congress Cataloging-in-Publication Data
Greenspan, Stanley I.
    Infant and early childhood mental health : a comprehensive, developmental approach /
by Stanley I. Greenspan, Serena Wieder.—1st ed.
        p. ; cm.
    Includes bibliographical references and index.
    ISBN 1-58562-164-1 (pbk. : alk. paper)
    1. Infant psychiatry. 2. Child psychiatry. 3. Infants—Mental health. 4. Preschool
children—Mental health. 5. Toddlers—Mental health.
    [DNLM: 1. Child Development. 2. Early Intervention (Education)—methods.
3. Mental Disorders—diagnosis—Child, Preschool. 4. Mental Disorders—diagnosis—
Infant. 5. Mental Disorders—therapy—Child, Preschool. 6. Mental Disorders—therapy—
Infant. 7. Mental Health—Child, Preschool. 8. Mental Health—Infant.
WS 105 H815i 2005] I. Wieder, Serena. II. Title.
RJ502.5.G725 2005
618.92'89—dc22

                                                                    2005008194

British Library Cataloguing in Publication Data
A CIP record is available from the British Library.

CONTENTS

PART I
A COMPREHENSIVE MODEL
FOR INFANT AND EARLY
CHILDHOOD MENTAL
HEALTH

PART II
PRINCIPLES OF
ASSESSMENT AND
INTERVENTION

PART III
CLASSIFICATION, DIAGNOSIS, AND TREATMENT OF INFANT AND EARLY CHILDHOOD DISORDERS

PART IV
PREVENTION AND EARLY INTERVENTION

Introduction

The field of infant and early childhood mental health is relatively new and offers the prospect of not only early diagnosis and intervention but also prevention. The field covers both healthy functioning and emerging disorders. It includes pioneering studies on early emotional development by Spitz (1945), Erikson (1940), Bowlby (1951), Anna Freud (1965), and Murphy (1974); studies on individual differences by Ayres (1964), Escalona (1968), Murphy (1974), and Brazelton et al. (1974); and studies on caregiver and family dynamics and early intervention by Provence (1983) and Fraiberg and her colleagues (Fraiberg 1980; Fraiberg et al. 1987). It also includes a very detailed modern literature on normal emotional development, psychopathology in infants and young children, and preventive and early intervention. See Sander (1962), Ainsworth et al. (1974), Emde et al. (1976), Sroufe (1979), Stern (1974), Greenspan and colleagues (Greenspan 1979, 1989, 1997; Greenspan and Lourie 1981; Greenspan and Shanker 2004; Greenspan and Wieder 1998, 1999; Wieder and Greenspan 2001), and Shonkoff and Phillips (2000), among others, for a detailed review of this literature.

Even with such pioneers leading the way, it has remained a challenge to map completely the development of emotions and cognition and their relationship. It has also been difficult to construct a truly comprehensive developmental approach to intervention, one that takes into account all aspects of the infant's life, including individual differences in processing experience; developmental abilities; interactive patterns; and caregiver, family, cultural, and community dynamics. In the early 1970s, we had an opportunity to address this challenge. Joined by Reginald Lourie, we developed the Clinical Infant Development Program (CIDP) at the National Institute of Mental Health. CIDP was a comprehensive assessment and intervention program for infants and families with or at risk for a variety of developmental and emotional challenges. With the help of an advisory group that initially included Berry Brazelton, Selma Fraiberg, Sally Provence, Albert Solnit, and Peter Neubauer, we observed and charted children's early emotional milestones (in both healthy and pathological forms), motor and cognitive processing differences, and infant–caregiver and family interaction patterns. On the basis of our observations, we constructed a comprehensive approach to assessment, diagnosis, and intervention.

In 1977, the CIDP "gave birth" to ZERO TO THREE: National Center for Infants, Toddlers, and Families, and subsequently the Interdisciplinary Council for Developmental and Learning Disorders (ICDL). Our work at CIDP laid much of the foundation for *Diagnostic Classification of Mental Health and Developmental Disorders of Infancy and Early Childhood* (ZERO TO THREE Diagnostic Classification Task Force 1994); *Clinical Practice Guidelines* (Interdisciplinary Council for Developmental and Learning Disorders 2000); and more recently, *Diagnostic Manual for Infancy and Early Childhood Mental Health Disorders, Developmental Disorders, Regulatory-Sensory Processing Disorders, Language Disorders, and Learning Challenges* (Interdisciplinary Council for Developmental and Learning Disorders 2005). (See www.icdl.com and www.floortime.org.)

With ongoing clinical experience, we continue to refine this comprehensive developmental approach for children with severe developmental challenges and mental health problems (Greenspan 1981; Greenspan and Shanker 2004; Greenspan and Wieder 1999; Greenspan et al. 1987). This approach includes not only children with emotional and behavioral difficulties but also children with autism spectrum disorders as well as other disorders of relating and communicating, including severe language problems, severe regulatory problems, Down syndrome, fragile X syndrome, fetal alcohol syndrome, cerebral palsy, and even severe forms of attention-deficit/hyperactivity disorder. We are now in a position to truly redefine how we work with these children.

Earlier Models of Treatment and Education

Psychodynamic and Developmentally Informed Therapies

Dynamic interventions typically help children to express feelings through play and talk and to resolve core emotional conflicts. Another typical goal is to help parents who are unwittingly undermining their children's development to change problematic ways of perceiving and interacting with their children. Although dynamic approaches are helpful for some children at some ages, they cannot reach children who can neither speak nor engage in pretend play, including very young children and those with severe language problems. Some of the pioneers cited earlier designed interventions that made use of both psychodynamic understanding and developmental concepts but did not employ a comprehensive developmental model. Selma Fraiberg, for example, developed an "infant–parent psychotherapy" that helped parents resolve internal conflicts and distorted perceptions of their infants that originated in their own early childhood experiences and that prevented them from promoting the infants' healthy development (Fraiberg 1980; Fraiberg et al. 1987).

Behavioral Interventions

Behavioral interventions attempt to promote desired behaviors and to discourage less desirable ones. Behavioral interventions are used for a variety of symptoms. In its time, and for a long time, the behavioral approach was the only intervention approach available for children with autism spectrum disorders and other severe developmental delays. It offered the only alternative to ignoring or simply containing children's aggressive or withdrawn behaviors. An early report on this approach, from a nonexperimental research study of autistic children, was encouraging (Lovaas 1987). However, a more recent study, the only study of behavioral intervention with autistic children that has employed a clinical trial experimental design (i.e., random assignment of subjects to intervention and control groups), showed very modest educational gains and little or no difference in social and emotional functioning between the intervention and control groups (Smith et al. 2000). The behavioral approach made an important contribution by introducing intensity into educational and therapeutic work with children who have severe developmental challenges. Now, however, we can go beyond modifying behaviors and address the underlying developmental processes that are undermining the child's healthy development.

Teaching "Splinter Skills"

Other approaches involve teaching circumscribed cognitive skills to children with autism spectrum disorders and other severe developmental delays. For example, a teacher working with a 3-year-old who has no language might train him to identify shapes by having him match similar shapes in a rote and repetitive way. But this approach works only with isolated cognitive skills.

New Insights

Now, with new understanding of how the mind and brain function, we can employ a comprehensive developmental approach that integrates all the best information we have about how the mind and brain grow. Three insights serve as the cornerstones of a new way of working with infants and children with developmental problems.

1. *Social, emotional, language, and cognitive capacities, including the ability to regulate behavior, impulses, and mood, are all learned through interactive relationships that involve affective exchanges.* The mind and brain grow most rapidly in the early years as an outgrowth of interactions with caregivers. To promote healthy development, these interactions must have several critical features:

- Warmth and security
- Regulation, so that the child does not become overwhelmed
- Relatedness and engagement
- Back-and-forth emotional signaling and gesturing
- Shared social problem solving
- The use of ideas in a meaningful and functional way
- Thinking and reasoning

Most essential to a child's development are multiple interactions with caregivers that involve exchange of emotions and provide a fundamental sense of relatedness. When children are deprived of this relatedness, as we have seen in orphanages and other settings, they fail to grow. Their language and cognition do not develop well. We have seen in our clinical observations and our studies that even the simplest task, such as learning how to say "hello," is dependent on our emotions and our relationships.

The regulation of behavior, impulses, and mood is especially dependent on early relationships. In the early affective interchanges, infants and young children learn to read and respond to emotional and social signals that enable them to organize behavior, mood, and impulses. Emotions are also important when children must master abstract thinking—for example, understanding concepts such as *justice* or *fairness*. To learn such concepts, a child first has to have the experience of being treated fairly or unfairly. By giving a child six apples and then taking them away and giving them to his sister, one teaches him very quickly what unfairness is. The child can then label and abstract from that emotional experience, creating a category of things that are fair and things that are unfair. Without the lived experience, he cannot learn the concept. Every word in our language must be lived first in order to understand it. An apple is defined not only by its redness and roundness but also by how it tastes and what it feels like to throw it. Language, cognition, math, and quantity concepts are all learned through the affective experience of interactive relationships.

We cannot teach children in the old-fashioned ways anymore, particularly children with severe developmental delays and mental health problems. We must work on *relationships*: beyond the relationship between therapist or teacher and child, we must address the family's relationship patterns, because it is within the family as well as the larger community and cultural context that the child's relationships and emotional interactions occur. Intervention for infants and children with mental health problems and special needs must involve a broad relationship-, family-, and community-based approach.

2. *Variations exist in children's underlying motor and sensory processing (i.e., regulatory) capacities.* We have identified the important processing capacities that give rise to many children's worrisome behaviors. We understand how children differ in the way they process sounds (auditory processing and language), the

way they process what they see (visuospatial processing), and the way they plan and sequence actions (motor planning and sequencing). Visuospatial processing enables a child to search for and find a hidden object or to understand that "mommy is in the next room, and I'm here" and hence feel no panic about separation. When the child understands even more—for example, "I'm in school, and mommy is only a few minutes away"—he integrates visuospatial processing with a related concept of time. Some children have robust, age-appropriate processing abilities; in others, one or more processing capacities are impaired in some way.

We also find enormous variations in how well children can plan (and execute) actions. Some children can only bang an object against another object or a surface (a repetitive one-step action) or can only put a toy car in a garage and take it out (two steps). Other children in a similar age range can take the car out of the garage, take it to grandmother's house, make a tea party at grandmother's house, then bring the car back with some extra tea for mommy, who is sitting back at the original house (a complex idea involving more than six steps). This process is called *motor planning and sequencing*, an enormously important capacity for children. Many children with autism spectrum disorders have severe problems with motor planning and sequencing that underlie much of their repetitive behavior. If you cannot plan in sequence, you are going to repeat. Motor planning is extremely important in understanding such symptoms.

We have also observed that many of these children have differences in the way they modulate sensation. Some are very overreactive to things like sound and touch; they cover their ears upon hearing sounds that would not disturb most people, or they push away from people who try to tickle them. Other children crave sensory input and seek more touch or want more noise. Still others crave high levels of sensory input but easily get overloaded because they also have areas of oversensitivity. For these children, it is very hard to find the right sensory pattern to engage them and pull them into human interactions. We find that a lot of children who are self-absorbed are underreactive to stimuli such as touch and sound. Other children are very avoidant and keep running away from people, not because they do not love people but because they are hypersensitive to such stimuli. We need to look at the sensory modulation of each child to find the pattern that will pull that child into a relationship. By addressing the underlying processing differences, one can influence many behaviors and help the child function adaptively in a broad range of areas rather than just working on isolated cognitive skills or behaviors.

3. *A new road map of human development.* Our research has given rise to a new understanding of the early stages of human development. Historically, researchers, clinicians, and educators have thought of development in very isolated ways. For motor development, a timetable was pinpointed for sitting up,

for walking, and so on. In language development, age ranges were identified for making the first sound, speaking the first words, combining two words, and so on. In cognitive development, it was identified when a child searches for a hidden object, when a child can stack blocks in a certain way, and so forth. In social and emotional development, it was recognized when a child learns to greet others, when a child begins playing with peers, when a child will do some pretending. Separate lines of development were identified, considering each area separately as though they functioned independently of one another. For the child, however, these lines of development are intertwined. The child does not somehow isolate his motor skills from his language skills. He does not say, "Well, I'm a 4-year-old motorwise, only a 2-year-old languagewise, and only an 8-month-old socially and emotionally." The child integrates all these functions, much as the members of a basketball team play as an integrated unit. To evaluate a team's effectiveness, one cannot consider each player's skills and performance separately. It is the way in which the members play together that determines whether the team wins or loses.

Based on this understanding, we have developed a new road map illuminating the progressive development of the human "mental team": language, cognition, affect, and emotions. Six developmental stages, or functional emotional developmental capacities, have been identified that children must master in order to function adaptively. An understanding of these levels enables us to identify the underlying reasons (i.e., the missing or incompletely mastered functional capacities or levels) for a child's developmental delays or mental health symptoms. The six levels are

- *Level 1: Shared attention and regulation*
- *Level 2: Engagement and relating*
- *Level 3: Two-way intentional affective signaling and communication.* Back-and-forth emotional signaling involving gestures, smiles, smirks, nods, and so forth
- *Level 4: Long chains of coregulated emotional signaling and shared social problem solving.* Organization of affective gestures into a continuous flow of problem-solving interactions, as demonstrated when a child takes his mother by the hand, walks her to the refrigerator, bangs on the door, and points to the orange juice after mommy opens the door
- *Level 5: Creating representations (or ideas).* The emotional use of ideas in language (e.g., "Me hungry, juice please") or in pretend play (e.g., feeding and hugging dolls)
- *Level 6: Building bridges between ideas: logical thinking*

Each of these levels, or *core developmental capacities*, builds on those the child has already attained. For each of the six levels, we can identify the particular motor skills, language skills, and visuospatial processing skills that are needed to support the child's mastery of that level. This gives us an integrated picture of development. In assessing a particular child and his difficulties, we determine which levels he has mastered and which he has negotiated incompletely or not at all. We then determine how motor and sensory processing differences and family and community interactions have worked together to create the child's difficulties with one or more levels. Armed with this information, we can determine how best to intervene to help the child get on track developmentally.

A Developmental Biopsychosocial Model: The Developmental, Individual-Differences, Relationship-Based Model

The developmental, individual-differences, relationship-based (DIR) model builds on the three insights we have described. The **D** stands for *functional developmental level*: identifying where the child is in his development. The **I** stands for *individual differences* in sensory processing, sensory modulation, and motor planning. The **R** stands for *relationships*: What are the child's relationships with caregivers and others like now, and what patterns of affective interaction would best promote her healthy development?

The DIR model provides a framework for a comprehensive assessment of an infant or child and his family. It enables caregivers, educators, and clinicians to plan an assessment and intervention program that addresses the specific needs of each child and family. The DIR model is not an intervention but a method of analysis that helps clinicians and educators to organize many intervention components into a comprehensive program.

Sometimes, the DIR model is confused with "Floortime." *Floortime* is a specific component of a comprehensive, six-step intervention program based on the DIR model. It involves creating emotionally meaningful interactions that facilitate the child's mastery of the six functional developmental capacities described earlier. Other components of a DIR-based intervention program will vary depending on the child's and family's needs and may include semistructured problem solving, learning interactions, speech therapy, occupational therapy, peer play opportunities, educational programs, and other experiences.

The DIR model is a biopsychosocial framework to understand and organize programs of assessment and intervention for children with developmental delays and mental health problems. It has helped many children with special needs, including autism spectrum disorders, learn to relate to adults and peers with warmth and intimacy, communicate meaningfully with emotional gestures and words, and think with a high level of abstract reasoning and empathy (Greenspan and Wieder 1997; see also "Research Support for a Comprehensive Developmental Approach to Autism Spectrum Disorders and Other Developmental and Learning Disorders: The Developmental, Individual-Differences, Relationship-Based (DIR) Model" at http://www.icdl.com, accessed March 17, 2005).

Organization of This Book

In this book, we describe the DIR model, its theoretical underpinnings, and its use in understanding and treating a wide variety of infant and childhood developmental and mental health challenges.

Part I, "A Comprehensive Model for Infant and Early Childhood Mental Health," provides the reader with a thorough understanding of the DIR model. Chapter 1 ("A Developmental Biopsychosocial Model") describes the model in detail and further explores its theoretical and philosophical underpinnings. Chapter 2 ("The Functional Emotional Stages of Development") describes how biology and experience come together at each developmental stage to shape a child's relative mastery of the six core developmental capacities.

Part II, "Principles of Assessment and Intervention," focuses on principles of assessment and treatment. In Chapter 3 ("Assessment"), we first explain how to observe and analyze evidence of a child's functional emotional developmental stages and capacities. We then describe, step by step, how to conduct a comprehensive evaluation of a child and family. Chapter 4 ("Therapeutic Principles") compares DIR intervention approaches with traditional psychodynamic, behavioral, and developmentally informed interventions; instructs the reader in use of the assessment and intervention tool called "Floortime"; and describes a six-step intervention process. Chapter 5 ("Parent-Oriented Developmental Therapy") describes how to tailor interventions to different kinds of infants and children. Chapter 6 ("Clinical Strategies and Techniques for Different Types of Infants and Young Children") describes interventions that involve working primarily or substantially with a child's parents.

In Part III, "The Classification, Diagnosis, and Treatment of Infant and Early Childhood Disorders," we describe assessment and intervention strategies appropriate for different classes of childhood disorders: interactive disorders (Chapter 7); regulatory-sensory processing disorders (Chapter 8); and neurodevelopmental disorders of relating and communicating, such as autism (Chapter 9). Composite case illustrations at the end of each chapter elaborate the principles of clinical evaluation and intervention discussed.

Part IV, "Prevention and Early Intervention," describes a model for prevention and early intervention programs. In Chapter 10 ("Infants in Multirisk Families: A Model for Developmentally Based Preventive Intervention"), we present a model for a comprehensive preventive intervention program for infants and young children in families facing multiple challenges to healthy development. Chapter 11

("A Model for Comprehensive Prevention and Early Intervention Services for All Families") describes a model for programs to promote healthy emotional, social, and intellectual growth in all infants and young children. In each chapter, case examples illustrate the intervention methods described.

Infant and early childhood mental health is a rapidly growing field. In this work, we present a developmental, biopsychosocial model (the DIR approach) based on observations and research charting the developmental pathways to healthy and disordered emotional, social, and cognitive functioning. We show how this model can guide clinical work with infants and young children and their families. In addition, we describe how this model serves as a basis for the diagnostic classification and treatment of infant and early childhood mental health disorders as well as for working with multirisk families and organizing prevention and education programs.

References

Ainsworth M, Bell SM, Stayton D: Infant–mother attachment and social development: socialization as a product of reciprocal responsiveness to signals, in The Integration of the Child into a Social World. Edited by Richards M. Cambridge, England, Cambridge University Press, 1974, pp 99–135

Ayres AJ: Tactile functions: their relation to hyperactive and perceptual motor behavior. Am J Occup Ther 18:6–11, 1964

Bowlby J: Maternal Care and Mental Health. WHO Monograph No. 51. Geneva, Switzerland, World Health Organization, 1951

Brazelton TB, Koslowski B, Main M: The origins of reciprocity: the early mother–infant interaction, in The Effect of the Infant on Its Caregiver. Edited by Lewis M, Rosenblum L. New York, John Wiley and Sons, 1974

Emde RN, Gaensbauer TJ, Harmon RJ: Emotional Expression in Infancy: A Biobehavioral Study. Psychological Issues Monograph No. 37. New York, International Universities Press, 1976

Erikson EH: Studies in Interpretation of Play, I: Clinical Observation of Child Disruption in Young Children. Genetic Psychology Monograph 22. 1940, pp 557–671

Escalona S: The Roots of Individuality. Chicago, IL, Aldine, 1968

Fraiberg S: Clinical Studies in Infant Mental Health: The First Year of Life. New York, Basic Books, 1980

Fraiberg SH, Adelson E, Shapiro V: Ghosts in the nursery: a psychoanalytic approach to the problems of impaired infant-mother relationships, in Selected Writings of Selma Fraiberg. Edited by Fraiberg L. Columbus, OH, Ohio State University Press, 1987, pp 100–136

Freud A: Normality and Pathology in Childhood: Assessments of Development. New York, International Universities Press, 1965

Greenspan SI: Intelligence and Adaptation: An Integration of Psychoanalytic and Piagetian Developmental Psychology. Psychological Issues Monograph No. 47–48. New York, International Universities Press, 1979

Greenspan SI: Psychopathology and Adaptation in Infancy and Early Childhood: Principles of Clinical Diagnosis and Preventive Intervention. Clinical Infant Reports, No. 1. New York, International Universities Press, 1981

Greenspan SI: The Development of the Ego: Implications for Personality Theory, Psychopathology, and the Psychotherapeutic Process. New York, International Universities Press, 1989

Greenspan SI: The Growth of the Mind and the Endangered Origins of Intelligence. Reading, MA, Addison Wesley Longman, 1997

Greenspan SI, Lourie RS: Developmental structuralist approach to the classification of adaptive and pathologic personality organizations: infancy and early childhood. Am J Psychiatry 138:725–735, 1981

Greenspan SI, Shanker S: The First Idea: How Symbols, Language and Intelligence Evolved From Our Primate Ancestors to Modern Humans. Reading, MA, Perseus Books, 2004

Greenspan SI, Wieder S: Developmental patterns and outcomes in infants and children with disorders in relating and communicating: a chart review of 200 cases of children with autistic spectrum diagnoses. Journal of Developmental and Learning Disorders 1:87–141, 1997

Greenspan SI, Wieder S: The Child With Special Needs: Encouraging Intellectual and Emotional Growth. Reading, MA, Perseus Books, 1998

Greenspan SI, Wieder S: A functional developmental approach to autism spectrum disorders. J Assoc Pers Sev Handicaps 24:147–161, 1999

Greenspan SI, Wieder S, Lieberman A, et al: Infants in Multirisk Families: Case Studies in Preventive Intervention. Clinical Infant Reports No. 3. New York, International Universities Press, 1987

Interdisciplinary Council on Developmental and Learning Disorders Clinical Practice Guidelines Workgroup: Interdisciplinary Council on Developmental and Learning Disorders' Clinical Practice Guidelines: Redefining the Standards of Care for Infants, Children, and Families With Special Needs. Bethesda, MD, Interdisciplinary Council on Developmental and Learning Disorders, 2000

Interdisciplinary Council on Developmental and Learning Disorders Diagnostic Manual for Infancy and Early Childhood Workgroups: Interdisciplinary Council on Developmental and Learning Disorders Diagnostic Manual for Infancy and Early Childhood Mental Health Disorders, Developmental Disorders, Regulatory-Sensory Processing Disorders, Language Disorders, and Learning Challenges. Bethesda, MD, Interdisciplinary Council on Developmental and Learning Disorders, 2005

Lovaas OI: Behavioral treatment and normal educational and intellectual functioning in young autistic children. J Consult Clin Psychol 55:3–9, 1987

Murphy LB: The Individual Child. Publication No. OCD 74–1032. Washington, DC, U.S. Department of Health, Education, and Welfare, 1974

Provence S: Infants and Parents: Clinical Case Reports. Clinical Infant Reports No. 2. New York, International Universities Press, 1983

Sander L: Issues in early mother–child interaction. J Am Acad Child Adolesc Psychiatry 1:141–166, 1962

Shonkoff JP, Phillips DA (eds): From Neurons to Neighborhoods: The Science of Early Childhood Development. Washington, DC, National Academy Press, 2000

Smith T, Groen AD, Wynn JW: Randomized trial of intensive early intervention for children with pervasive developmental disorder. Am J Ment Retard 105:269–285, 2000

Spitz RA: Hospitalism: an inquiry into the genesis of psychiatric conditions in early childhood. Psychoanal Study Child 1:53–74, 1945

Sroufe LA: Socioemotional development, in Handbook of Infant Development. Edited by Osofsky J. New York, John Wiley and Sons, 1979

Stern D: Mother and infant at play: The dyadic interaction involving facial, vocal, and gaze behaviors, in The Effect of The Infant on Its Caregiver. Edited by Lewis M, Rosenblum L. New York, Wiley, 1974

Wieder S, Greenspan SI: The DIR (developmental, individual-difference, relationship-based) approach to assessment and intervention planning. ZERO TO THREE 21:11–19, 2001

ZERO TO THREE Diagnostic Classification Task Force: Diagnostic Classification of Mental Health and Developmental Disorders of Infancy and Early Childhood. Arlington, VA, ZERO TO THREE: National Center for Clinical Infant Programs, 1994

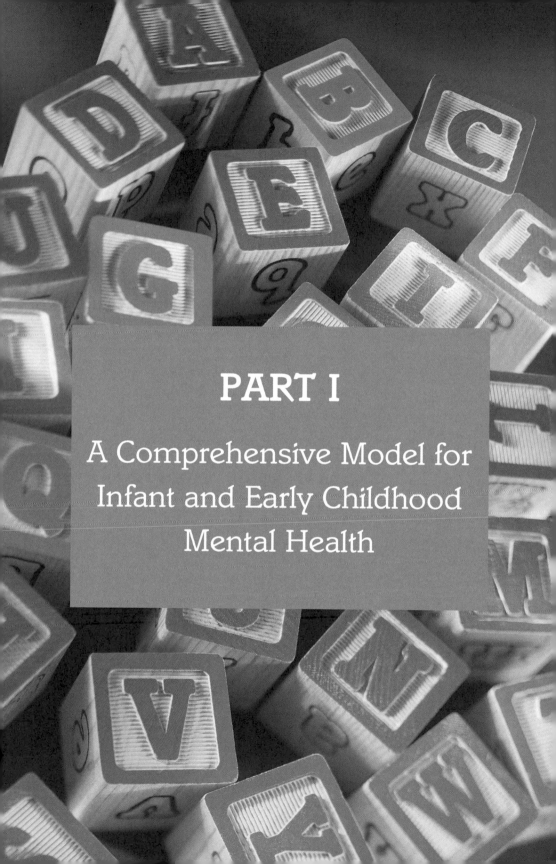

PART I

A Comprehensive Model for Infant and Early Childhood Mental Health

1

A Developmental
Biopsychosocial Model

*The Developmental, Individual-Differences,
Relationship-Based (DIR) Approach*

Our approach to assessment and treatment encompasses three dynamically related influences that work together to direct human development:

1. *The biological and genetic makeup that the infant brings into the world.* This includes relative strengths or weaknesses in auditory processing and language, visuospatial processing, motor planning and sequencing, and sensory and affective modulation. Children's processing capacities mediate the way they interact with those around them.
2. *The social environment, including family dynamics and cultural characteristics, in which the child resides.* Family, cultural, and other environmental factors help shape the thoughts, feelings, and behaviors that caregivers and others bring to their interactions with him or her.
3. *These interaction patterns with others are shaped by the child's biological and genetic makeup (1) and the child's social environment (2); these interaction patterns determine the extent to which the child masters or fails to master several of the six core developmental capacities.* The core developmental capacities include self-regulation, relating to others, preverbal two-way affective communication, and the use of symbols. Successful mastery of these capacities is reflected in adaptive emotional and behavioral functioning; lack of mastery or incomplete mastery results in developmental problems or symptoms.

3

As described in the Introduction, we call our approach to assessing and under-standing the role of these factors in the development of infants and young children the *developmental, individual-differences, relationship-based (DIR) model*. In this model, **D** stands for the core developmental capacities the child needs to master; **I** refers to individual differences, which are the expression of the child's unique bi-ology (genetic, constitutional, and maturational components); and **R** describes the child's relationship with caregivers, family members, and the larger culture.

The goal of assessment is to understand as much as possible about D, I, and R. This understanding sets the stage for intervention, in which the strategy is to tailor interactions with the child, including therapeutic interactions, to his or her individual processing differences (i.e., unique biology). The goal of intervention is to facilitate mastery of each of the core functional emotional developmental capac-ities (e.g., engagement, affect signaling, and symbol formation). Using this model, a clinician can help children and families deal with and overcome emotional and cognitive lags, constrictions, and deficits—as well as associated symptoms—and foster adaptive development.

Functional Emotional Developmental Capacities

The infant or young child's functional emotional developmental level reveals how the child uses everyday functioning to integrate all capacities (social, motor, cog-nitive, language, spatial, and sensory) to carry out emotionally meaningful (i.e., functional) goals. Evidence for the existence of functional emotional develop-mental levels is reviewed elsewhere (Greenspan 1979, 1989, 1992, 1997, 2002; Greenspan et al. 2001; Wieder and Greenspan 2001). Functional capacities in-clude the ability to

1. Attend to multisensory affective experience and, at the same time, attain a calm, regulated state (e.g., looking at, listening to, and following the move-ment of a caregiver).
2. Engage with and display preference and affection toward familiar caregivers (e.g., greeting mother, father, or regular babysitter with joyful smiles).
3. Initiate and respond to two-way presymbolic gestural communication (e.g., trading smiles and vocalizing back and forth with a parent).
4. Organize chains of two-way social problem-solving communications (i.e., open and close several "circles of communication" in a row), maintain commu-nication across space, organize behaviors and affects into purposeful patterns, integrate affective polarities, and synthesize an emerging presymbolic sense of self and other (e.g., taking dad by the hand to get a toy on the shelf).
5. Create and use ideas as a basis for creative or imaginative thinking, giving meaning to symbols (e.g., engaging in pretend play, using words—"Juice!"— to meet needs).

6. Build bridges between two or more ideas. This ability is the basis for logic, reality testing, thinking, and judgment (e.g., engaging in debates, opinion-oriented conversations, or elaborate, planned pretend dramas).

This list reflects the child's progression through developmental stages or levels; each capacity builds on the ones previously attained. A child must first learn to attend and engage before he or she can exchange a series of coos and smiles with the mother. No stage is ever finished, however. The capacities already attained continue to be strengthened and refined. As children grow, they ideally learn to focus attention for longer periods. Their relationships continue to become more subtle and reciprocal. Emotional signaling becomes richer, deeper, and broader.

Each stage involves the simultaneous mastery of what are ordinarily thought of as emotional abilities and cognitive, or intellectual, abilities. A baby learns "causality" through the exchange of emotional signals (by smiling, she can make her parents smile back). This lesson is both emotional and cognitive. In fact, from the earliest moments of life, even our simplest physical experiences have an emotional valence. The sound of mother's voice is not a neutral auditory sensation but is experienced as soothing or aversive, depending on the mother's pitch and emotional tone and the infant's inborn sensitivity to sound. Father's touch is both a tactile sensation and a comforting, or overstimulating and upsetting, experience. At each developmental stage, new cognitive skills are learned from emotional interactions with caregivers.

We call the six core capacities "functional" for two reasons. First, they enable the child to interact with and comprehend his or her world. Second, they orchestrate many other capabilities. For example, as children learn to signal with emotions, in the first year of life, their emotions determine whether they will reach for something (i.e., use the motor system and muscles) and what kinds of vocalizations they will employ (one sound to indicate "I like that," another to say "I don't like that"). Emotions also lead them to search for and find the hidden toy in mommy's hand. Only a desirable toy will be searched for. Searching and finding develop the infant's perceptual-motor and visuospatial problem-solving skills. From early on, therefore, infants' emotions orchestrate the different parts of their minds, enabling the parts to work together in an integrated manner. We call the six core capacities "emotional" to highlight the role of emotions in organizing developmental processes.

Individual Differences in Sensory Modulation, Sensory Processing, and Motor Planning

Biologically based individual differences are the result of genetic, prenatal, perinatal, and maturational variations. The following individual differences can be observed in infants and young children:

1. Sensory modulation, including under- and overreactivity to touch, sounds, sights, smells, tastes, and movements
2. Sensory processing, including auditory processing, language processing, and visuospatial processing. Processing includes the ability to register, decode, and comprehend sequences and abstract patterns.
3. Sensory-affective processing, or the ability to process and respond to affect. This includes the ability to link symbols and actions with emotions and intent. This processing capacity may be especially relevant for individuals with autism spectrum disorders (Greenspan and Wieder 1997, 1998).
4. Muscle tone
5. Motor planning and sequencing, or the ability to purposefully organize a sequence of actions or symbols, including symbols in the form of thoughts, words, visual images, and spatial concepts

Relationships and Interactions

The family, community, and culture in which an infant is embedded will combine with her unique biologically based processing style to shape the kinds of human interactions she experiences. The interaction patterns between the child and her caregivers and family members bring the child's biology into the larger developmental progression. Developmentally appropriate interactions mobilize the child's intentions and affects. They broaden the child's range of experience at each level of development, helping the child move from one functional developmental level to the next. In contrast, interactions that ignore or fail to match the child's functional developmental level or individual differences can undermine progress. For example, a parent who is by nature aloof and taciturn may be unable to fully engage an infant who is by nature underreactive and self-absorbed. This child may not experience enough lively, warm interactions to develop the ability to focus attention and engage emotionally with others.

Understanding how biologically based processing differences and family/caregiver patterns influence each core functional emotional developmental capacity has allowed us to describe the developmental pathways that lead to mental health or to various disorders. This understanding has also helped us to discover methods of early identification and intervention that can help an infant return to an adaptive developmental pathway before problems become chronic. A recent study of more than 15,000 families by the federal government's National Center for Health Statistics showed that including items about functional emotional developmental capacities in a health survey led to the identification of approximately 30% more infants at risk than were identified by earlier surveys that asked only about developmental or emotional problems. Most of these children were not receiving intervention services (Simpson et al. 2003).

Assessment and Treatment Planning Using the DIR Model

An assessment encompassing all aspects of the DIR model requires several sessions with the child and family. It also includes a biomedical evaluation and consultation with other professionals, such as speech pathologists, occupational and physical therapists, teachers, and mental health colleagues. The assessment leads to construction of a functional emotional developmental profile describing the child's six functional emotional developmental capacities (as well as three additional, more advanced capacities, which we describe in Chapter 3, "Assessment"); his or her biologically based processing differences; and the patterns of interaction available to the child at home, in school, with peers, and in other settings.

The profile serves as a basis for determining the specific kinds of experiences the child and his or her family need in order for the child to acquire missing developmental capacities or strengthen underdeveloped ones. The profile thus guides the clinician in creating interventions tailored to the individual child, as opposed to the all-too-common practice of placing children into existing intervention programs based on broad, nonspecific diagnostic criteria. Treatment planning addresses all elements of the DIR model: developmental competencies, individual processing differences, and relationships with family, teachers, peers, and others who play important roles in the child's life.

The functional approach enables the evaluating clinician to consider each of the child's functional challenges separately, explore different possible explanations for them, and resist the temptation to assume prematurely that difficulties are tied together as part of a syndrome. For example, hand flapping is exhibited by children with a variety of motor problems when they become excited or overstimulated. Many conditions, including cerebral palsy, autism, hypotonia, and dyspraxia involve motor problems and, at times, hand flapping. Yet this symptom is often assumed to be uniquely a part of autism. Over time, the functional approach to assessment may help clarify which symptoms are truly unique to particular syndromes, leading to new classifications.

The DIR model emphasizes early, presymbolic levels of functioning. It is in the early developmental stages—associated with the first four functional emotional capacities—that the basic structures of personality are being built. A person's ability or inability to test reality, interact socially, form relationships, control behavior, regulate moods, integrate emotional polarities such as love and anger, and form a sense of self that is cohesive rather than fragmented all have roots in this period of life. A child's personality organization can be thought of as the stage on which his or her current drama—relationships, concerns, wishes, fantasies, feelings—unfolds. An accurate picture of the construction and contours of this stage is essential if we are to fully understand the drama.

The assessment and treatment planning process and the contents of the functional emotional developmental profile are described in detail in Chapter 3, "Assessment."

A Developmental Biopsychosocial Approach

As we have described, the DIR approach attempts to understand the developmental steps or organizations leading to mental health and mental illness. It takes into account biology as well as the experiences of the individual. Not only do biology and experience interact, but at each stage of development they interact in different ways. Between the biologically based characteristics a baby might inherit and his or her behavior as an adult lie many intermediary developmental levels of organization, each of which builds competencies, vulnerabilities, or full-blown disorders.

This building process is especially complex because biology and experience interact bidirectionally. At each developmental stage, experience can alter not only behavior but also the underlying biology of the organism. Learning experiences, for example, change the physical structure of the synapses used by the brain when it converts experience into long-term memory. Extra experiences with one sensory pathway or another increase the neuronal connections in that pathway. In the other direction, certain physical characteristics of the organism tend to invite certain types of experiences. A "floppy" baby with low muscle tone who is underreactive to sound and touch will be somewhat unresponsive, and many parents will respond to the baby's unresponsiveness with a lack of involvement, making the baby even more withdrawn. If we change the direction of this process once again, and the caregiver woos the underreactive baby into especially pleasurable nurturing interactions by being highly energetic and persistent, this same baby becomes outgoing, assertive, curious, and delightful. In our clinical work, we have observed differences in social, language, and cognitive outcomes for such children, depending on how the caregiving environment responds to their inborn characteristics.

Neither biology nor experience, then, is destiny. The baby with low muscle tone can successfully or unsuccessfully negotiate his early capacity for forming relationships. This step will then form the foundation for either intimacy and trust or self-absorption and, perhaps, suspiciousness. The toddler with an inborn tendency to be emotionally labile can experience further and more dramatic mood swings if his caregiver is habitually too intrusive or too withdrawn. With caregivers who can sensitively "upregulate" and "downregulate" their emotional interactions with the child, he will gradually internalize the ability to regulate his own moods.

As we can see from these examples, a baby's biological and genetic makeup does not act directly on her behavior or intrapsychic experience; rather, it influences the ways in which the baby is able to interact with others. Relative strengths or weaknesses in such areas as auditory and language processing, visuospatial processing, and sensory and affective modulation will play a mediating role in the ease or difficulty a child has in relating to those around her. The child brings inborn characteristics to each relationship; caregivers and others in her environment bring their cultural patterns and family dynamics, including their own individual histories. These factors combine to produce the interactions that will, over time, result in the child's relative mastery or nonmastery of what we have labeled the functional emotional developmental capacities. Will the child develop the ability to focus her attention on sights and sounds, and then learn to exchange a series of smiles with her parents? Will the child later learn to communicate using words and ideas? The kinds of interactions regularly available to the child will determine whether she progresses smoothly and adaptively through each successive stage or develops difficulties and disorders along the way.

The DIR Model and Philosophies of Mental Health and Illness

Unfortunately, few children (or adults) who access mental health services ever receive a truly comprehensive, developmentally guided assessment and intervention program. In most cities in the United States and in the world, assessment and treatment are likely to focus far more narrowly on presenting symptoms and observable behaviors. Funding limitations, together with the increased power of managed care companies to control the delivery of health care, have helped shape the current trend toward rapid assessment and time-limited treatment.

A model of mental health and illness that considers only symptoms and behaviors fails to provide a framework for evaluating the adequacy of treatment outcomes. If we limit ourselves to observable phenomena, how are we to determine whether a given treatment improves or undermines a person's capacity to engage in meaningful relationships? Whether it furthers or limits his ability to experience, as well as express, the full range of human feelings, including empathy, compassion, anger, curiosity, loss, and sadness? An overly narrow, phenomenological system of classification, however reliably used, may not pass the fundamental test of validity: it may not actually capture the phenomena it purports to address.

To adequately describe and explain human functioning, we must consider the full range and depth of what it means to be human. Evidence from developmental studies of individuals (Greenspan 1997; Greenspan and Shanker 2004) indicates that human beings

- perceive, move, attend, and self-regulate
- interact, read, and respond to social and emotional cues and experience and express a wide range of emotions such as love, assertiveness, grief, sadness, jealousy, and empathy

- form a sense of self that incorporates many different interaction patterns
- form a sense of self that integrates different wishes, feelings, and emotional polarities, such as love and hate
- regulate mood, behavior, and impulses and engage in ongoing social coregulation of these
- create internal representations, or symbols, that include feelings and wishes, impersonal ideas, and a growing sense of self and others
- categorize internal representations, differentiating between reality and fantasy, self and others, and multiple feelings and wishes; modify wishes and feelings by means of defense mechanisms and coping capacities; and make use of internal representations in self-observation, reflection, and judgment
- broaden and deepen these capacities with each new stage of adaptive development.

To be valid, therefore, any model must address these fundamentally human capacities. All have adaptive developmental sequences and are compromised to varying degrees in different kinds of psychopathology. But how do we define health and pathology? What does it mean to be mentally healthy? Does it mean to be free of symptoms? To have warm, satisfying relationships? To be able to cope with expected stresses? To be successful in one's career? To be joyful and happy?

Does mental health include the ability to tolerate deep levels of loss and sorrow when life's circumstances challenge us? To carry a high moral and ethical standard that can survive even group pressure?

We would answer *yes* to all of the above. As a developmental biopsychosocial approach, the DIR model defines the steps or stages that individuals must master in order to attain the many qualities and capabilities that make up "mental health." As a biopsychosocial model, it offers the promise of understanding internal psychological dynamics while also addressing objective symptoms and other observable, empirically verifiable phenomena.

This model has enabled us to characterize not only healthy development but also the major mental health disorders, enabling early identification as well as prevention. Developmental pathways leading to major depression, bipolar disorder, and other major psychiatric disorders are described in subsequent chapters.

Conclusion

The DIR model builds on a considerable foundation of infant and early childhood research. It provides a comprehensive developmental approach that works with the child's functional emotional developmental capacities, biologically based individual processing differences, and relationships with parents and caregivers as well as the larger context of family and culture. It guides both assessment and intervention and enables parents to facilitate the emotional and cognitive growth of their infants and young children, even those with significant problems. The goal of the DIR model is not merely to help the child overcome presenting problems but rather to enable the child to return to an adaptive developmental pathway.

References

Greenspan SI: Intelligence and Adaptation: An Integration of Psychoanalytic and Piagetian Developmental Psychology. Psychological Issues, Monograph No. 47–48. New York, International Universities Press, 1979

Greenspan SI: The Development of the Ego: Implications for Personality Theory, Psychopathology, and the Psychotherapeutic process. New York, International Universities Press, 1989

Greenspan SI: Infancy and Early Childhood: The Practice of Clinical Assessment and Intervention With Emotional and Developmental Challenges. Madison, CT, International Universities Press, 1992

Greenspan SI: The Growth of the Mind and the Endangered Origins of Intelligence. Reading, MA, Addison Wesley Longman, 1997

Greenspan SI: The Secure Child: Helping Our Children Feel Safe and Confident in an Insecure World. Cambridge, MA, Perseus Publishing, 2002

Greenspan SI, Shanker S: The First Idea: How Symbols, Language and Intelligence Evolved From Our Primate Ancestors to Modern Humans. Reading, MA, Perseus Books, 2004

Greenspan SI, Wieder S: Developmental patterns and outcomes in infants and children with disorders in relating and communicating: A chart review of 200 cases of children with autistic spectrum diagnoses. Journal of Developmental and Learning Disorders 1:87–141, 1997

Greenspan SI, Wieder S: The Child With Special Needs: Encouraging Intellectual and Emotional Growth. Reading, MA, Perseus Books, 1998

Greenspan SI, DeGangi GA, Wieder S: The Functional Emotional Assessment Scale (FEAS) for Infancy and Early Childhood: Clinical and Research Applications. Bethesda, MD, Interdisciplinary Council on Developmental and Learning Disorders, 2001

Simpson GA, Colpe L, Greenspan SI: Measuring functional developmental delay in infants and young children: prevalence rates from the NHIS-D. Paediatr Perinat Epidemiol 17:68–80, 2003

Wieder S, Greenspan SI: The DIR (developmental, individual-difference, relationship-based) approach to assessment and intervention planning. ZERO TO THREE 21:11–19, 2001

2

The Functional Emotional Stages of Development

The Cornerstone of the DIR Model

The developmental, individual-differences, relationship-based (DIR) model recognizes six early stages of development corresponding to the six core capacities described in Chapter 1 ("A Developmental Biopsychosocial Model"). At each successive stage, the infant or child organizes sensory and emotional experience in increasingly complex ways. We refer to these as *levels of development*. For each level, we first consider the adaptive patterns that characterize that level. We then separately examine the two interrelated dimensions of sensory organization and affective organization.

Level 1: Shared Attention and Regulation (0–3 Months)

Adaptive Patterns: Self-Regulation

At birth or shortly thereafter, the infant is capable of initial states of regulation to organize his or her experience in an adaptive fashion. The early regulation of arousal and physiological states is critical for successful adaptation to the environment. It is important in the modulation of sleep–wake cycles and cycles of hunger and satiety. It is needed for mastery of sensory functions and for learning how to calm oneself and respond emotionally to one's environment. It is also important

13

for regulation of attention (Als et al. 1982; Brazelton et al. 1974; Field 1981; Sroufe 1979; Tronick 1989). Self-regulatory mechanisms are complex and develop as the result of physiological maturation, caregiver responsiveness, and the infant's adaptation to environmental demands (Lachmann and Beebe 1997; Lyons-Ruth and Zeanah 1993; Rothbart and Derryberry 1981; Tronick 1989).

During a baby's early months, the caregiver provides sensory stimulation through activities such as play, dressing, and bathing. When the infant is distressed, the caregiver normally soothes her to help her return to a calm, organized state (Als 1982). Parent and infant engage in an interactive process of mutual coregulation: the infant uses the parent's physical and emotional state to organize herself (Feldman et al. 1999; Sroufe 1996). This synchronization of states lays the groundwork for the infant's later ability to be emotionally attuned to other people. It is the precursor to social referencing and preverbal communication.

During this early stage of life, the infant is learning to tolerate the intensity of arousal and to regulate his internal states so that he can maintain an interaction while gaining pleasure from it (Sroufe 1979). This has been called *affective tolerance*, or the ability to maintain an optimal level of internal arousal while remaining engaged in the stimulation (Fogel 1982). At first, the parent must act to help regulate the infant's arousal level; once the infant can regulate himself, the parent works to facilitate his self-regulating responses. Brazelton et al. (1974) observed how mothers attempt to synchronize their behavior with their infants' natural cycles. For example, a mother generally reduces her facial expressiveness when her baby gazes away from her but will maintain her expressiveness when the baby looks directly at her (Kaye and Fogel 1980).

An infant who does not develop affective tolerance may withdraw from arousing stimuli. As a result, he may have difficulty forming and maintaining relationships. Field (1977, 1980) proposed an "optimal stimulation" model of affect and interaction. If the mother provides too much or too little stimulation, the infant withdraws. The optimal level varies considerably from one infant to another, depending on the infant's threshold for arousal, tolerance for stimulation, and ability to self-regulate arousal.

Adaptive Patterns: Attention and Interest in the World

In order to perceive the world outside themselves, infants have to want to look and listen. They may have an innate tendency to find human faces and eyes of interest. Klaus and Kennell (1976) described how newborn babies, if allowed to be in close physical contact with the mother right after birth (and anesthesia has not been used), will immediately begin crawling up her belly to find the breast. Infants seem to be born primed to take interest in their world. From the earliest moments of life, however, the infant requires a relationship to fulfill this potential. The rhythmic, near-synchronous patterns of movement and vocalization between infant and caregiver enable the infant to begin attending to and appreciating the world. In fact, this process begins prenatally. The mother becomes attuned to the fetus's movement patterns and responses to sound and other stimuli, and she begins to fantasize about her new baby. Their emotional relationship has already begun.

Through repeated interactions with the caregiver, a baby gradually becomes more and more interested in sights, sounds, touch, and other stimuli. She begins discriminating between different stimuli. However, just as infants can fail to develop affective tolerance, they can fail to become invested in the world outside themselves. In order to elicit the baby's interest and attention, the stimulation the caregiver provides must generally be emotionally pleasurable. If it is aversive, the baby will withdraw or shut down.

What is pleasant for one infant, however, may be aversive to another. Each infant has her own ways of responding to sights, sounds, smells, touch, and movement. Some babies are highly sensitive and require gentle soothing. Others are underreactive and require more energetic wooing. Some babies discern patterns of sights and sounds quickly, others more slowly. Some will immediately turn toward a new sound or sight, whereas others take longer to notice. The infant therefore depends on her caregiver's ability to fit gaze, voice, and way of moving to her unique way of taking in and responding to the world.

The positive impact of pleasurable stimulation, and the detrimental effects of too much aversive stimulation, on the baby's ability to attend to the world suggests that from the beginning of life, emotions play a critical role in our development of cognitive faculties. In observational studies of healthy and developmentally challenged infants, we have observed that every sensation, as it is registered by the child, also gives rise to an affect or emotion (Greenspan 1979, 1989, 1997). In other words, the infant responds to the sensation's emotional as well as its physical impact. A blanket may feel smooth *and* pleasant or itchy *and* irritating, a toy bright red *and* intriguing or boring, a voice loud *and* inviting or jarring. As a baby's experiences multiply, sensory impressions become increasingly tied to feelings. We call this the *dual coding* of experience.

Humans begin this coupling of phenomena and feelings at the very beginning of life. Infants only days old react to sensations emotionally, preferring the sound and smell of their mothers, for example, to all other voices and scents. They suck more vigorously when offered sweet liquids. By 4 months of age, a child can react with fear to the sight or voice of particular persons who have scared him. In order to understand how and why this dual coding varies from infant to infant, we must first consider the infant's organization of sensory experience.

Sensory Organization

Biologically based variations in sensory and motor functions influence the ability of an infant to simultaneously self-regulate and take an interest in the world. Despite widely held, and long-held, assumptions that we all experience sensations such as sound or touch in more or less the same way, significant variations are now known to exist in the ways that individuals process even very simple sensory information. This observation was initially made years ago by Jean Ayres (1964), a pioneer in occupational therapy, and the issue continues to be discussed in the occupational therapy literature.

Each sensory pathway may be hyperarousable (e.g., the baby overreacts to normal levels of sound, touch, or brightness) or hypoarousable (e.g., the baby hears and sees but gives no sign of emotional or behavioral responses to routine sounds or sights). In addition, subtle information processing impairments can be present in each pathway, whether or not that pathway is hyper- or hypoarousable. Problems in the functioning of a pathway can limit the range of sensory experience available to the infant. In our research and clinical work, we have observed babies who brighten up or calm in response to visual experience but have difficulty responding to sound. When presented with auditory stimuli, they may be relatively unresponsive, become overexcited, or appear confused. (A 2-month-old baby may be defined as confused when, instead of looking toward a normal, high-pitched maternal voice and becoming alert, she makes random movements—suggesting that she has indeed heard the sound—yet repeatedly looks past the person making the sound and continues moving randomly.) Other babies appear to have no problems with vision and hearing but have a more difficult time using touch and movement to regulate themselves and connect with their world. Such babies often become irritable in response to even gentle stroking and become hyperaroused when held vertically, calming down only when held horizontally. Still others can calm down only when rocked to their own heart rate, their respiratory rate, or their mother's heart rate. The roles of proprioceptive and vestibular pathways in infant psychopathology are very important areas for future research.

Not only do infants use several sensory pathways, they also integrate experiences across the senses (Spelke and Owsley 1979). Some infants can use each pathway but have difficulty, for example, integrating vision and hearing. They can brighten up in response to a sound or a visual cue, but they cannot turn and look at a stimulus offering visual and auditory information simultaneously. Instead, they appear confused and may even actively avert their gaze or go into a pattern of extensor rigidity.

Another variety of processing disorder may impair the infant's ability to connect a new stimulus with stored images or action patterns. An infant who cannot integrate new sights, sounds, or other sensory information with previous experiences will have ongoing difficulties making sense of his experience.

An infant's experience of sensory pathways is usually observed in sensorimotor patterns. Turning toward a stimulus or brightening and becoming alert can be thought of as motor "outputs." Some babies have trouble integrating their sensory experience with motor output. Most obvious are the difficulties experienced by babies with severe motor impairments, but it is possible to observe more subtle impairments in such basic abilities as nuzzling in the corner of mother's neck or relaxing to rhythmic rocking. Escalona's (1968) classic descriptions of infants with multiple sensory hypersensitivities require further study as part of a broader approach to understanding subtle impairments in each sensory pathway as well as in higher levels of sensory integration.

Affective Organization: The Dual Code

Because of inborn differences in sensory processing, the emotional experience of a stimulus will vary from infant to infant. Differences in sensory reactivity can make the same sound—for example, a high-pitched voice—strike one person as exciting and invigorating but another as piercing and shrill. A gentle caress may tickle one person but painfully startle another, like a touch on sunburned skin. Each of us, over time and quite unwittingly, creates a personal and sometimes quite idiosyncratic "catalog" of integrated sensory and affective experience.

Furthermore, each of an infant's sensory experiences occurs in the context of a relationship that gives it additional emotional meaning. Nearly all her early feelings, positive and negative, involve the caregivers on whom she depends for survival. Having a bottle, for example, might mean the bliss of love and satiation with a warm, generous mother or fear, hunger, and frustration with a stiff, peremptory attendant who snatches the nipple away on schedule.

The emotional quality of an infant's experience, therefore, is shaped by his sensory organization and the nature of his interactions with caregivers. Impairments in sensory processing and integration, together with maladaptive child–caregiver interactions, may result in the child's inability to organize experience of entire "affective themes," such as dependency or aggression. A baby with a tendency toward hyper- or hypoarousal may have difficulty experiencing joy, pleasure, or exploration, especially if his caregivers are unable to adapt their style of interaction to his needs. Instead, he may become withdrawn and apathetic or disregard entire sensory realms while overfocusing on others (for example, staring for a long time at an inanimate object while ignoring the humans around him).

Sensorimotor dysfunction can profoundly affect a child's emotional and relational experience. Children with sensorimotor dysfunction typically have trouble using the range of sensory experiences available to them for learning; as a result, they may be unable to organize purposeful, goal-directed movement and socially adaptive behavior. These difficulties often cause such children to respond maladaptively in forming emotional attachments. For example, tactile hypersensitivity, high muscle tone, or poor muscle coordination may cause a baby to arch away from her mother when she is held or breastfed; this tendency will affect her mother's ability to respond warmly and consistently, especially if the baby's sensorimotor problems have not been identified and the mother interprets the baby's behavior as deliberate avoidance or evidence of her own inadequacy. An older child with low muscle tone or poor sensorimotor feedback may have problems sequencing actions, a high need for physical contact, or inappropriate affect during interactions with others. As a result, the child may suffer emotionally because she cannot successfully play with her peers.

Some investigators have explored sensory, motor, and affective differences in the context of research on temperament. Temperamental differences have been shown to influence children's intrapsychic development and ways of relating to others (Campos et al. 1989). Temperamental qualities characterized as "difficult," for example, have been linked to later psychopathology (Thomas and Chess 1984). (An infant with a difficult temperament has irregular body functions, unusually intense reactions, a tendency to withdraw from new situations, a generally negative mood, and a tendency to adapt slowly to change [Thomas et al. 1968].) The difficult temperament may create problems in self-regulation and infant–caregiver interactions. It is important to remember, however, that neither sensory nor temperamental characteristics alone necessarily predict psychopathology. The effects of such inborn characteristics can be mediated by the attention of a sensitive, responsive caregiver. A caregiver who feels impatient with or threatened by the infant's sensory or temperamental sensitivity and who reacts with abuse or withdrawal may encourage the infant's reliance on ineffective patterns of behavior and further damage the infant's ability to self-regulate. Even when an infant is constitutionally quite competent at self-regulation, a caregiver can fail to draw the infant into a regulating relationship. Dysregulation may occur, for example, if the caregiver is exceedingly depressed or so self-absorbed that he or she does not soothe or woo the new infant.

We have seen how the emotional quality of the infant's experience influences her ability to master the core competencies of this stage of self-regulation and interest in the world. As the infant grows and explores her world, emotions will help her comprehend even what appear to be purely physical or mathematical concepts. She learns "too hot," "too cold," and "just right" through chilly or comforting bottles, pleasant or painful baths. More complex ideas have a similar basis in feelings. "A lot" is a bit more than makes the child happy; "too little" is less than she expected. "More" is another dose of pleasure or of discomfort. "Near" is snuggled next to mother in bed. "Later" is a frustrating stretch of waiting.

Although time and space eventually take on objective parameters, the emotional component persists. Before a child can count, she must have attained an emotional grasp of *quantity* and *extent*. In our clinical work with children facing various challenges who could nonetheless count and even calculate, we found that numbers and computations lacked meaning to them. We had to provide them with an emotional experience of quantity by, for example, arguing with them about how many pennies or candies they should receive.

Level 2: Engagement and Relating (2–7 Months)

Adaptive Patterns

Once the infant has achieved some capacity for self-regulation and interest in the world, he has a greater ability to respond to his environment and form relationships. With warm nurturing, he becomes progressively more interested and invested in his parents or other primary caregivers. By 2–5 months, he can exchange joyful smiles and coos with his mother and experience a deep sense of intimacy. This capacity for engagement is supported by the infant's inborn ability to selectively focus on the human face and voice and to process sensory information (Meltzoff 1985; Papousek 1981; Papousek and Papousek 1979; Stern 1985).

A baby's experience of his primary caregiver as a special person who brings joy and comfort as well as a little annoyance and unhappiness furthers not only his emotional development but also his cognitive development. He begins learning to discriminate the pleasures of human relationships from his interests in the inanimate world. His joy and pleasure in his caregivers enable him to detect and decipher patterns in their voices. He begins to discriminate their emotional states and interpret their facial expressions. His early experience of emotional engagement and attachment starts him on a lifelong journey of learning to recognize patterns and organize perceptions into meaningful categories.

In forming his first intimate relationships, the baby is also beginning his first lesson in becoming a social being. This experience is the cornerstone of functioning as part of a family, group, or community and later in an entire culture and society.

The early quality of engagement between the infant and his caregivers has implications for later attachment patterns and behavior (Ainsworth et al. 1974; Bates et al. 1985; Belsky et al. 1984; Grossmann et al. 1985; Lewis and Feiring 1987; Miyake et al. 1985; Pederson et al. 1990). *Attachment* was described by Bowlby (1969) as the emotional bond between an infant and his primary caregiver. The infant is biologically prepared to use the primary caregiver as a secure base while exploring the environment, returning to the caregiver for comfort when experiencing challenges. The concept of attachment has been expanded to include the infant's capacity to regulate emotions and levels of arousal within the context of the parent–child relationship (Sroufe 1996). When the infant feels distressed, he signals his caregiver; a sensitive and responsive caregiver reads the infant's signals and responds by helping him attain a calm and regulated state.

Atypical attachment patterns can have a negative impact on children's emotional, cognitive, and interpersonal development (Carew 1980). Longitudinal studies have found that securely attached children tend to have better emotional adaptability, social skills, and cognitive functioning (Cassidy and Shaver 1999).

During the school-aged and adolescent years, children who were securely attached as infants were more likely to be accepted by their peers and were better able to form close friendships (Sroufe et al. 1999). A secure attachment seems to provide a protective mechanism for children whose families experience a high level of stress (Egeland and Kreutzer 1991). The key element that underlies a secure attachment is sensitive and responsive caregiving (Ainsworth et al. 1978; De Wolff and van IJzendoorn 1997).

Note that *attachment* has a specific research meaning in studies such as those just cited. In clinical work as well as considerations of normative development, however, it is useful to consider a broader meaning of the word. This involves the overall pattern of relating between an infant and caregiver, including depth of pleasure and range of feelings experienced in the relationship. The processes that define relationships go significantly beyond definitions used in research paradigms (Greenspan 1997).

Sensory Organization

Some babies can adaptively employ all their senses to experience highly pleasurable feelings in their relationships with primary caregivers. The baby with a beautiful smile, looking at and listening to mother, experiencing her gentle touch and rhythmic movements, and responding to her voice with synchronous mouth, arm, and leg movements is perhaps the most vivid example. Clinically, we observe babies who cannot employ their senses to form emotional bonds. In the most extreme cases, the baby actively avoids sensory—and, therefore, emotional—contact with others. She avoids human sounds, touch, and even scents by chronic gaze aversion, recoiling, flat affect, or random and nonsynchronous patterns of brightening and alerting. Other babies can use one or another sensory pathway to experience a pleasurable human relationship but cannot orchestrate the full range and depth of sensory experience. Such a baby might, for example, listen to mother's voice with a smile but avert her gaze and look pained at the sight of mother's face.

Affective Organization

Primary relationships form the context in which the infant can experience a wide range of "affective themes"—comfort, dependency, and joy as well as assertiveness, curiosity, and anger. A healthy 4-month-old can become negative but also may quickly return to his mother's loving smiles and comforting. However, infants and children can already be constricted in their emotional range. Rather than evidencing joy, enthusiasm, or pleasure with their caregivers, they may wear a flat, uninterested expression. Rather than showing periodic assertive, curious, protesting, or angry behavior, they may exhibit only compliance and shallow smiles.

Babies can also evidence a limitation in the stability of their affective organization. Some babies, after hearing a loud noise, cannot quickly resume their engagement with mother. If the environment is frequently disruptive or for other reasons the child's development continues to be disordered, early attachment difficulties may occur. If severe enough, these may form the basis of an ongoing deficit in the baby's capacity to form human connections and to develop the basic personality structures that depend on internalization of relationship experiences.

Level 3: Two-Way Intentional Affective Signaling and Communication (3–10 Months)

Adaptive Patterns

Beginning in the middle of the first year, humans engage in intentional, nonverbal communication. The infant uses facial expressions, arm and leg movements, vocalizations, and spinal posture to engage in back-and-forth emotional signaling with caregivers. This process can be thought of as opening and closing circles of communication. The 6-month-old smiles eagerly at her mother, gets a smile back, then smiles again. By smiling again, the infant is closing a circle of communication. By 8 months, most infants can participate in many of these exchanges in a row.

The infant's ability to use voice and body to purposefully communicate with others plays a critical role in his cognitive development. His two-way emotional signaling with caregivers helps him begin to differentiate between perceptions and actions. It leads to his earliest sense of causality and logic. A smile and squeal of glee directed at father gets a happy expression and sound from him; playfully grabbing his nose causes dad to say, "toot-toot!" From this point onward, causality and logic can play a role in all new learning. For example, the baby will gradually begin applying his emerging sense of logic to the spatial world and the purposeful use of his body. A dropped rattle falls to the ground, and the baby follows it with his gaze. If his father hides the rattle, the baby will look at and touch his father's hand that just hid the object. This emerging sense of causality can be considered the beginning of the baby's appreciation of "reality," his understanding of the world as purposeful rather than random. Contrary to the theories of Piaget (1962), who contended that the infant first develops mental schemes of causality in relationship to the inanimate world, we believe that a sense of causality emerges in the emotional experience of two-way communication and is then generalized to the inanimate world.

Distortions in the emotional communication process—such as those that can occur when parents project their own feelings onto their infant or respond to the infant's vocalizations and gestures in a mechanical, remote manner—can prevent the infant from learning to appreciate cause-and-effect relationships in the arena of feelings. A baby who does not experience shared warmth, closeness, or compassion may never learn how these feelings are elicited in one person by another. This kind of impairment can develop even in an infant who seems to be developing a sense of causality regarding inanimate objects and spatial relationships.

Through repeated engagement in reciprocal, purposeful communication, the baby increasingly experiences her own willfulness and sense of purpose. Her consciousness of herself and the world is growing as she gradually differentiates self from other, the physical world from the emotional world, and a sense of purpose or agency from a swirling sea of sensations, feelings, and responses. The baby's early participation in reciprocal communication helps her begin to distinguish between the "me" who is smiling or cooing and the one who is "not me." At this stage, however, the "me" and "not me" are not defined in the baby's mind as whole persons. The baby's "self" is felt to exist only in terms of the smiles or sounds she is exchanging—that is, each "part" of her that is involved in the communication is experienced as a separate entity. In the next developmental stage, these parts of the self will come together.

Sensory Organization

Some babies are unable to orchestrate their sensory experience in the service of purposeful nonverbal communication. A loving glance or smile from mother does not elicit a look, smile, vocalization, or body movement from the baby. Perhaps this baby perceives the visual stimuli offered but is unable to organize his perceptions or responses and as a result either looks past his mother or makes random movements. Some babies can engage in purposeful communication using one sensory pathway but not another. For example, when presented with an object, the baby may look at it with interest and then examine it. When presented with an interesting sound, however, the same baby does not respond vocally or reach toward the source of the sound but instead behaves chaotically, flailing his limbs and banging his head. A baby who can use his sense of touch in an organized manner may touch his mother's hand in response to mother gently stroking his stomach, whereas a baby with problems processing tactile experience may respond with random or chaotic movements that appear unrelated to the gentle stimulus.

As we can see from these examples, compromises in sensory processing may limit the strategies available to the infant for engaging in purposeful communication. Motor characteristics, such as high or low muscle tone or lags in motor development or motor planning, can affect the infant's ability to signal her feelings and wishes. As a result of such compromises, certain sensory or motor pathways may never become organized at the level of purposeful two-way communication, thus never becoming available to the infant as modes of learning about cause and effect. As we discuss later, these sensory organizational lags have implications for the baby's affective development as well.

At this developmental stage, we begin seeing a shift from proximal to distal modes of communication. *Proximal modes* involve direct physical contact, such as holding, rocking, and touching; *distal modes* involve communication that occurs across space through visual stimuli, auditory cuing, and emotional signaling. A crawling 8-month-old can maintain an emotional connection with his caregiver through reciprocal glances, vocalizations, and emotional gestures. Some babies, however, continue to rely primarily on proximal modes for a sense of security and connection. Early limitations in negotiating space, as we discuss later, can affect the baby's ability to construct internal representations of human relationships.

Affective Organization

In healthy emotional development, the full range of emotions evident in the attachment phase will also be played out in purposeful, two-way communication between the infant and her caregivers. An 8-month-old can experience causality in the area of dependency (she reaches out or makes other overtures to be held and cuddled). She smiles with pleasure at being touched, unless she has a tactile sensitivity. She communicates curiosity and assertiveness as she reaches for the rattle in her babysitter's hand, expresses anger and protest as she intentionally throws food on the floor, and looks at her mother as if to say, "What are you going to do now?" Eight-month-olds can even express defiance, which they often do by biting or butting their heads, because they have better control over their mouths, heads, and necks than over their arms and hands.

When the caregiver fails to respond to the baby's signal, we have observed that the baby's affective-thematic inclinations may fail to become organized at this developmental level. That is, the baby's feelings do not become differentiated from his caregiver's but remain synchronous, as in the attachment phase, or shift from synchronicity to a more random quality. Perhaps the baby can experience a full range of emotions, but these do not become organized into purposeful cause-and-effect interchanges.

A lack of reciprocal responses from caregivers causes many babies to develop a flat affect and a hint of despondency or sadness. This can happen even to babies who have previously exhibited joyfulness and adaptive attachment. In some of these cases, it seems that the baby becomes flat and subdued because caregivers continue to offer only more primitive forms of relatedness instead of advancing to the kinds of interactions that the baby is now capable of. The baby, failing to get a response to her purposeful attempts at communication, does not experience the sense of efficacy that comes from making an impact on other people. Most interesting are the subtle cases in which the baby can reciprocally communicate certain feelings and themes, such as pleasure and dependency, but not others, such as assertiveness, curiosity, and protest. We can imagine how such uneven development occurs as a result of the baby's own temperament and the consequences of expressing each type of feeling in her specific environment. For example, parents who are uncomfortable with closeness and dependency may fail to engage their baby in back-and-forth communication in this domain, while readily engaging her in the less intimate areas of assertion and protest. The baby's own affective-thematic "sending power," combined with the varying responses her communications elicit, may have important implications for how she internally differentiates emotions as well as for how she organizes her internal experience at the symbolic or representational level later on.

Level 4: Long Chains of Coregulated Emotional Signaling and Shared Social Problem Solving (9–18 Months)

Adaptive Patterns

During the second year, the infant makes momentous strides. He begins taking a more active role in developing and maintaining reciprocal relationships with his parents (Bell 1977; Goldberg 1977; Reingold 1969). His interactions with them become increasingly complex (Cicchetti and Schneider-Rosen 1984; Greenspan and Porges 1984; Talberg et al. 1988; Tronick and Gianino 1986). His communication is still largely preverbal, yet he can organize a long series of problem-solving interactions. He takes his father by the hand, gestures with his eyes and hands toward the kitchen door, leads him into the kitchen and up to the refrigerator, and points to the juice carton inside. Assuming his caregivers are able to read his signals and respond to them appropriately, the child increasingly develops the ability to use and respond to social cues, eventually achieving a sense of competence as an autonomous being in relationship with significant others (Brazelton and Als 1979; Lester et al. 1985).

In taking a parent by the hand to go to the refrigerator, a child is learning pattern recognition in several domains. These include her own feelings and desires; the action patterns involved in taking her father's hand, getting to her destination, and getting the object she wants; the visuospatial patterns involved in going from one room to the next and then to the shelf where the juice resides; the vocal patterns needed to get her father's attention; and the social patterns involved in working together with parents toward a common goal. Pattern recognition involves perceiving how the pieces fit together. It enables the child to move beyond isolated, piecemeal actions and to create increasingly elaborate, integrated combinations of emotions and behavior.

As the baby organizes his emotions and behavior into patterns, an early sense of self is forming. At the previous stage, through his involvement in purposeful, two-way communication, he began to distinguish between "me" and "not me." As his repertoire of emotional signaling becomes richer and he begins to discern patterns in his own and others' behavior, he adds these observations to the map delineating himself and others as people. He learns that his mother usually responds when he makes friendly requests but not when he's fussy. His father loves to rough-house but will not sing lullabies. Grandma lets him do things neither parent would allow. Which actions reap affection and approval? Which yield only rejection or anger? Is he worthy of care, attention, and respect? Are those around him also worthy?

As the child improves her ability to imitate others, she begins copying not just discrete actions but large patterns encompassing several actions. She puts on her mother's hat, picks up her purse, hangs it over her own shoulder by the strap, and walks around the house in imitation of her mother's stride. Her ability to discern and create patterns, together with her growing capacity for complex signaling, now enables her to negotiate multiple relationships at the same time. She can send a mischievous grin to dad and immediately follow it with an irritated glance at mom. The toddler's capacities for problem-solving communication, multiple relationships, and rapid learning of whole patterns through imitation lay the foundation for her ability to participate in groups, beginning with her family and moving outward to her community, society, and culture.

Pattern recognition, ideally learned first through social interactions, can then be applied to the physical world as well. Turning this shiny silver knob causes water to gush out of a faucet; holding your palm under the water causes splashing and spills and may bring mother running to turn off the water. Seeing the world in patterns increases understanding of how it works, enabling the child to have expectations and make predictions and thus increasing his sense of mastery. The ability to recognize and organize patterns is an essential component of intelligence, one that the child will build on the rest of his life.

The toddler is simultaneously strengthening several other abilities. More complex vocalizations are emerging, and the child may develop a private language as a prelude to learning the family's language. She develops a more elaborate sense of physical space and improves her visuospatial problem-solving as she learns to search the house for desired toys or people. These developmental gains occur because physical space is now invested with emotional meaning through the pursuit of emotional goals.

Similarly, through interactive play, the child rapidly learns to plan and sequence actions. Given a new toy truck, he may load it, unload it, move it to one side of the room, then back to the other side.

Well before she acquires language and symbols, therefore, the typical child has developed the basic skills that will enable her to learn about her world. She has become a scientific thinker, figuring out and implementing new solutions all the time. She is learning not only about her family and the physical world but also about her culture. Through increasingly complex, emotionally laden chains of interaction with her caregivers, she obtains continual, often unspoken cues and feedback informing her what is good and bad, what is acceptable and unacceptable. Is defiance permissible? Is it better to be aggressive or passive? What's the correct way to greet another person? All of these cultural attitudes and patterns can be learned even before symbolic thought is eminent.

Sensory Organization

A baby's organization of behavior into increasingly complex patterns can be viewed as a task that involves coordinated and orchestrated use of the senses. To reach this level of development, the baby has to be able to process sights and sounds, use reciprocal motor gestures, and comprehend spatial relationships. A toddler who can use vision and hearing to perceive various vocal and facial gestures, postural cues, and complex emotional signals from others is able to extract relevant information and use it in interactions. A toddler who cannot incorporate certain sensory experiences as part of his early cognitive and affective abstracting abilities (Werner and Kaplan 1963) may show signs of a very early restriction in sensory information processing.

Balanced reliance on proximal and distal modes of communication becomes even more important during this stage of development. By looking, listening, and vocalizing across space, a mobile toddler can enjoy her freedom while maintaining her connection with her caregiver. She does not have to tolerate a great deal of insecurity because she can "refuel" (Mahler et al. 1975) distally, moving closer for a cuddle or other proximal contact when necessary. Some children, however, have trouble using distal modes to remain in contact and need to stay physically close to the caregiver. Although this reliance on proximal modes of communication may reflect feelings of insecurity generated by an ambivalent primary caregiver, limitations in the child's own sensory organization can also make important contributions to this pattern.

As a child develops his capacity for complex problem-solving interactions and pattern recognition, he increases his ability to modulate his sensory experience. He is less likely to become overwhelmed or underaroused by sensory stimuli because he can actively participate in shaping his experience of these. He can reach out for just a bit more touch, vocalize to hear just a bit more sound. He can use looks, hand gestures, or body posture to slow down an interaction that has started to become overwhelming.

Affective Organization

As the toddler strings together long chains of back-and-forth communication, her interactions encompass a range of emotions. A healthy toddler may start with a dependent interaction such as cuddling and kissing her parents; shift to an enjoyable, giggly interchange with them; and then jump down and assertively dash into a room she knows is off limits, inviting pursuit. When the parents respond by saying, "No, you can't go in there!" protest and negativism may emerge. Under optimal circumstances, the interaction might close with the toddler back in the playroom, sitting on a parent's lap, enjoying her favorite book. Here the child has gone full circle, suggesting she has made connections between the many affective themes.

The toddler's growing capacity for pattern recognition, developed through repeated experiences of emotional interaction, enables him to become increasingly sophisticated at distinguishing between emotions. He learns to tell approval from disapproval, acceptance from rejection. He begins to use this ability in increasingly complicated social situations. Is his mother's tense face a signal that she is angry with him? The child begins to respond differently to people depending on their emotional tone. For example, he may pull away from a situation that feels undermining. The intuitive ability to decipher human exchanges by picking up emotional cues before any words have been exchanged becomes a "supersense" that often operates faster than our conscious awareness. This supersense is the foundation of our social life.

In a very young infant, anger is explosive, and sadness feels like it will go on forever. Daily loving exchanges and struggles with sensitive caregivers will gradually enable the toddler to turn these raw, extreme emotional reactions into feelings and behavior that are more regulated and modulated. Once a child can exchange rapid, back-and-forth emotional signals with her caregiver, she is able, in a sense, to negotiate how she feels. If she is annoyed, she can make a sound or hand gesture expressing this. Her mother may come back with a gesture indicating, "I understand," or "OK, I'll get your snack more quickly," or perhaps, "Can't you wait just one more minute?" Whatever her response, the child gets immediate feedback that helps her modulate her own response. Her frustration may be tempered by the sense that mother is going to do something to help, even if she cannot do it immediately. Just the sound of mother's voice signals that she is getting that bottle ready, and it is coming soon. If the mother can use a soothing voice and gradually calm the toddler, she will learn not to get so frantic. With a fine-tuned reaction rather than a global and extreme one, she will not need to have a tantrum to register annoyance; she can do it with an expressive glance. Even when an emotionally healthy toddler does escalate to a real tantrum, she does not jump from 0 to 60 in 1 second.

For various reasons, a child may lack the experience of nurturing exchanges that enable him to learn to regulate and modulate feelings. Perhaps he has a motor problem that prevents him from gesturing and signaling well. Perhaps his motor skills are normal but one or both parents are too intrusive and anxious, or too self-absorbed and distant, to respond appropriately to his signals. Such a child gets no feedback fitting his emotional expressions, and he comes to learn that his emotional signals will not lead to a response. His expression of feelings, therefore, never becomes part of a signaling system. It is simply an isolated expression of feeling.

Without the modulating influence of an emotional interaction, the child's feeling may grow more intense, or she may give up and become passive and self-absorbed. In either case, the child is left with only global feelings of anger or rage, fear or avoidance—the sorts of feelings characteristic of very young infants in the early months of life. One of us (S.G.) often sees such children in his practice. In many cases, the children continually hit or bite. The parents seek help, expressing concerns about "aggression" and often requesting that their child be medicated. If the parents are given coaching on how to read the child's signals and respond consistently and calmly, however, within a few months these children can become well-regulated, highly energetic toddlers.

If parents continue to respond inappropriately or not at all, however, the child can become even more vulnerable. Left in the clutches of raw, powerful emotions, many children tend to become more anxious and fearful. When caregivers tune out, freeze up, or slow down too much in response to fierce anger from their infants and toddlers, the child may feel a sense of loss, which can increase her tendency to depression. When anger and impulsive behavior are met by abrupt withdrawal or a single intense, punitive reaction, the child's aggression and impulsiveness tend to increase.

At this developmental stage, children who do have sufficient experience of modulating interactions will begin to develop a more integrated sense of themselves and others. Somewhere between 18 and 24 months of age, a child can experience "me" as no longer just the smile or vocalization or feeling of the moment but as a whole person. Emotional polarities are united in that whole person: the "me" who feels happy is the same person who another time feels angry. "Nice mommy" is no longer experienced as a completely separate person from "frustrating mommy."

Our research on early emotional signaling is shedding some light on the genesis of gender differences. Although individual boys and girls vary considerably, as a group girls tend to develop more empathy and earlier language skills than boys. Prevailing theories state that these gender differences result from differences in the brain structures or hormones of human males and females. Our hypothesis is that, instead, preverbal learning experiences are responsible. Beginning in the cradle, we teach boys and girls differently.

We believe that girls develop deeper empathy and earlier language skills because adults engage female infants and toddlers in longer preverbal emotional "conversations" than they do boys. As a group, boys tend to be more active as babies, inviting shorter bursts of back-and-forth signaling and more roughhousing or other physical play. By regularly engaging girls in longer chains of communication, we enable them to better recognize, modulate, and regulate a wide range of emotions. These abilities lead to earlier symbolic and language skills as well as empathy and concern for others.

Is it any wonder that a child with more extensive early experience in navigating her emotional terrain will grow up better able to understand and express how she feels? Or that a boy who missed out on extensive early emotional interchanges might have some of the deficits or problems we think of as typically male, such as an inability to acknowledge his feelings, a strong desire to separate his emotional world from his rational one, or a habit of using withdrawal or explosive action to discharge uncomfortable feelings?

Our studies of autism also suggest an important role for the affective problem-solving interactions that are a hallmark of this developmental phase. Children with autism, we believe, have a biologically based difficulty in connecting emotion to their emerging capacity to plan and sequence their actions. Histories and video-tapes of autistic children's interactions during their formative years show that although some of the children could engage with caregivers and minimally signal emotions, they never got to the point of being able to take a parent by the hand to find a toy or to open and close 50 circles of affective communication. They were thus blocked from moving to higher developmental levels. Using symbols mean-ingfully, for example, requires investing symbols with regulated and integrated emotions: "Mom" is understood as the total of one's emotional experiences with mother. Fortunately, extra practice with meaningful emotional interactions can help children master such interactions and move on developmentally. In a chart review of 200 children with autism spectrum disorders, we found that a compre-hensive program to develop this capacity could help the majority of them master goal-directed emotional interactions; become meaningfully verbal, empathic, cre-ative, and reflective; and have solid peer and family relationships (Greenspan and Wieder 1997).

Level 5: Creating Representations (or Ideas) (18–30 Months)

Adaptive Patterns

Assuming the toddler has had plenty of opportunity for emotional interactions, toward the end of her second year she can more easily separate perceptions from actions and hold freestanding images, or representations, in her mind. Related to the ability to create internal representations is the capacity for "object perma-nence." Object permanence, which is relative and advances through a series of stages, involves the toddler's ability to recall that an object hidden from view still exists and to search for it (Gouin-Decarie 1965). Internal sensations and unstable images gradually become organized in the child's mind as multisensory, emotion-ally laden images that can be evoked and are somewhat stable (Bell 1970; Fenson and Ramsay 1980; Gouin-Decarie 1965; Piaget 1962). This capacity is somewhat fragile between 16 and 24 months, but it soon becomes a dominant mode in or-ganizing the child's behavior.

As the child learns to control his tongue, other mouth muscles, and vocal cords, he can begin forming words to label internal representations. If he has had a broad range of emotionally relevant experiences, he will now be able to create a broad range of meaningful labels or symbols.

As a child acquires new words, the words become meaningful to the degree that they refer to lived emotional experiences. When children are neurologically capable of speaking but do not learn to create emotionally meaningful images and symbols, the result is very different. The child could see a picture of a chair and say, "chair." She could also complete rote memory tasks. Yet she would be unable to say, "Mommy, come play with me!" or "I don't like that!" Such a child would never develop meaningful spoken language. Nor would she understand written language. She might learn to read and regurgitate back a series of words, such as "red hat, green hat, blue hat," but would be unable to tell you the meaning of a story or the motives of its characters.

The development of language moves through several levels:

1. *Words accompany actions.* The child bangs on a table, saying "hit!" He cannot yet use ideas or words in place of actions.
2. *Words are used to convey bodily feeling states.* "My muscles are exploding." "Head is aching."
3. *Action words conveying intent are used in place of actions.* "Hit you!"
4. *Words are used to convey emotions, but the emotions are treated as real rather than signals.* The child says, "I'm mad!" or "I'm hungry," rather than "I feel mad" or "I feel hungry." In the first case, the feeling state demands action and is very close to action; in the second, the words are a signal for an internal experience, a signal that makes possible a consideration of many possible thoughts and actions.
5. *Words are used to signal feelings, as in the second case above, but these are mostly global, polarized feeling states ("I feel awful," "I feel good.").* The prevalence of polarized feeling words continues throughout this developmental stage and can also characterize stage six, when children begin using logic to make connections between ideas. If it persists into later childhood, however, it can indicate a constriction in the child's mastery of these two levels of development.

Although we have emphasized the child's acquisition of words, which is a cornerstone of most intellectual endeavors, the capacity to construct symbols occurs in many domains. It gives rise to higher levels of intelligence in all of them. The child can now form visuospatial representations, as when a preschooler builds a toy house and describes what goes on in each room. She can plan and sequence actions symbolically, as when she runs a toy bus from the house to the school to pick up some children.

In addition, the child can now use symbols to manipulate ideas in his mind without actually having to carry out actions. This gives him tremendous flexibility in reasoning and thinking, because he can now solve problems mentally.

The child's ability to construct symbols enables her to share meanings with others, which in turn facilitates her ability to describe herself and to understand the difference between herself and others. Her consciousness of "me" and "not me" now involves internal images rather than simply integrated behavior patterns, as in the previous stage. Her development of perspective coincides with the early stages of empathy and prosocial behavior (Butterworth 1990; DesRosiers and Busch-Rossnagel 1997; Meltzoff 1990; Pipp-Siegel and Pressman 1996; Stern 1983).

Symbols, however, do not create consciousness. Rather, they provide a new way of labeling and expanding consciousness. Symbolization and language build on a sense of self and the outer world that was already well established. When the presymbolic experience of emotional signaling and problem-solving is insufficient to provide a beginning emotional knowledge of the world, as we see in some children with autism, the child cannot use words as true symbols. Instead, they are empty containers of memorized scripts.

Sensory Organization

A person's mental representation, or idea, of an object or person is a multisensory image that integrates all the object's physical properties as well as levels of meaning abstracted from the person's experiences with the object. The object is at once a visual, auditory, tactile, olfactory, vestibular, and proprioceptive object as well as one that is involved in various emotional and social experiences. Therefore, the range of senses and sensorimotor patterns a child employs in relationship to his world is critical. If the child's range, depth, or integration of sensory experiences of objects in the world is limited, his construction of representations will be limited as well.

Affective Organization

A child who has reached the level of representational thinking now has the tools she needs to label and interpret feelings rather than simply act them out. A verbal 2½-year-old displays this interpretive process when she says, "Me mad" or "Me happy." Because many children have language delays, however, pretend play is an even more reliable indicator of the ability to label and interpret. A child who as yet says little can already present a vivid picture of her representational world by pretending her dolls are feeding each other, hugging each other, or fighting with each other.

Between ages 2 and 5, children who are able to experience and communicate emotions symbolically develop the capacity for higher-level emotional and relational experiences. They develop the capacity for empathy. Their loving feelings toward themselves and others become more consistent and better able to survive separations and affect storms such as anger. Later on, they will become able to experience loss, sadness, and guilt.

Level 6: Building Bridges Between Ideas: Logical Thinking (30–48 Months)

Adaptive Patterns

At this level, the child moves beyond having discrete internal images and labeling them. He now develops the ability to make logical connections between two ideas or feelings. Instead of simply knowing, and saying, "Me mad!" he can think, and say, "I'm mad because you hit me." He learns to make a variety of logical connections, including understanding how one event leads to another ("The wind blew and made the tree fall down"); how events are connected across time ("That girl let me play with her doll yesterday, I bet she will tomorrow, too" or "If I'm bad right now, I'll get in trouble later"); and how events are connected across space ("Mom is not here beside me, she's down in the basement"). He learns to use ideas to understand his feelings: "I'm happy now because Sally's coming over to play").

The ability to make such connections is the basis for a whole host of capacities associated with healthy mental functioning. A child who can make logical connections will be able to differentiate her own feelings, making increasingly subtle distinctions between emotional states. She will be able to say whether she is feeling angry or merely frustrated. Her earlier experiences of back-and-forth communication have already helped her feel the difference between "me" and "not me." The capacity for logical connection takes this process to the next level, making reality testing possible by enabling the child to categorize experiences into those originating inside herself ("make-believe") and those originating outside ("real"). Similarly, she can begin to understand the relationships between her own thoughts, feelings, or actions and those of other people. This makes it possible for her to reason, argue with others, and answer "why" questions. It forms the basis of new social skills, such as following rules and participating in groups.

Because the child can now understand the logical connections between different feeling states, his sense of self becomes more complex and sophisticated. Not only does he realize that "angry me" and "happy me" are the same person, he is able to reflect on how these parts of himself relate to each other: "When you don't let me do what I want, I'm mad. When you're nice to me, I'm happy and then I'm nice back."

Sensory Organization

The child is now learning to understand what she hears, sees, touches, tastes, and smells in a more complex way. She faces the challenge of categorizing sensory information along many dimensions—past, present, and future; closer and farther away; appealing and distasteful—and thinking about the relationships among her sensory and emotional experiences. To meet these challenges, the child needs to be able to organize information coming from each sensory pathway, and her sensory pathways need to work together smoothly. Any impairment in sensory processing will likely compromise her ability to make meaning of her sensory experience. For example, if she cannot distinguish between certain sounds, she will have trouble understanding words. If she confuses different spatial images with one another, she will be unable to think in a clear and organized manner about what she sees. If she has poor short-term memory for either auditory or spatial symbols, she will lose important information before her mind can combine and compare it with other information in order to abstract meanings. In turn, such impairments in the ability to think abstractly will compromise the child's very ability to categorize her experience.

What he needs to be able to categorize, of course, are not just simple, static sensory stimuli but complex emotional and interpersonal experiences that keep changing over time. Sensory processing difficulties, if not addressed, can cause people to spend much of their lives confused, unable to make sense of themselves or their world.

Affective Organization

At this developmental stage, we observe the child's experiences and expression of affective themes become broader and deeper. The child's relationships and pretend play show an increasingly wide range of themes, including dependency and closeness, pleasure, excitement, curiosity, aggression, self-control, and the beginnings of empathy and consistent love. One frequently sees a child of this age repeatedly enact a scene in which one doll feeds or hugs another. Over time, assuming the child is experiencing a healthy range of parental interactions, the dramas the child initiates will expand to include scenes of dolls experiencing separation, competition, aggression, injury, death, recovery, and more.

Simultaneously, the child's pretend play and use of language are becoming increasingly complex, showing a growing understanding of causality and logic. The content of play may be fantasy, but the stories make logical sense: a prince slays a dragon *because* the dragon stole a treasure or kidnapped a princess. In conversation, a 3½-year-old child can correctly use the words "but" and "because" and argue in lawyerly fashion: "I can't eat that food because it looks icky and it will make me sick."

In our discussion of Level 1, self-regulation and interest in the world, we argued that from the beginning of life, all experience has an emotional component. The child's capacity for logical thinking, like his earlier developmental capacities, arises out of emotional experience, resulting as it does from his repeated interactions with primary caregivers. Parents have to be able not only to engage their child in such interactions, but to interpret and name the child's feelings correctly and consistently from day to day. For example, if a child frequently plays with toy guns and the parents see this as aggression on one day, an expression of sexuality the next day, and an indication of the child's need for closeness on the third day, their responses will vary widely and will likely confuse the child. The child may never develop a stable, realistic sense of what behavior and feelings mean. Similarly, some parents regularly project their own feelings onto their child, with the result that the child ends up sharing his parents' confusion about which feelings emanate from inside him and which belong to other people. Formation of a realistic understanding of the world can also be compromised if parents consistently fail to set limits, depriving the child of feedback that would let him learn the logic of action and consequence, cause and effect.

In contrast to the views of Freud (1900/1958) and Mahler et al. (1975), children do not appear to go through a distinct period of magical thinking followed by one of reality-oriented thinking. Instead, the ability to separate magical from realistic thought seems to develop gradually, through repeated experiences of getting logical, meaningful feedback from parents or other caregivers.

The ability to see the world realistically and logically is critical not only in human relationships but also in the ability to succeed at what are commonly thought of as purely cognitive or academic tasks, such as learning math and reading. As we will see in our later discussions of assessment and treatment, a thorough evaluation of a child with attention or learning disabilities often reveals that these academic problems have their roots in the child's early emotional interactions. Coaching parents on how to interact in healthier ways, as well as addressing any sensory impairments affecting the child's ability to interact, can result in impressive gains in academic skills.

Advanced Levels of Development

If a child masters the functional emotional capacities associated with Levels 1–6, she is able to move on to more advanced ways of thinking and experiencing: multicause and triangular thinking; gray-area, reflective thinking; and an internal standard of thinking. These are addressed briefly in Chapter 3 ("Assessment"). The DIR model defines additional levels that can be reached in adolescence and adulthood. (For a brief description of these levels, see Table 11–1, Functional Emotional Developmental Levels From Infancy to Adulthood, in Chapter 11, "A Model for Comprehensive Prevention and Early Intervention Services for All Families.")

References

Ainsworth M, Bell SM, Stayton D: Infant–mother attachment and social development: socialization as a product of reciprocal responsiveness to signals, in The Integration of the Child Into a Social World. Edited by Richards M. Cambridge, England, Cambridge University Press, 1974, pp 99–135

Ainsworth M, Blehar M, Waters E, et al: Patterns of Attachment: A Psychological Study of the Strange Situation. New York, Lawrence Erlbaum and Associates, 1978

Als H: Patterns of infant behavior: Analogs of later organizational difficulties? In Dyslexia: A Neuroscientific Approach to Clinical Evaluation. Edited by Duffy FH, Geschwind N. Boston, MA, Little, Brown, and Co, 1982, pp 67–92

Als H, Lester BM, Tronick E, et al: Towards a research instrument for the assessment of preterm infants' behavior (APIB), in Theory and Research in Behavioral Pediatrics. Edited by Fitzgerald H, Yogman MW. New York, Plenum Press, 1982, pp 35–132

Ayres AJ: Tactile functions: their relation to hyperactive and perceptual motor behavior. Am J Occup Ther 18:6–11, 1964

Bates JE, Maslin LA, Frankel KA: Attachment, security, mother–child interaction, and temperament as predictors of problem behavior ratings at age three years. Monogr Soc Res Child Dev 50:167–193, 1985

Bell R: Socialization findings re-examined, in Child Effects on Adults. Edited by Bell R, Harper L. New York, John Wiley and Sons, 1977

Bell SM: The development of the concept of the object as related to infant–mother attachment. Child Dev 41:219–311, 1970

Belsky J, Rovine M, Taylor DG: The Pennsylvania Infant and Family Development Project, III. The origins of individual differences in infant–mother attachment: maternal and infant contributions. Child Dev 55:718–728, 1984

Bowlby J: Attachment and Loss. London, Hogarth, 1969

Brazelton TB, Als H: Four early stages in the development of mother–infant interaction. Psychoanal Study Child 34:349–369, 1979

Brazelton TB, Koslowski B, Main M: The origins of reciprocity: the early mother–infant interaction, in The Effect of the Infant on Its Caregiver. Edited by Lewis M, Rosenblum L. New York, John Wiley and Sons, 1974

Butterworth G: Self perception in infancy, in The Self in Transition: Infancy to Childhood. Edited by Cicchetti D, Beeghly M. Chicago, IL, Chicago University Press, 1990

Campos J, Campos R, Barrett K: Emergent themes in the study of emotional development and emotion regulation. Dev Psychol 25:394–402, 1989

Carew JV: Experience and the development of intelligence in young children at home and in day care. Monogr Soc Res Child Dev 45:1–115, 1980

Cassidy J, Shaver PR: Handbook of Attachment. New York, Guilford, 1999

Cicchetti D, Schneider-Rosen K: Toward a transactional model of childhood depression. New Dir Child Dev 26:5–27, 1984

De Wolff MS, van IJzendoorn MH: Sensitivity and attachment: a meta-analysis on parental antecedents of infant attachment. Child Dev 68:571–591, 1997

DesRosiers FS, Busch-Rossnagel NA: Self-concept in toddlers. Infants Young Child 10:15–26, 1997

Egeland B, Kreutzer T: A longitudinal study of the effects of maternal stress and protective factors on the development of high risk children, in Life-Span Developmental Psychology: Perspectives on Stress and Coping. Edited by Green AL, Cummings EM, Karraker KH. Hillsdale, NJ, Lawrence Erlbaum and Associates, 1991, pp 61–84

Escalona S: The Roots of Individuality. Chicago, IL, Aldine, 1968

Feldman R, Greenbaum CW, Yirmiya N: Mother–infant affect synchrony as an antecedent of the emergence of self-control. Dev Psychol 35:223–231, 1999

Fenson L, Ramsay D: Decentration and integration of play in the second year of life. Child Dev 51:171–178, 1980

Field T: Effects of early separation, interactive deficits, and experimental manipulation on infant–mother face-to-face interaction. Child Dev 48:763–771, 1977

Field T: Interactions of high risk infants: quantitative and qualitative differences, in Current Perspectives on Psychosocial Risks During Pregnancy. Edited by Sawin D, Hawkins R, Walker I, et al. New York, Brunner/Mazel, 1980, pp 120–143

Field T: Gaze behavior of normal and high-risk infants during early interactions. J Am Acad Child Psychiatry 20:308–317, 1981

Fogel A: Affect dynamics in early infancy: affective tolerance, in Emotion and Early Interaction. Edited by Field T, Fogel A. Hillsdale, NJ, Lawrence Erlbaum and Associates, 1982

Freud S: The Interpretation of Dreams (1900), in The Standard Edition of the Complete Psychological Works of Sigmund Freud, Vols 4 and 5. Translated and edited by Strachey J. London, Hogarth Press, 1958

Goldberg S: Social competence in infancy: a model of parent–infant interaction. Merrill-Palmer Q 23:163–177, 1977

Gouin-Decarie T: Intelligence and Affectivity in Early Childhood: An Experimental Study of Jean Piaget's Object Concept and Object Relations. New York, International Universities Press, 1965

Greenspan SI: Intelligence and Adaptation: An Integration of Psychoanalytic and Piagetian Developmental Psychology. Psychological Issues, Monograph No. 47–48. New York, International Universities Press, 1979

Greenspan SI: The Development of the Ego: Implications for Personality Theory, Psychopathology, and the Psychotherapeutic Process. New York, International Universities Press, 1989

Greenspan SI: Developmentally Based Psychotherapy. Madison, CT, International Universities Press, 1997

Greenspan SI, Porges SW: Psychopathology in infancy and early childhood: clinical perspectives on the organization of sensory and affective-thematic experience. Child Dev 55:49–70, 1984

Greenspan SI, Wieder S: Developmental patterns and outcomes in infants and children with disorders in relating and communicating: a chart review of 200 cases of children with autistic spectrum diagnoses. Journal of Developmental and Learning Disorders 1:87–141, 1997

Grossmann K, Grossmann KE, Spangler G, et al: Maternal sensitivity and newborns' orientation responses as related to quality of attachment in Northern Germany. Monogr Soc Res Child Dev 50:233–256, 1985

Kaye K, Fogel A: The temporal structure of face-to-face communication between mothers and infants. Dev Psychol 16:454–464, 1980

Klaus M, Kennell J: Maternal–Infant Bonding: The Impact of Early Separation or Loss on Family Development. St. Louis, MO, CV Mosby, 1976

Lachmann FM, Beebe B: The contribution of self- and mutual regulation to therapeutic action: a case illustration, in The Neurobiological and Developmental Basis for Psychotherapeutic Intervention. Edited by Moskowitz M, Monk C, Kaye C, et al. Northvale, NJ, Jason Aronson, 1997, pp 94–121

Lester BM, Hoffman J, Brazelton TB: The rhythmic structure of mother–infant interaction in term and preterm infants. Child Dev 56:15–27, 1985

Lewis M, Feiring M: Infant, maternal and mother–infant interaction behavior and subsequent attachment. Child Dev 60:831–837, 1987

Lyons-Ruth K, Zeanah C: The family context of infant mental health, I: affective development in the primary caregiving relationship, in Handbook of Infant Mental Health. Edited by Zeanah C. New York, Guilford, 1993, pp 14–37

Mahler MS, Pine F, Bergman A: The Psychological Birth of the Human Infant: Symbiosis and Individuation. New York, Basic Books, 1975

Meltzoff A: The roots of social and cognitive development: models of man's original nature, in Social Perception in Infants. Edited by Field TM, Fox NA. Norwood, NJ, Ablex Publishing, 1985, pp 1–30

Meltzoff A: Foundations for developing a concept of self: the role of imitation in relating self to other and the value of social mirroring, social modeling, and self practice in infancy, in The Self in Transition: Infancy to Childhood. Edited by Cicchetti D, Beeghly M. Chicago, IL, Chicago University Press, 1990, pp 139–164

Miyake K, Chen S, Campos J: Infant temperament, mother's mode of interaction, and attachment in Japan: an interim report. Monogr Soc Res Child Dev 50:276–297, 1985

Papousek H: The common in the uncommon child, in The Uncommon Child. Edited by Lewis M, Rosenblum L. New York, Plenum, 1981, pp 317–328

Papousek H, Papousek M: Early ontogeny of human social interaction: its biological roots and social dimensions, in Human Ethology: Claims and Limits of a New Discipline. Edited by Foppa K, Lepenies W, Ploog D. New York, Cambridge University Press, 1979, pp 456–489

Pederson DR, Moran G, Sitko C, et al: Maternal sensitivity and the security of infant–mother attachment: a Q-sort study. Child Dev 61:1974–1983, 1990

Piaget J: The stages of intellectual development of the child, in Childhood Psychopathology. Edited by Harrison S, McDermott J. New York, International Universities Press, 1962, pp 157–166

Pipp-Siegel S, Pressman L: Developing a sense of self and others. ZERO TO THREE 17:17–24, 1996

Reingold H: The social and socializing infant, in Handbook of Socialization Theory and Research. Edited by Goslin D. Chicago, IL, Rand McNally, 1969, pp 779–789

Rothbart MK, Derryberry D: Development of individual differences in temperament, in Advances in Developmental Psychology, Vol. 1. Edited by Lamb ME, Brown AL. Hillsdale, NJ, Lawrence Erlbaum and Associates, 1981, pp 37–86

Spelke ES, Owsley C: Intermodal exploration and knowledge in infancy. Infant Behav Dev 2:13–27, 1979

Sroufe LA: Socioemotional development, in Handbook of Infant Development. Edited by Osofsky J. New York, John Wiley and Sons, 1979, pp 462–516

Sroufe LA: Emotional Development: The Organization of Emotional Life in the Early Years. New York, Cambridge University Press, 1996

Sroufe LA, Egeland B, Carlson E: One social world: the integrated development of parent–child and peer relationships, in Relationships as Developmental Context: The 29th Minnesota Symposium on Child Psychology. Edited by Collins WA, Laursen B. Hillsdale, NJ, Erlbaum, 1999, pp 241–262

Stern D: The early development of schemas of self, of other, and of various experiences of 'self with other,' in Reflections on Self Psychology. Edited by Lichtenberg J, Kaplan S. Hillsdale, NJ, The Analytic Press, 1983, pp 49–84

Stern D: The Interpersonal World of the Infant: A View From Psychoanalysis and Developmental Psychology. New York, Basic Books, 1985

Talberg G, Couto RJ, O'Donnell ML, et al: Early affect development: empirical research. Int J Psychoanal 69:239–259, 1988

Thomas A, Chess S: Genesis and evolution of behavioral disorders: from infancy to early adult life. Am J Psychiatry 141:1–9, 1984

Thomas A, Chess S, Birch HG: Temperament and Behavior Disorders in Children. New York, New York Universities Press, 1968

Tronick EZ: Emotions and emotional communication in infants. Am Psychol 44:112–119, 1989

Tronick EZ, Gianino AF Jr: The transmission of maternal disturbance to the infant. New Dir Child Dev Winter:5–11, 1986

Werner H, Kaplan B: Symbol Formation. New York, Wiley, 1963

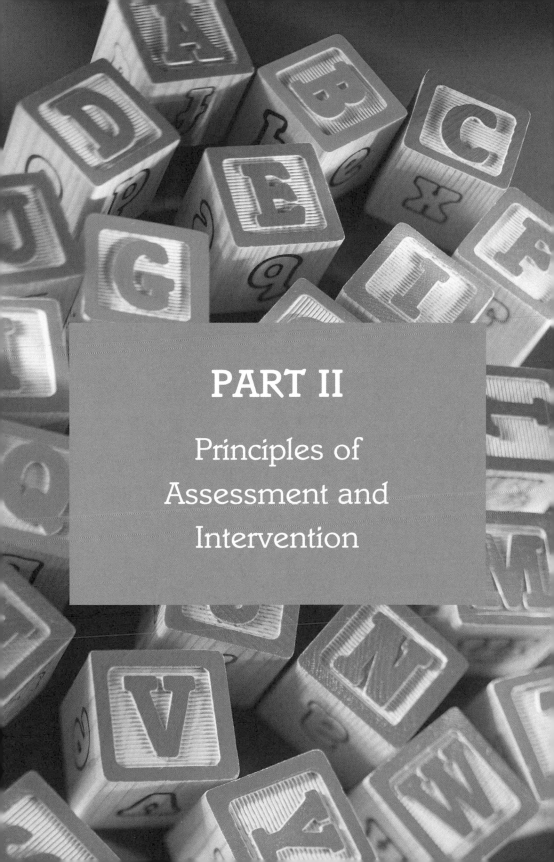

PART II

Principles of
Assessment and
Intervention

3

Assessment

Recall from Chapter 1 ("A Developmental Biopsychosocial Model") that assessment using the developmental, individual-differences, relationship-based (DIR) approach produces a *functional emotional developmental profile* that describes the child's functional emotional developmental capacities; his biologically based sensory and motor processing differences, and the patterns of interaction available to him within the family, community, and culture. For review, and so this chapter can stand on its own for teaching purposes, the DIR model is summarized in Figure 3–1. As illustrated, we can visualize the child's constitutional characteristics on one side and his environment on the other. Both sets of factors operate through the child–caregiver relationship, pictured in the middle. Child–caregiver interactions shape how the child organizes his experience at each of the six developmental levels and thus how well he masters the capacities associated with each level.

In this chapter, we first explain how to observe and interpret each element of the DIR model. How can a clinician meeting a child (or an adult) for the first time tell whether this individual has attained age-appropriate capacities for attending, relating, and communicating? Whether her sensory and motor functions are supporting or hindering her attainment of these capacities? Whether the interpersonal interactions available to her are supporting or undermining her development? Using clinical examples, we illustrate what each element of the DIR model "looks like." We then describe the formal assessment process step by step.

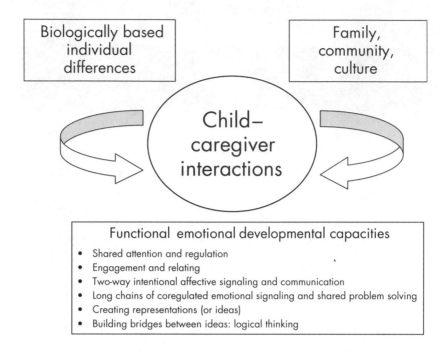

FIGURE 3–1. The developmental, individual-differences, relationship-based (DIR) model.

How to Observe the Functional Emotional Developmental Capacities

Overview

The clinician should evaluate how the child has negotiated each of the six developmental levels, determining whether the child demonstrates a deficit, a constriction, or an instability at one or more levels. A *deficit* occurs when the child has not mastered the level at all, as in the case of a toddler who, based on his age, should easily be able to engage in two-way nonverbal communication but has not begun doing so. A *constriction* occurs when the child has mastered a level in relation to some emotional themes but not others. Perhaps a toddler can use two-way nonverbal communication to negotiate assertiveness and exploration, pointing at a toy and vocalizing to entice a parent to play. The same child, however, withdraws or cries in a disorganized way when he wants to be dependent or close instead of reaching out or crawling into a parent's lap. When assessing whether the child shows constrictions at each level, the clinician should consider the following areas of expected emotional range: dependency, closeness, and pleasure; assertiveness, exploration, and curiosity; anger; self-limit-setting (for children older than 18 months); interest in and collaboration with peers (for children older than 2 years); participation in a peer group (for children older than 2½ years); empathy (for children older than 3½ years); stable forms of love (for children older than 3½ years); and the ability to deal with competition and rivalry (for children older than 3½ years).

Some children achieve a level with one parent but not the other, or with one substitute caregiver but not another. If a given relationship shows evidence of being secure and stable enough to support a certain developmental level, but the child has not reached that level within the relationship, then the child also can be said to have a constriction at that level.

If the child has generally mastered the capacities associated with a particular level but loses those capacities under the slightest stress, such as fatigue, mild illness, or playing with a new peer, then the child can be said to have an *instability* at that level.

Level 1: Shared Attention and Regulation

An infant or child who has difficulty attending, focusing, or maintaining a calm, alert state will provide evidence of these difficulties. Does the child seem to have trouble seeing you or hearing you? Does she seem to hear you but have difficulty turning toward you and making eye contact? Does she fail to react to a light touch on the shoulder, as though she felt no sensation at all? Or is she, in contrast, hypersensitive, perhaps recoiling at the light touch as though she has been slapped?

The clinician who keeps in mind the list of biologically based sensory and motor characteristics from Chapter 1 ("A Developmental Biopsychosocial Model") will have a useful framework for observing an infant's or child's regulatory capacities. To review, these characteristics are

1. sensory modulation, including hyper- or hyporeactivity in each sensory pathway
2. sensory processing, including the ability to register, decode, and comprehend sequences and abstract patterns in each sensory pathway
3. sensory-affective processing, or the ability to process and respond to affect
4. muscle tone
5. motor planning and sequencing, or the ability to purposefully organize a sequence of actions or symbols.

As indicated earlier, sensory reactivity can be observed clinically. How does the child react not only to sights, sounds, and touch but also to movement through space? In each sensory modality, how well does the child seem to process, or take in and decode, stimuli? Does a 4-month-old seem able to take in a complicated pattern of information or only a simple one? Is a 4½-year-old unable to make sense of a sequence of spoken words or to follow complex directions? Is a 3-year-old advanced in talking and language comprehension, but slower in visuospatial processing?

In the clinician's office, a child who understands spatial patterns poorly may forget where the door is or have a hard time picturing in his mind that mother is only a few feet away in the waiting room. In addition to lacking mental pictures of spatial relationships, such a child may also have difficulty comprehending the emotional "big picture." If mother is angry, he may feel as though the earth is opening up and he is falling in, because he cannot hold in his mind the bigger picture: mother is angry now, but she was nice before and probably will be again.

As we can see from this example, a child with a lag in visuospatial processing may become overwhelmed by the emotion of the moment. This reaction is often intensified when the child also has precocious auditory-verbal skills and is sensitive to every emotional nuance. The child becomes overloaded and does not have the ability to put the pieces together and comfort herself by making sense of her experience. Thus the clinician needs not only to evaluate each sensory pathway but also to compare the child's auditory-verbal processing skills with her visuospatial processing skills.

Observing how a child sits, crawls, hops, or runs; maintains his posture; holds a crayon, scribbles, or draws; and makes rapid alternating movements will provide a picture of the child's gross motor and fine motor systems. Shaking the child's hand reveals whether he has adequate hand–eye coordination. Can he meet the clinician's hand with his own? The child's security in regulating and controlling his body plays an important role in how he uses gestures to communicate and how he regulates emotions such as dependency (can he readily move closer or farther away from another person?) and aggression (can he control his hand that wants to hit?). His motor skills will also strongly influence his overall physical confidence and sense of self.

These sensory and motor capacities are not only constitutional but also maturational factors, because they may change as a person develops. The constitutional and maturational variables we have been discussing can be thought of as "regulatory factors." When they contribute significantly to difficulties with attending, remaining calm and organized, or modulating emotions or behavior, the resulting disorder of behavior, affect, or thought can be considered a "regulatory disorder" (Greenspan 1992). Parents, teachers, and clinicians sometimes attribute regulatory disorders to "lack of motivation" or emotional conflicts. The child who fails to respond to others' gestures or words is assumed to be globally distractible or preoccupied with her own thoughts, when in reality she may have a very specific processing disorder. Observing the child carefully and obtaining a thorough history of her self-regulatory patterns will enable the clinician to separate constitutional and maturational variations from other factors and to determine how several factors may be operating together to produce the child's symptoms.

Level 2: Engagement and Relating

People offer evidence of their way of relating from the moment one greets them in the waiting room. A child who strides into the office and goes straight to the toys, ignoring the clinician, is different from one who looks at the clinician with a twinkle in his eye, points to the toys, and waits for a warm, accepting smile. Most clinicians have a great deal of experience in assessing and monitoring the quality of relatedness. Sometimes, however, a clinician focusing on a child's specific ideas or thoughts will ignore the overall quality of engagement, missing the child's general indifference, negativity, or aloofness.

Level 3: Two-Way Intentional Affective Signaling and Communication and Level 4: Long Chains of Coregulated Emotional Signaling and Shared Social Problem Solving

Levels 3 and 4 both involve organized patterns of behavior and intentional, nonverbal gestures and emotional signals that can be directly observed. These gestures include facial expressions, arm and leg movements, vocalizations, and spinal posture. Complex, self-defining gestures involving the opening and closing of many circles of communication in a row (30 or 40) should emerge in the second year of life. This capacity is seen thereafter in complex nonverbal interactions in which patterns are communicated and comprehended.

The clinician should note whether a child initiates communicative gestures and if she in turn responds to the clinician's countergesturing with gestures of her own. The physician should especially note the range of emotions the infant, toddler, or preschooler can express and respond to as part of this pattern of back-and-forth gesturing. For example, some toddlers or preschoolers will comprehend and respond to emotional gestures dealing with pleasure and dependency but not with assertiveness or aggression (and vice versa). Observing a child's emotional range at this preverbal level provides important information regarding the foundations of a child's emotional life. Difficulty at this level suggests a more fundamental limitation in the experience and comprehension of age-expected emotions than simply difficulty at the verbal level. Therefore, observe carefully not only whether the toddler or young child interacts in a back-and-forth way but also the different emotions she can bring into this nonverbal dialogue. For the verbal preschool child, the clinician who focuses only on a child's words may miss an underlying, critical lack of organized gestural communication ability. The "spacey" child who floats in and out of the room or misreads the implied social rules of the playroom and hides toys, ignoring the therapist's facial expressions and sounds, is displaying her inability to fully process organized nonverbal communication. The adult who regularly misreads the intentions of others, perceiving assertiveness as anger or independence as rejection, is displaying the same limitation.

Level 5: Creating Representations (or Ideas)

Level 5 involves the elaboration and sharing of meanings. A young child's ability to symbolize experience is illustrated in pretend play, whereas an older child or an adult may explicitly discuss concerns or anxieties. In an initial interview, one child stages pretend dramas featuring hurricanes or children getting injections, perhaps communicating his fears about this new relationship. A child whose play involves dolls being fed and everyone being happy may be expressing a different set of expectations. An adult who spends much of his initial session recounting past relationships that have led to disappointment may be giving the message that he expects the clinician will disappoint him as well.

The capacity for symbolization can also be displayed in subtle spatial communications, such as building complicated towers or houses with passages in them. Some older children and adults communicate complex ideas and feelings through artwork. However ideas are expressed, the clinician can discern the depth and range of emotional themes represented. Does the person communicate only shallow, repetitive dramas or rich, deep ones involving a wide range of emotions?

A child or adult who has not achieved the ability to symbolize will act out behaviors and feelings rather than represent them symbolically. In a clinical interview, can a child say, "I'm mad" or represent anger by creating scenes of soldiers or animals fighting, as opposed to actually hitting or throwing a tantrum? Can she express dependency by having two dolls hug each other, or does she need to hug the therapist or grab toys and try to take them home?

Level 6: Building Bridges Between Ideas: Logical Thinking

As logical bridges between ideas are established, various types of reasoning and appreciation of reality emerge, including the ability to deal with conflicts, find prosocial outcomes, and distinguish reality from fantasy (Dunn and Kendrick 1982; Flavell et al. 1986; Harris et al. 1991; Harris et al. 1994; Wolf et al. 1984; Wooley and Wellman 1990). At this level, a child can make connections between different ideas and feelings ("I am happy because you took me to the playground").

A child who has successfully negotiated this developmental level does not simply have ideas but can communicate ideas to another person and build on the other person's responses. Some people only communicate their own ideas. In both childhood dramas and adult conversations, they talk but do not easily absorb, incorporate, or reply to other people's ideas and comments. For example, whenever a 4-year-old girl came home from preschool, she played out scene after scene of being a princess, letting her mother hold her imaginary robe, but made no response to her mother's casual questions, such as "What does the princess want me to do next?" and "Who did you play with at school today?" Other individuals display just the opposite tendency, diligently following instructions or listening to others but rarely elaborating their own feelings or ideas. Both tendencies, of course, can be directly observed in an evaluation session.

Children who can create logical bridges begin to negotiate their relationship with the clinician not simply through pretend play but in a more reality-based way: "Can I play with this truck?" "What will you do if I kick this dollhouse over?" The child may ask if he and the clinician can play after the session is over. A child who negotiates about bringing parents into the playroom or expresses curiosity about where the clinician lives and what his family is like is clearly displaying the capacity to use words or symbols in a logical, interactive way. An adult who shifts between free association and logical reflection or who wonders aloud about how two of his feelings are connected is displaying the same capacity.

Level 6 can be further assessed as one looks at the way in which the child organizes the content of her communications. The organization of topics reveals the degree to which a person has an age-appropriate capacity for reality testing and organized thinking or communicating. Are there logical links connecting the topics a person discusses? With a child, of course, the degree to which such links can be expected varies with age. In a 4-year-old, we would not be surprised by the partial absence of logical links; in a 2½- to 3½-year-old, we would be even less surprised. In children of 6, 7, or 8, however, we expect a greater capacity to form logical bridges.

One can also learn about the child's mastery of levels 5 and 6 by noting whether and how he describes his own feelings. A child who can describe feelings is showing true representational ability, as opposed to one who can only describe behaviors. The child who simply says, "I went to the toy store and bought some matchbox cars. Then I came home and played with the cars" is different from one who says, "I was so excited when I got those cars, I couldn't wait to get home and play with them. I've been wishing for that yellow one for so long, ever since I saw one like it at Brian's house."

The ability to symbolize feelings can occur at three levels. At the first level, children (or adults who have never advanced beyond this level) tend to talk only about undifferentiated feeling states that have a physical ring to them: "My tummy hurts." At a slightly more advanced level of symbolization, one may hear global descriptors: "I don't like that," "I feel good," "I feel bad." At the third level, one hears what we generally think of as "feeling words"—happiness, anger, rage, despair, excitement. The person can say, "When my teacher said that about me, I felt really happy and excited" or "When my friend made fun of me in front of all those people, I felt so embarrassed and angry." Many 4-year-olds can reach this level. Along with more differentiated affect descriptions, one looks for whether the child can put different descriptions together into meaningful patterns. If the child has two dolls fight, are there reasons for their fight? Perhaps the child explains that they are mad at each other because one doll hid the other's favorite toy. Such a child is clearly demonstrating an ability to build logical bridges.

Besides looking for such logical links, the clinician also looks at how the child applies those logical links to a broad range of themes. Is her thematic range broad or narrow? In her play and talk, does she address dependency but leave out aggression or curiosity entirely? Does she focus only on aggression, but leave out dependency? Which particular emotions and themes can the child address at the developmental level of building bridges between ideas?

A sudden disruption in a developing theme often indicates that the child has touched on an area that triggers anxiety. For example, a 9-year-old boy asks the evaluating clinician, "Do you have a basketball? I like to play basketball," and proceeds to talk for a time about how he loves to play but has no friends to play with, nor will his father play basketball with him. In response to the therapist's occasional question, he elaborates on the issue of his loneliness. His statements are organized in the sense that they flow logically from one to the other and center on the theme of his desire for greater closeness.

The boy next asks the therapist if she will play basketball with him. When she asks how he envisions that happening, he gleefully says that they could go to the schoolyard and play one-on-one. Immediately following this remark, he asks, "Can people die of heart attacks?" The therapist wonders aloud why that thought occurred to him, and the child responds, "There was a car accident and people had their arms and legs cut off. Can robbers get into a building and steal?" Here we see an abrupt shift from the interwoven themes of basketball, the wish for closeness, and feelings of isolation to fragmented statements about heart attack, physical injury, and things being stolen. A breakdown in thematic organization is signified by the absence of the connecting links that one would expect from a 9-year-old. Although the clinician cannot yet know for sure what triggered the breakdown, she might hypothesize that by imagining playing basketball with her, the child touched on some anxiety about intimacy.

One can learn a great deal by noting the sequence of themes that arise during a child's evaluation session. For example, suppose a child plays with the father doll, darts over to the other side of the room and gets a toy gun, frantically shoots it at the dartboard, then goes back to the doll and pretends to shoot its arm off. Thus the child works a new theme—using the gun for violence—into the old drama. He presents a picture of apprehension and anxiety; the theme is temporarily disrupted, but the child later returns to it. He has armed himself but still comes back into the doll "family." The sequence may suggest that he was concerned with some danger for which he felt a gun would be protective. One might hypothesize that this child is more concerned with bodily damage than with separation or a more global loss.

By looking at disruptions in a child's play patterns, gestures, verbalizations, and quality of engagement, one can begin to determine whether the child is anxious and to seek clues about the sources of her anxiety. One looks for a shift from a higher developmental level to a lower one, a shift from a more adaptive to a less adaptive pattern within a single level, or a sudden narrowing of the thematic or emotional range. The first kind of shift is displayed by a child who switches from talking about anger to throwing toys around and by the 9-year-old boy described earlier who switches from a logical conversation (level 6) to the fragmented expression of discrete thoughts without clear connections (level 5). The second kind of shift is seen in a boy who, in his gestures, starts out interacting in a warm and assertive, even empathic way. He respects the interviewer's wishes when told what objects he can and cannot touch in the playroom. Suddenly, the boy becomes more indifferent or impersonal, or perhaps he begins interacting in a purely aggressive or clinging manner. He has continued engaging in two-way, nonverbal communication (levels 3 and 4) but has shifted from an adaptive to a maladaptive pattern. This child has also exhibited the third kind of shift, switching from expressing a broad range of emotions (warmth, assertiveness, empathy) to a more narrow, rigid pattern (just aggression or just neediness).

How to Observe and Evaluate Constitutional-Maturational Characteristics

As described earlier in our discussion of level 1, in many cases a child's sensory and motor functioning can be assessed through direct observation. An instrument to clinically assess aspects of sensory functions in a reliable manner has been developed and is available (DeGangi and Greenspan 1988, 1989). In some cases, the initial observation will indicate that referral for neurological evaluation or psychological testing is appropriate. For example, if an 8 year old girl shows excellent gross motor coordination in her ability to run, skip, and throw a ball, but she has trouble writing letters or completing other fine motor tasks, the clinician may refer her for psychological testing to determine whether she has some minimal dysfunction or immaturity of the central nervous system.

By comparing one's observations of the child in the clinical setting with reports from teachers and parents—or with direct observation of the child in school or other settings—one can begin to assess the functional cause of the child's difficulties. For example, suppose a child whose teacher has labeled him "learning disabled" initially seems to display good fine motor coordination and sensorimotor integration during the assessment session. When some anxiety-arousing topic is touched on, however, the child suddenly "falls apart" and can no longer follow directions or write legibly. Such a pattern suggests that emotional issues are interfering with otherwise intact physical and sensory processing capabilities.

How to Observe and Evaluate Family, Community, and Cultural Patterns

During the assessment process, the clinician will have two sources of information about how the child's relationship with her parents contributes to her organization of experience at each developmental level. In interviews with the parents, the clinician will ask questions and obtain descriptions of the family's history and relationships. Equally important, however, is the opportunity to observe first-hand how the parents relate to the child, to each other, and to the clinician. The clinician will be able to get some sense, from the ways in which the parents relate and communicate, of how well each of them has mastered each developmental level; these observations, in turn, will suggest what kinds of developmentally appropriate or inappropriate interactions these parents are able to offer their child. Family patterns are discussed further in the next section on the formal assessment process.

The interviews with the parents and with the child, if he is verbal, provide an opportunity to gather information about the child's other important relationships, beginning with siblings and moving beyond the immediate family. Perhaps the parents have difficulty engaging their child in complex pretend play or an organized, logical exchange of ideas, but a favorite aunt, a grandparent, or a devoted teacher sometimes plays that role. Asking parents and child, "Outside the immediate family, who would you say are the important people in Johnny's life?" will give you some idea of the child's supports, if any, beyond his family. Another way to get a feel for the community in which the child is embedded is to complete an "eco-map" (Hartman 1978) with the family, showing all the people and institutions (e.g., school, church, sports teams) that play major roles in the family's life, with notes as to how parents and child describe each relationship. In the event that the assessment includes direct observation of the child in school or another setting, the clinician will, of course, be able to observe some of these relationships first-hand.

Specific cultural norms and expectations may play a critical role in the child's way of negotiating the six developmental levels. For example, suppose a child is growing up in a religious or ethnic community in which the expression of certain emotions or themes (e.g., aggression, sexuality) is generally frowned upon. That child may appear to have a constriction in her ability to address these themes at one or more developmental levels. Some religious sects forbid the reading of fairy tales, and a few proscribe fiction entirely. One might anticipate that children raised in such communities would appear constricted in their ability to fantasize or engage in pretend play or that such mental activities would be fraught with conflict. In order to form a good alliance with the family and develop an appropriate treatment plan, the clinician must take the time to learn about possible cultural sources of its members' style of relating, thinking, and communicating.

The Process of Clinical Assessment

As mentioned in Chapter 1 ("A Developmental Biopsychosocial Model"), an extremely thorough assessment is necessary to determine how constitutional and maturational factors, environment, and social interactions combine to produce a

---

TABLE 3–1. Formal assessment process using the DIR model

I. Presenting complaints and review of child's current functioning, including

    A. Each functional emotional developmental capacity

    B. Each sensory and motor processing capacity

    C. Relevant contexts (e.g., at home, at school, with caregivers, siblings, and peers)

II. Developmental history, including history of items reviewed in session I

III. Family dynamics and caregiver functioning

IV. Child and child–caregiver observations: two or more 45-minute sessions

V. Biomedical evaluations as needed (e.g., electroencephalogram, metabolic work-up, genetic studies, nutritional assessment)

VI. Speech and language evaluation

VII. Formal motor and sensory processing evaluation, including

    A. Motor planning and sequencing

    B. Sensory modulation

    C. Perceptual-motor capacities

    D. Visuospatial capacities

VIII. Evaluation of cognitive functions, including neuropsychological and educational testing

IX. Mental health evaluations of family members and family dynamics and assessment of family needs

---

Note. Steps V–IX should be carried out only if necessary to answer specific questions arising from steps I–IV.

particular child's competencies and presenting symptoms. Assessment using the DIR model requires several sessions with the child and family and may include consultations with other professionals such as speech pathologists, occupational and physical therapists, and teachers. Such consultations, including referrals for structured testing, are conducted only as needed to answer diagnostic questions raised by the child and family evaluation sessions.

Table 3–1 provides an outline of the formal assessment process. We now discuss selected elements of the assessment.

Presenting Complaints

Many clinicians spend an entire session on "presenting complaints." In our clinical work, we generally suggest to the parents of an infant or preverbal child that they bring the child with them to this first session. Although we spend most of the time talking with the parents, we have our eyes on the child, and we watch the spontaneous interactions between them. If the child is verbal, we ask the parents to leave him at home for the first meeting, if possible, so that they can speak freely.

We begin by asking the parents, "How can I help?" We listen closely as they describe the child's "problem." If we ask a question, it is generally to clarify something they have said or to ask for elaboration: "Can you give me some examples of Susan's fights in school?" "How is this different now from the way it was 6 months ago?" "When wasn't this a problem?" We want to know when the problem started, how it evolved, and its nature and scope. If a 2½-year-old is hitting her playmates, we want to find out if she behaves this way with all peers or only with certain children. We want to get a sense of what may have precipitated the problem and what may contribute to it. Was there a change in the family around the time the problem began, such as father getting a new job with longer hours? Were the parents experiencing new marital tension? Was the child reaching new developmental milestones, gaining new abilities that, paradoxically, placed additional stresses on her?

To create a supportive environment in which parents feel free to spontaneously tell their story and elaborate on their own feelings, we strive to be unstructured. We avoid yes-or-no questions and checklists. We are attempting to establish rapport with the family and begin a collaborative process. In our experience, the same developmental capacities we have described in children—attention and engagement, two-way gestural communication, the sharing of meanings, and the linking of meanings—can be achieved between an empathic clinician and the parents seeking help. The way the clinician relates to the parents provides a model of how they will be encouraged to relate to their child. A clinician who asks hurried yes-or-no questions provides a highly untherapeutic model. It usually takes parents a long time to decide to seek the help of mental health professionals. They should be able to tell their story without being rushed or repeatedly interrupted.

It is important to encourage the parents to describe all areas of the child's current functioning. Whatever the presenting complaint, we want to know about the child's other capacities. Has he attained the age-appropriate developmental levels? If so, does he seem to have constrictions or instabilities at any level? Can an 8-month-old, for example, engage in purposeful two-way exchanges? Is a 4-month-old engaging, with wooing smiles and vocalizations? Can a 2½-year-old engage in pretend play and use words to get his needs met? At each developmental level, how comfortable does the child seem with dependency, assertiveness, anger, and other age-appropriate themes? In listening to the parents' stories and in watching the child, if he is present, we look for indications of the child's sensory, language, cognitive, and motor functioning. We listen for evidence of the child's ability to retain information and follow commands, his word retrieval and word association skills, his fine and gross motor skills, and his motor planning and sequencing skills. Toward the end of the session, we may fill in gaps in our information by asking specific questions about these factors.

Some clinicians wait till after the session to write down what the parents have said. Others write during the session, which need not be an interference as long as the clinician pauses throughout to make good contact with the parents. We prefer to take detailed notes during the first 15 or 20 minutes because we want as much information as possible in the parents' own words.

By the end of this first session, we have a sense of the child's developmental level, the range of emotional themes she can handle, and the degree of support or hindrance she experiences from her sensory, language, cognitive, and motor abilities. We also form an impression of the support she gets from her parents. We observe how the parents communicate and organize their thinking, the quality of their engagement with the child and with us, their emotional availability, and their interest in the child. We have a good sense of their relative comfort with each major emotional theme.

Developmental History

In the second session, we meet with the parents alone to construct a developmental history of the child. (If, however, urgent marital or family problems have burst out during the initial session, these must become the focus of the second session. Perhaps the parents could not tell you their story without yelling at each other, or a parent is clearly experiencing severe depression or other mental health symptoms. These problems will need the clinician's attention first.)

Again, we usually start the session in an unstructured manner, inviting parents to describe how their child's development unfolded. We encourage them to alternate between what the child was like at different stages of life and what they felt was going on in the family at each stage. We try to start by finding out how, or if, the couple planned for the child, then progress through their experience of the pregnancy, delivery, and postpartum period. We then cover each of the developmental stages in the DIR model that a child of this age would be expected to have mastered.

Family Dynamics

In the third session, we meet with the parents to explore in greater depth the functioning of the caregiver and family at each phase of the child's life. Some clinicians just beginning to work with children and families feel reluctant to ask parents about difficulties in their marriage or relationship. However, we have found that an open and supportive approach can elicit relevant information without alienating the parents. We might ask, "What can you tell me about yourselves as a couple, and as a family?" By following the parents' lead, we try to develop a picture of their relationship, the careers of each parent, the parents' relationships with each of their children, the relationships among their children, the parents' relationships with their own families of origin, and the family's friendships and other community ties. In addition, we are interested in certain aspects of each parent's family history. Does either family have a history of mental illness, learning disabilities, or other atypical developmental patterns?

Some families do not hesitate to discuss marital difficulties or other problems. Some will describe "power struggles" or other kinds of conflict between their child and one or both parents. At this point, we are likely to ask, "Does this same pattern occur in other family relationships—for example, between mother and father?" We inquire whether either or both parents experienced similar struggles in their families of origin.

By considering the information provided verbally by the parents, and by observing how they relate to one another and to us, we try to get a sense of how the family's style of interacting furthers or hinders the child's development. Sometimes, we discover that the family as a whole functions in a very fragmented, presymbolic way. They gesture, "behave at" each other, overwhelm each other, or withdraw from each other, but they never negotiate at a symbolic level. That is, they do not share ideas or meanings with one another. In some such cases, each individual in the family is capable of functioning at a symbolic level, but something about the family dynamics "cancels out" this ability. We want to know how the family as a whole handles major emotional themes such as dependency, excitement, sexuality, anger, assertiveness, empathy, and love. We want to get a sense of how the family and its subsets—the parents and each parent–child dyad—dealt with these emotional themes at each of the child's developmental stages.

Child and Caregiver Observation Sessions

In the next two sessions, we focus on the child. (Many clinicians prefer to observe the child first, before exploring family dynamics. The sequence is not critical.) With an infant, we may tell each parent, "Show me how you like to play with, or be with, your baby." If the parent asks, "What do you want me to do?" we reply "Anything you like." When scheduling the first observation appointment, we tell parents they may use the toys in our office or bring a special toy from home.

We first observe each parent playing in an unstructured way with the child for 15 or 20 minutes. We look for the child's developmental level, the range of emotional themes addressed in the parent–child play at each level, and the support that the child is able to derive from his sensory, language, cognitive, and motor skills. We also watch for the ways in which each parent supports or undermines the child's developmental capacities and emotional range. After we watch each parent separately, we ask the parents to play together with the child. We observe how they interact as a group. For some families, the group situation is particularly challenging.

Toward the end of the first observation session, we briefly join the group. We do some preliminary coaching of the parents and begin to play with the child ourselves. We spend more time doing these things in the second session. We want to see how the child relates to a new person. We try to determine what kinds of interactions will bring out the highest level at which she can function. For example, suppose a child is repetitively moving a truck back and forth in a withdrawn, self-absorbed way. We will suggest to the parents that they entice her into a more interactive mode by joining her in trying to move the truck, or ask mother to make a fence with her hands in front of the truck, or have father pick up another car and announce, with great joy and enthusiasm, "Here I come!" Sometimes, marching or jumping with an aimless child or lying next to a passive, withdrawn child and offering a back rub or a tickle will draw the child in.

If a 3-year-old shows signs of symbolization and the parents do not appear to support this capacity, we coach or direct them to initiate pretend play with the child. If an 8-month-old is being overstimulated, we try to introduce more organized, cause-and-effect interactions between parents and child. If a 4-month-old looks withdrawn, we try to engage him by flirting. We work hands-on with an infant to explore his tactile sensitivity, muscle tone, motor planning, and preference for patterns of movement in space.

With children who can hold a conversation and can handle separation from their caregivers, we may start the first observation session by meeting with the child alone. Some children start by standing in the middle of the room and looking us over while we look at them. If we can tolerate 10 or 15 seconds of ambiguity and do not rush to control the situation (for example, by asking, "Do you want to play with the toys?"), the child will tell us a great deal about herself by what she does next. One child may proceed to become self-absorbed, another to ask questions about our toys, and still another to talk about her family. A child who looks around and says, "I heard there were toys here. Where are they?" is showing herself to be an organized, intentional person who understands why she is here. Some 4-year-olds talk to us throughout the session, engaging in an almost adult-to-adult dialogue about school or home, nightmares or worries, or subjects of interest to the child. Others quickly become aggressive or overly familiar, wanting to jump on us or wrestle.

In our time with the child alone, we observe how he relates to us, how intentional he is in using gestures, and how quickly he sizes up the new situation without words. We try to determine his emotional range and how he deals with anxiety. We note his general state of health and mood, his expressive and receptive language skills, his gross and fine motor skills, and his visuospatial problem-solving skills (for example, can he search for a toy?). We assess his core developmental capacities: how well he attends; engages; initiates purposeful, two-way nonverbal communication; opens and closes a series of circles of communication to solve problems; creates and expresses ideas; and links ideas logically. If the child has mastered these six capacities, we assess whether he has reached three additional, more advanced ways of organizing experience:

1. *Multicause and triangular thinking.* For example, the child can figure out several reasons why something is happening, rather than just one, and can hold in his mind at least three possible views of the same thing.
2. *Gray-area, reflective thinking.* For example, a child can weigh and judge the relative causes of events.

3. *An internal standard of thinking.* The child has developed a sense of self that is fairly stable and from which he can form opinions, make judgments, and reflect on what he is learning.

We next focus on the content of the child's play or conversation. What is on this child's mind? What topics may be causing conflict or anxiety?

Case Formulation: The Functional Emotional Developmental Profile

After learning about the child's current functioning and history, assessing family dynamics, and observing the child and family firsthand, we should have a convergence of impressions. If a clear picture is not emerging, we may need to spend another session or two developing the history or observing further.

Our assessment results in a written profile of the child and family that addresses each element of the DIR model. The profile describes the child's relative mastery of each functional emotional developmental capacity, beginning with the degree to which she can remain calm and attentive while processing and responding to a variety of sensations in an organized way. In addressing each developmental capacity, the profile should describe strengths and achievements as well as deficits, constrictions, and instabilities. This section of the profile can be thought of as a thorough description of the stage on which the child's particular drama—her relationships, anxieties, conflicts, and symptoms—unfolds. The stage may be solid or have gaping holes (developmental deficits). It may be stable or unstable. It may be wide and deep enough to accommodate a complex, emotionally rich drama or too narrow and cramped for anything more than a very simple performance.

The next section of the profile is an evaluation of the child's constitutional-maturational characteristics, the family and cultural patterns surrounding the child, and the contribution of each to the interactions the child experiences.

The profile provides a "road map" for planning interventions that fit the child's needs. By identifying the developmental deficits, constrictions, or instabilities that underlie the child's symptoms, the profile indicates *what* must change—that is, which functional emotional developmental capacities must be taught or strengthened if symptoms are to be resolved. By providing an understanding of how the child's typical interactions have produced his developmental strengths and limitations—and by describing how biology and experience have combined to influence these interactions—the profile will indicate *how* the necessary changes can be accomplished. What alterations need to be made in the kinds of interactive experiences available to the child? To accomplish this, what accommodations need to be made to address the child's biological and genetic characteristics and his information processing style? What changes should parents, teachers, and the child himself be helped to make in their ways of responding and communicating? In short, what courses of action will best help this child move up the developmental ladder?

The case illustration that follows provides an example of the assessment and case formulation process and shows how the information gleaned from an assessment can be used to plan effective interventions for the child and family.

Clinical Illustration

Five-month-old Lucy's crying spells, which lasted up to half an hour, prompted her parents to bring her for an evaluation. Her mother explained that when she attended a parent support group with her daughter, "Lucy stares for a few minutes at other babies and mothers and then gets bent out of shape and cries and cries and cries; she needs constant attention." At home, Lucy required constant holding to keep her from crying, and in a new environment, such as a friend's house, Lucy would get "wound up" and would not settle down until she got home.

The pregnancy had been unremarkable in terms of mother's physical health; however, because Lucy was turned in the wrong position, she was born by cesarean section, with the cord wrapped around her neck. She was 8 pounds, 9 ounces at birth, had an Apgar score of 9/9, and seemed healthy and alert. She was soon turning toward mother's voice and easily engaging with it, and even engaging with mother's facial expressions. Lucy was breastfed for 3 months, then weaned and bottle-fed with a milk-based formula augmented by rice cereal, peaches, and strained vegetables. On the growth charts, Lucy was in the 75th percentile for weight and the 90th percentile for height.

Lucy had slept through the night, from 6 P.M. until 6 A.M., and took as many as three 1-hour naps during the day. Yet as she grew older, she became irritable and had a harder time sleeping. She had progressed through her motor milestones; by 5 months of age, she could sit by herself, reach for her cup with both hands, and roll over both ways. At her happiest, Lucy played peek-a-boo, smiled, and vocalized, seeming more attentive to her mother's voice than to her facial expressions; she gave her mother broad smiles and remained engaged with her for 5–10 seconds or more before taking time out. Lucy preferred high-pitched noises to low-pitched ones, startled easily at loud noises, and cried up to 20 minutes when scared.

Lucy's father had a seizure disorder secondary to an occipital lobe trauma he had sustained in an automobile accident. He had some blurry vision from medication but no progressive difficulties. Both parents worried about the seizure disorder. Mother reported being such a "nervous wreck" that she feared it was affecting the baby. She worried about her ability to be a good mother and about whether Lucy would be okay. Mother confessed to being a nervous kind of person, with a tendency to anxiety and depression; she had been in therapy and had taken antidepressants intermittently.

Mother felt that both parents played with Lucy well, but that the father was more gentle. "I am so stressed," she explained, "that I didn't want to hold her or look at her sometimes. I'm afraid that I didn't bond with her, that I wasn't excited enough with her, too scared that I would do something wrong. I was afraid the medication for my depression was off and that would make me do something wrong."

Mother went on to say that Lucy was easily "startled by strangers" and could get very upset when the family had company. "I can't calm her down," she said. "Sometimes I feel like hitting her when she is demanding and crying uncontrollably. I worry about this and worry I'll go out of control." Mother was a careful, cautious person, with no history of acting impulsively with adults or children. However, she feared that she would lose her temper like her own mother, a very intrusive and aggressive woman who could easily say "I hate you" and mean it. The maternal grandparents were Holocaust survivors, and mother felt that their experience still influenced her and would in turn influence her own children.

In the office, Lucy was very attentive and responsive when interacting with each parent—smiling, vocalizing, and looking around—and focused equally well on both. She also smiled and flirted with the clinician quite easily. Mother stayed within an inch or two of Lucy, rather than giving her some room, and whenever Lucy vocalized, mother made several sounds immediately, so Lucy had little time to take over the interaction. As she talked to her, mother kept touching and holding Lucy to try and calm her; Lucy did not have a few seconds to calm down before mother started rubbing her back, stroking her feet, or rocking her in different rhythms. Even when Lucy sat with her father, mother distracted herself from me by engaging with Lucy, saying, "Oh my! I think I better go hold her. She looks like she is going to cry."

Father's interactions were gentle and gave Lucy more room. He seemed a bit depressed and preoccupied, and his rhythm was a little too slow for a bright, responsive baby. Lucy would do two or three actions in sequence, such as taking an object and holding it out to her father, but rather than take the object, father would keep trying to get her to repeat a sound he had made. When the clinician pointed out that Lucy had moved on to a new behavior, father looked puzzled and took a bit longer than normal to shift gears. Later, he admitted that he was still very absorbed by the effects of his accident; he worried that he might have a seizure and hurt Lucy. He said that he had been somewhat depressed, and he thought that the seizure medication might be dulling his appreciation of his daughter.

Upon examining Lucy, the clinician noted that she had good motor tone in her extremities and responded with pleasure to being touched. She responded to the clinician's facial expressions and vocalizations by brightening, looking, and vocalizing back, much as she had with her mother. While holding Lucy, the clinician spoke loudly to mother, who was sitting across the room; Lucy started crying, showing the sensitivity to loud noises mother had reported. She also showed evidence of being excruciatingly sensitive to sudden movements, especially in the vertical direction. As the clinician played with her, Lucy started to cry if he moved a toy abruptly, but if his movements were very gradual, allowing her to be visually in charge of the action, she was less likely to get upset.

The clinician suggested that the parents help Lucy take better control of her world by using her solid abilities for shared attention and engagement and beginning abilities for two-way communication. This would involve shifting from more proximal modes of communication to more distal modes such as vocalization and visual cuing, especially when Lucy was upset. He discussed with the parents Lucy's need for more time to calm herself and take the lead in play. Mother appreciated the insight that she needed to slow down her own rhythm and deal differently with her anxiety. Father seemed to feel better about the situation, too, particularly after sharing his feelings about the accident and fears of hurting Lucy, and he was able to review his medical history more realistically. Both parents were pleased to know that Lucy was so competent.

The clinician recommended that the parents have special play times with Lucy to practice and coach each other on their interactive skills, because they complemented each other well. Father, who had been extremely independent in his own family, was more sensitive to Lucy's need for independence, letting her do more things on her own. Mother was so cued into Lucy that she could point out missed opportunities for interaction. We practiced a little in the office, and the parents coached each other quite successfully. (Whereas tense parents could make each other more anxious by looking over each other's shoulders during childrearing, parents with a solid marriage, as these two had, can relax each other by exchanging support and reassurance.)

The clinician discussed how mother could break down interactions into circles of communication. Before responding to Lucy, she would have to figure out what Lucy was trying to do, which would keep her from doing several things before Lucy had finished one. Mother needed to practice saying to herself, "Okay. Now Lucy is making funny sounds at me, or trying to get me to look at the ball." Then she could respond appropriately. With practice, mother learned how to gain that split second she needed to read Lucy's signals and follow her lead.

Mother was also coached to give Lucy time to use her considerable strengths to calm herself down. In addressing Lucy's sensitivity to loud noises and sudden changes in her environment, the clinician followed the principle of breaking new challenges into small steps by helping the parents offer Lucy gradual exposure to new or changing experiences. For example, parents and clinician hid a ball in one hand to see whether Lucy became curious, and experimented with whether she would follow an object that traveled from high up down to her level on the floor, first slowly, then gradually faster. With these exercises, she could learn to be more flexible, using her vision and hearing to find objects and deal with a changing environment, especially a changing human environment. The clinician suggested that, in a new place, rather than putting Lucy immediately in the midst of a new group of six or seven parents and children, mother could first spend time with Lucy and perhaps one other person in a corner of the room so Lucy would not feel overwhelmed, then slowly introduce her to the group. The key was to be very gradual with Lucy without overprotecting her.

In a follow up meeting 1 month later (when she was almost 7 months old), Lucy showed good progress. She was taking a stronger lead in interactive play, and she would lie on her stomach and slither a little instead of just sitting up. Mother was much more relaxed and able to let Lucy take the lead, and father had a better rhythm of interaction. When Lucy made faces at him, cooing and reaching for his nose, father smiled and giggled back. When he commented on her curiosity about his nose, he used a vocal rhythm in tune with hers. He then offered her his hand, and she played with his fingers, a very nice interaction. Mother was still a little tense when Lucy cried, and grabbed her too quickly, but was better at trying to talk to her and use facial expressions first. Sometimes, she would attempt to calm Lucy down by pointing at things out the window, rather than just frantically rocking her.

Mother reported that at other people's houses, taking Lucy into a calm corner first seemed to work: Lucy still cried but was able to calm down. At home, however, Lucy still had trouble entertaining herself and always wanted to see mother in the same room. She tolerated playing on the floor for only a minute or two while mother stayed nearby, talking to her, and then she would demand to be picked up. Progress in this area was slow, but Lucy's ability to play independently gradually improved.

As the clinician watched Lucy interact with her parents and with him, he saw that she was still too passive and that her mother was still moving in too quickly. They again discussed letting Lucy assert herself more. Now that she could move on her tummy, he demonstrated getting down face-to-face with her and putting objects in front of her that she could work toward, encouraged with lots of affect cues. Mother worried, "Isn't she going to be in pain when she has to reach for something she can't quite get?" The clinician stressed the importance of Lucy getting some exercise and assured mother that Lucy's groans and even cries were more often signs of hard work than signs of discomfort.

Lucy continued to sleep and grow well. She was now in the 75th percentile for weight and the 99th percentile for height. The clinician saw her again when she was 9 months old, and her progress continued slowly but steadily. She was beginning to search for things she could not see, and she crawled confidently when going after her toys. Mother was learning to play without moving in too quickly, and father, who had by this point been reassured by his doctors that he did not need medication anymore, was much more relaxed, warm, and engaged with Lucy. He had improved in the rhythms of his vocalizations and motor gestures.

Mother's primary concern at this visit was Lucy's anger, which was more evident now that she was asserting herself. Mother associated Lucy's anger with her own childhood experience of her mother's terrifying anger: "I'm not going to be intimidated by my daughter, just like I was by my mother." She wanted to calm Lucy down before she got angry. The clinician discussed how mother's fear that Lucy would be like her own mother was understandable—given the family tradition and Lucy's behavior—but also premature, because Lucy was so young. He also talked about anger being a legitimate human emotion, just like love and warmth and assertiveness. Lucy would sometimes need to practice her protesting ability, just as she sometimes needed to reach out to be picked up. These ideas seemed to ease mother's concern.

Lucy continued to do well, becoming a competent and assertive toddler. When frustrated or under stress she could still become passive and needy, and mother could still become anxious and overprotective when stressed. But overall, they had moved confidently from the shared attention and engagement stage to flexible two-way communication encompassing a broad range of behaviors and emotions.

It was agreed that the parents would call the clinician as needed from this point on. He pointed out to mother that Lucy's confident engagement, her great ability to attend and focus, and her mastery of two-way communication, but he also emphasized that the family would need to continue negotiating the issue of assertiveness over the next few years. As Lucy became more comfortable being assertive, mother's anxiety about aggression would likely be triggered. Mother recognized the need to resist her own tendencies.

Lucy's parents contacted the clinician again when Lucy was about 27 months old. By telephone, mother expressed concern that she was falling into a pattern of making her daughter "too passive." They brought Lucy in for a visit; she was a highly verbal little girl, capable of nice pretend play with dolls and organized themes. Her warm, deep engagement, pleasurable smiles, and two-way gestural communication demonstrated that she was still able to share attention, and she was building good representational and symbolic capacities into these tendencies. However, watching mother and Lucy play, the clinician observed that mother's worry was in fact justified; she had a tendency to try to control the rhythm of symbolic play, much as she had done with Lucy's presymbolic play.

For example, when mother asked, "What do you want to do now?" Lucy answered, "Play some more." Lucy then had the dolls drink juice, adding, "Drink juice and play." There was a little chair in the office, and Lucy said, "Let's bring a chair." Mother responded with a friendly, "What for?" Lucy paused for a second, and mother jumped in: "Oh, I know. The chair will be for this doll. Let's make this doll the mommy, and this doll the baby, and the mommy will give the baby some juice. Here, you be the mommy." As mother took charge, Lucy's expression of pleasure decreased. She looked spacey and sad, and she became a bit passive. Rather than doing as mother suggested, Lucy knocked over a doll and turned to do something else, as if trying to get away from mother. Mother said, slightly anxiously, "Oh, this doll fell down. She must be hurt. Let's get the doctor." Lucy passively reached for the doll and mimicked her mother's vocalizations, saying, "Fix doll." Her enthusiasm waned as mother continued to take charge.

The clinician intervened, telling mother he could see how hard it was for her to let Lucy fully take the lead, now that Lucy was using a wide vocabulary and her marvelous imagination. Mother said that her "secret wish" was for Lucy "to perform." When the clinician asked what the impetus was for this wish, mother reiterated her earlier fear of "being a bad mother," and said, "I'll prove I'm a good mother by making Lucy do what she should." He commented that she might best prove herself a good mother by helping Lucy to think for herself. Lucy had to learn to use ideas to guide her play; this would help her to control her behavior better. Mother smiled; she had heard this advice before. The clinician said that he was just reminding her of some earlier principles, which her feelings made it hard for her to follow. She again associated Lucy's competence with her own mother's dominance, adding, "Lucy is so competent now that at times I feel she is smarter than me." She obviously felt somewhat threatened by Lucy's use of ideas; under the guise of encouraging Lucy's competence, she was inadvertently playing out an unconscious wish to make sure her daughter would not dominate her.

As mother and daughter played some more, mother relaxed and started to follow Lucy's lead. Lucy took charge, a smile returning to her face. They looked through some toys, Lucy tentatively asking, "What's this?" and "What's that?" Once she saw that mother was not taking over, she arranged some of the toys into a theme, "Who lives in this house?" She said, "Maybe this person lives in a house," or "That person lives in a house." She looked at mother to see if she would interfere, but mother just said, "Oh yes, I can see where this one lives in a house. What are they going to do next?" Lucy soon had a whole family living in a house, with each member deciding which bedroom to have and who would sit where around the table. She was obviously starting her play with a safe theme around order and finding one's place; it was nice to see her take the lead.

Parents and clinician discussed additional ways to give Lucy opportunities for increased assertiveness. Mother revealed that Lucy was a little cautious with some of her more assertive friends, and the clinician suggested exposing her to a wider variety of companions so that she could learn to interact with the more assertive ones. A follow-up visit was arranged for 1 month later to monitor Lucy through this new stage of development.

In summary, Lucy had only slight constitutional contributions to her mild regulatory difficulty: sensitivity to loud noises, being moved rapidly in space, things moving rapidly toward or away from her, and transitions to new situations. More significant was the environmental factor of an extremely anxious mother (who had good reason to be anxious, given her family history as the child of Holocaust survivors). The mother's depressive ideation, in particular her fear of being a "bad" mother, made her very overprotective as she tried desperately to be a good mother. This was played out with Lucy in the developmental stage of two-way communication: mother made communication a one-way affair by overcontrolling her daughter and moving in too quickly. She interfered with Lucy's ability to calm herself and to take initiative in their communication. Compounding the problem was the anxiety of both parents about the father's seizure disorder. Sharing his worries about injuring his child allowed father to move from less available, noncontingent relatedness to greater empathy and availability.

A series of four sessions had helped this family negotiate two-way communication during infancy and early toddlerhood. When the issue of assertiveness came up again during Lucy's preschool years (when she started using representational capacities, emotional ideas, and the beginning of emotional thinking), they were able to come back again. The clinician remained available in a preventive capacity, because the issue of assertiveness was likely to come up again at further developmental junctures.

References

DeGangi GA, Greenspan SI: The development of sensory functioning in infants. Phys Occup Ther Pediatr 8:21–33, 1988

DeGangi GA, Greenspan SI: The assessment of sensory functioning in infants. Phys Occup Ther Pediatr 9:21–33, 1989

Dunn J, Kendrick C: Siblings. Cambridge, MA, Harvard University Press, 1982

Flavell JH, Green FL, Flavell ER: Development of knowledge about the appearance–reality distinction, with commentaries by M.W. Watson and J.C. Campione. Monogr Soc Res Child Dev 51:1–87, 1986

Greenspan SI: Infancy and Early Childhood: The Practice of Clinical Assessment and Intervention With Emotional and Developmental Challenges. Madison, CT, International Universities Press, 1992

Harris PL, Brown E, Marriott C, et al: Monsters, ghosts, and witches: testing the limits of the fantasy–reality distinction in young children. British Journal of Developmental Psychology 9:105–123, 1991

Harris PL, Kavanaugh RD, Meredith MC: Young children's comprehension of pretend episodes: The integration of successive actions. Child Dev 65:16-30, 1994

Hartman A: Diagrammatic assessment of family relationships. Soc Casework 59:465–476, 1978

Wolf D, Rygh J, Altshuler J: Agency and experience: actions and states in play narratives, in Symbolic Play. Edited by Bretherton I. Orlando, FL, Academic Press, 1984, pp 195–217

Wooley JD, Wellman HM: Young children's understanding of realities, nonrealities, and appearances. Child Dev 61:946–964, 1990

4

Therapeutic Principles

Having completed the assessment and created the functional emotional developmental profile, we are now ready to design and implement an intervention program to teach missing developmental capacities, expand constricted capacities, and strengthen unstable ones. To fully understand the special features of our developmental approach, let us first consider more traditional approaches to infant and child therapy and how these differ from the interventions we propose.

Traditional Approaches to Child Therapy

Psychodynamic Therapy

Dynamic interventions with children typically involve several goals. A therapist may help a child put feelings into words through play and talk. If 3-year-old Susie makes one puppet bite another, the therapist might wonder out loud if the first puppet is mad at the second. If Susie then elaborates on how the first puppet wants to bite and hit the second, the therapist might conclude that she has successfully verbalized her feelings.

Another typical goal is to help children resolve core emotional conflicts. If a young child makes one doll bite another doll, then has the first doll act very fearful or disorganized, the therapist might infer that the child is playing out a conflict between aggression and fear, and that withdrawal and disorganization are her solutions to this conflict. The therapist might then try to help the child understand that there are two different feelings involved, "mad" and "scary," thus helping her resolve the conflict.

The therapist will also try to help parents refrain from undermining their children's development. A clinician may determine that parents are unwittingly too permissive or punitive, that they are abusive or neglectful, or that they subtly put pressure on their child by drawing her into their marital conflicts. Treatment goals would include helping the parents to change these patterns of behavior.

Dynamic approaches, although helpful for some children at some ages, cannot reach children who can neither speak nor engage in pretend play. This group includes children under the age of 2 years and older children whose developmental delays or emotional challenges interfere with the age-appropriate use of language. Furthermore, even children or adults who can use symbols will exhibit a range of healthy functioning and challenges at the earlier, presymbolic developmental levels. Dynamic therapy, focusing as it does on symbolic representation of feelings and conflicts, does not offer a way to address these earlier levels. How can therapists help children attend and focus better, become more engaged and connected with others, and become more intentional and reciprocal in their communication? Furthermore, how can they help parents and teachers not simply to avoid behaving in damaging ways but to actively promote children's healthy development? How can therapists help caregivers create experiences that harness and develop their children's emotional and intellectual capacities at all developmental levels? The developmental, individual-differences, relationship-based (DIR) approach to treatment, as we will see, offers interventions to address these issues.

Behavioral Therapy

Behavioral interventions are designed to promote behaviors that are deemed appropriate and desirable and to discourage less desirable behaviors. This process occurs through "discriminative learning" in which the child comes to associate certain targeted behaviors with positive reinforcement and certain other behaviors with negative reinforcement or with no reinforcement. In addition, a behavior therapist helps a child master complex tasks by "shaping," or breaking a single task into its component parts, each of which is taught individually and given positive reinforcement.

Behavioral approaches offer a means of understanding why a child may persist in certain behaviors (for example, he may be receiving less-than-obvious positive reinforcement for them) and how complex behaviors can grow from simpler ones. However, the focus on isolated units of behavior tends to obscure more fundamental developmental deficits. What is one to do when the main challenge for a child is not so much a specific set of behaviors but failure to master an entire developmental capacity?

Suppose a child habitually pinches, pokes, and hits other children. It might help to positively reinforce cooperative behavior by providing praise, candy, or stars when this child shares a toy with someone and to negatively reinforce the aggressive behavior with a "time out" or other sanction. A more skillful behavioral intervention might involve initially rewarding even the simplest piece of cooperative behavior—a kind look, an instance of sitting briefly next to someone else without poking—and waiting until the child is consistently accomplishing this simple action before reinforcing progressively more complex positive behaviors.

If the child's aggressive behavior is part of a larger developmental failure, however, he may never have learned how to relate warmly to other people. There may be no difference in his mind between a human being and a chair; both can be kicked when he feels aggressive. (This deficit is often found in sociopathic individuals who have experienced severe and prolonged emotional deprivation early in life.) He has never learned how to empathize with other people because he has little positive feeling for them, and he has never learned how to regulate his aggressive impulses because he lacks a basic capacity to see that his own behavior can have an impact on other people. It is not that he does not care whether he behaves aggressively; he does not understand the concept of social consequences.

For such a child, the first step is to help him master a sense of engagement. All subsequent learning will depend on him being part of an intimate, trusting relationship. If this goal is sacrificed, more will be lost than gained. An intervention that focuses on behavior alone without considering the more fundamental developmental challenge—e.g., an intervention that uses isolation as negative reinforcement and very concrete rewards, such as candy, as positive reinforcement—may actually work against the goal of fostering the child's ability to engage and relate.

The second goal for such a child would simply be to foster two-way communication and thus an understanding of cause and effect. A child who sees himself and the world as aimless needs to master these core competencies before he can appreciate the consequences of his interactions. Once he has mastered them, he might well be able to benefit from systematic feedback that relies not on specific behaviors but on a great deal of warmth and empathy, along with firm limits. Such an approach would be consistent with behavioral principles but would not be so mechanical or systematic as to undermine the child's achievement of basic developmental capacities.

As another example, consider the child who will not take turns. It would be easy to systematically reinforce turn taking. However, if the child's behavior stems from a more basic inability to understand two-way communication and the nature of his impact on the world, this narrow behavioral approach might miss the boat, preventing him from learning to experiment with ways of interacting and to assess the feedback he gets from others.

Another limitation of behavioral approaches is that children may become dependent on concrete reinforcers. A child may want stars and candy but not seem to care much about people. The child's focus on "primitive" reinforcers (Greenspan 1975) may constitute more of a problem than the particular behaviors he evidences. Similarly, a child who focuses on not just primitive but also very generalized reinforcers, or who does not distinguish among reinforcers, will present a special challenge. Such a child may behave as he does because he feels rewarded by circumstances most children would not find rewarding. The child who enjoys other people's discomfort, who craves things rather than relationships, or who feels rewarded by any form of attention rather than specifically by praise or respect, lacks the developmental capacities that would enable him to derive pleasure from age-appropriate rewards. In such circumstances, a broad developmental approach rather than a narrow behavioral one is indicated.

Developmentally Informed Therapies

Several intervention approaches have made use of developmental concepts but have not used a comprehensive developmental model. Selma Fraiberg (Fraiberg 1980; Fraiberg et al. 1987) pioneered an approach that involved understanding how parents' perceptions of their infant or young child shaped their interactions with the child; the parents' perceptions, or misperceptions, were seen as stemming from their own early childhood experiences. Through "infant–parent psychotherapy," Fraiberg and her colleagues helped parents gain insight into this process and resolve internal conflicts that prevented them from interacting in ways that fostered their child's optimal development. Fraiberg's model, although a seminal contribution to the field, did not include much focus on infants' individual physiological and constitutional qualities or how these influence caregivers' perceptions, family dynamics, and infant–caregiver interactions.

In addition to Fraiberg, several other individuals and programs laid the foundations for the field of comprehensive, developmentally based treatment. Sibylle Escalona (1968), Lois Murphy (1974), Jean Ayres (1964), and T. Berry Brazelton (Brazelton and Cramer 1990) described individual differences in the ways infants and children respond to sensory stimulation and plan motor activities. Sally Provence (1983) and her colleagues conducted pioneering studies showing how family support programs, based on an understanding of many aspects of infant and early childhood functioning, could be helpful. Several other pioneering projects involved early intervention with varying degrees of cognitive and social support, showing the impressive results that could be obtained by intervening early in children's development. Such intervention programs, which include those of Ron Lally (Honig and Lally 1981; Lally et al. 1988), David Olds (1984), The Abecedarian Project (Berrueta-Clement et al. 1984), and the Ypsilanti Project (Ramey and Campbell 1984; Ramey and Ramey 1998; Schweinhart et al. 1983), have been shown to improve educational outcomes and reduce social dropout rates, delinquency, teenage pregnancy, and other problems.

The DIR Approach to Intervention

The DIR approach does not contradict psychodynamic or behavioral therapies but instead incorporates elements of these into a more comprehensive developmental approach that can be applied not only to child therapy but also to intervention in family relationships and in educational settings. The DIR approach, unlike the traditional therapies, addresses all six core developmental capacities that children need to learn in order to function and thrive. It addresses children's need to develop each capacity in a stable and wide-ranging manner so that they can use all six capacities to experience and explore a wide range of feelings within their relationships and can access these capacities even when under stress. The biopsychosocial nature of the DIR approach also sets it apart from traditional therapies. Unlike dynamic or behavioral approaches, the DIR approach addresses each child's unique information processing and motor characteristics as well as family dynamics and interactional patterns at home, at school, and in other relevant settings.

Putting the DIR Approach Into Practice: An Introduction to "Floortime"

The cornerstone of the DIR approach to intervention is what we call "Floortime." This term is a sort of shorthand for a set of principles that guide the application of the DIR model in therapeutic interactions, in family relationships, and in educational settings. The most fundamental principle of Floortime is that of engaging an infant or child in interactions that mobilize his six core developmental capacities. Technically, Floortime is a period of unstructured, spontaneous play or talk in which the adult follows the child's lead, tuning in as closely as possible to the child's interests and rhythms and attempting to respond in ways that support and amplify whatever themes the child seems to be expressing. With infants and very young children, the adult needs literally to get down on the floor with the child. With older children, one might be playing basketball, walking in the woods, talking on a couch, or sharing in some other activity. Regardless of the activity, the goal of Floortime is to build a warm, trusting relationship in which shared attention, interaction, and communication are occurring on the child's terms. A parent, educator, or therapist can engage a child in this way; a comprehensive therapeutic program may involve all three. Because the basic Floortime processes are the same, we describe these processes in general terms, with occasional references to the special challenges faced by the therapist in serving as a consultant to the parents.

In many cases, the first therapeutic goal is getting the parents to engage in regular Floortime with their child. The diagnostic workup may indicate that one-on-one therapy is also needed. The diagnostician may observe certain limitations in the way the parents engage their child or discover that the youngster is particularly challenging due to her constitutional-maturational characteristics. In such cases, the therapist will incorporate the principles of Floortime into the direct therapy while helping the parents learn to implement the same principles in their relationship with the child. Direct therapy will include traditional psychotherapeutic interactions as needed—for example, helping a verbal child see the connections between one feeling and another or between feelings and behavior—but these should also be built on the principles of Floortime.

The therapist will work to help the parents discover how to interact with their child in ways that harness or strengthen the child's capacities for attention and engagement; two-way communication; symbolic representation of feelings, ideas, and intentions; and organization, differentiation, and connection of meanings. Furthermore, the therapist helps the parents to assist their child in applying each of these capacities to a broad range of age-appropriate emotions—pleasure, dependency, excitement, aggression, self-control, empathy, and more mature types of love.

The therapist will spend some of the time actively coaching parents, suggesting that they try a particular approach or going through the motions of Floortime with them. It is best to get down on the floor with the parents, sometimes whispering into their ears, sometimes wondering aloud why they are trying something one way rather than another, sometimes offering a few ideas that they can use to discover how it feels to engage their child in a new way. All the principles of Floortime apply to working with parents: capture their attention, engage them, do not lecture, and help them use symbolic representations ("ideas") to comprehend the Floortime process.

A second facet of consulting involves discovering and working with the parents' difficulties in engaging their child in Floortime. The therapist must be aware of the parents' emotions and conflicts and clarify for the parents how these affect their interaction with the child. For example, one needs to bring out the feelings of the mother who is unable to deal with her child's aggression because it frightens her or the father who fears intimacy and therefore wants only to roughhouse rather than engage in slower and more dependency-oriented kinds of play. Such clarification can be achieved on the floor and in sessions alone with the parents, when they can feel freer to discuss their reactions to the child's Floortime. Sometimes, revealing chitchat takes place off to the side of the play, as a parent talks about his own background while playing with his child.

Global difficulties, or deficits (e.g., a fear of relating and interacting), will inhibit a parent from engaging in a whole developmental realm with the child, whereas more focal anxieties and conflicts allow a parent to engage in some emotional realms but not in others. For example, someone who is anxious about sexuality, excitement, or aggression may suddenly become controlling during play with the child when such themes emerge.

These challenges notwithstanding, parents who are motivated by warmth and concern and have the potential for growth can be mobilized by their strong desire to help their children. In learning to address their child's developmental challenges, the parents make developmental progress as well.

The therapist may determine that his special skills as a "Floortimer" are necessary for a child who is very avoidant, is overly reactive, has difficulty staying focused, or easily becomes agitated. Other candidates for direct intervention include children who become paralyzed with anxiety, have overwhelming fears, become fragmented and lost in fantasy, evidence difficulties in processing information, or have conflicts that need to be gently teased to the surface. The therapist will want to coach himself in much the same way he coaches the parents, paying attention to his own tactics. For example, "How am I trying to simplify my gestures or words for this child with an auditory processing difficulty?" The therapist will need to pay attention to his own emotional reactions: "Why do I get so bored and avoidant when Johnny tunes me out or becomes repetitive in his play?" The therapist may conduct direct intervention with one or both parents present, alone with the child, or both, depending on the needs of the child and family.

A teacher's Floortime will have much in common with that of parents, including the therapist's role as consultant. Teachers, however, often work simultaneously on additional educational goals and generally work with small groups. Examples of educational applications of Floortime are described later.

Floortime is an assessment approach as well as a therapeutic strategy. After completing the initial evaluation, the clinician should continue to use his Floortime experiences with the child to refine his diagnostic impressions and revise therapeutic goals accordingly.

Floortime, although a technique, is also a general philosophy of relating to children. The core developmental capacities of attention and engagement; two-way communication; the symbolic representation of meanings; and the organization, differentiation, and connection of meanings can be fostered, or undermined, in all interactions between child and caregivers. Most intervention plans will begin with the establishment of regular Floortime between parents or other key caregivers and the child. The strengthened relationships they build through Floortime will be necessary for all subsequent interventions to succeed.

In the next three sections, we describe how to use Floortime to foster each of the six core developmental capacities. We then describe a series of additional interventions that can be implemented after Floortime has begun to yield results.

Floortime, Level 1: Shared Attention and Regulation, and Level 2: Engagement and Relating

A parent, teacher, or therapist working with a child needs to figure out how to pull the child in. The adult needs to ask him- or herself, "How do I get this child to look at me, listen to me, be calm in my presence, and feel emotionally connected to me?" In most relationships, these first steps—what we might call "good chemistry"—are accomplished without the parties even thinking about them. Many challenging children, however, have a hard time with them.

For Floortime to succeed, the adult must get down on the floor with the child (or follow an older child's lead in some other shared activity); be patient and relaxed (a nervous, jittery adult cannot help a child feel calm and focused); and try to capture the child's emotional tone. It is important to resist the natural tendency to want another person's tone to match our own or our idea of an appropriate tone. Instead, the adult needs to find ways to let the child know he is being understood. Words are not always necessary; one's way of looking at the child, or the tone and rhythm of one's voice, can provide an effective mirror. With a verbal child, one might say, for example, "Gee, I can tell you are feeling kind of tired today," in a tone of voice that conveys warmth and acceptance.

The adult needs to be aware of his or her own feelings—warmth and enjoyment as well as irritation, anger, or feeling overwhelmed—because these will affect his or her ability to tune in to the child's feelings. A depressed caregiver, for example, may convey a flat, empty emotional tone and talk or gesture very slowly, with long pauses. Children often find it hard to attend to and engage with someone in such a state. The caregiver's tone of voice also communicates a great deal. A warm, compelling, expectant tone of voice confidently invites the child to engage. Some parents, in contrast, have an anxious, hesitant way of speaking that seems to say, "I know you won't even look at me." Tone of voice is an important parameter for the therapist to consider in coaching the parents and in sessions with the child.

Sensory Pathways and Motor Patterns

Remember that each of us takes in information through all sensory pathways. When an adult's intuition fails to enable him or her to engage a child, it is necessary to examine each sensory pathway to determine what information processing characteristics may be affecting the child's ability to attend, self-regulate, and engage. This is, of course, a continuation of the process begun during the assessment phase. As we observe the child and try different ways of interacting during Floortime, we refine our initial hypotheses and fine-tune our approach. We may discover, for example, that in order to mirror a particular child's emotional tone we must keep in mind that this child prefers soft, gentle sounds and startles easily at loud or sudden noises. We may be able to help parents understand that their child cannot help stiffening up or flinching if they approach her with sudden movements or unexpectedly clap a hand on her shoulder. The parents of a child who is underreactive to sound can be taught that their child may be unable to process a quietly spoken question; instead, they must capture her attention by speaking in an animated, excited manner.

The child's motor characteristics will also shape the way he attends and engages. Parents and teachers often complain about the "fidgety" child who cannot seem to sit still and may continually touch objects or put them in his mouth. Some of these children actually crave touch and can focus better if given worry beads or other safe objects to fiddle with. Some also have a strong need for motor discharge. For example, a child may have trouble reading and comprehending a story while sitting in a chair because it takes all his concentration just to sit still; his body *needs* to move. An understanding teacher may discover that the child has a much easier time completing the task if he is allowed to simultaneously walk around and fidget with some unbreakable objects in the classroom. By responding to him in this way, instead of berating and lecturing him about the need to sit still, the teacher not only enables the child to attend and take in information but gives him the experience of empathy and warmth as well.

In addition to the child's senses and motor tendencies, it is important for the adult to respect the child's natural pace. Some children—even if they crave a lot of sensory input—are slow to form relationships. Others are quicker to warm up to a new person. Some babies reach eagerly for a parent who returns from work at the end of the day, whereas others take longer to reconnect. The child's pace and rhythm are determined, in part, by her way of using her motor system to carry out complex actions. The first sign of a motor planning problem is often seen in the baby who cannot cuddle or figure out how to get her neck into the crook of her mother's neck. Related to motor planning are variations in the way children use their muscles. If a child's muscle tone is excessively loose or tight, she will be unable to get her muscles to do what she wants them to, and this impairment will shape how she responds to her world. For example, suppose an adult is holding up a colorful stuffed toy for a baby to see, but the baby just keeps looking and pointing slightly past the object. An adult who is impatient and does not recognize the muscle tone problem may think the baby is not interested. If the baby grabs the adult's nose instead of the toy, the adult may feel attacked. This baby is not bored, distractible, or aggressive; she just cannot control her head and arm movements. Parents, therapists, and other caregivers need to be aware that such a child is in fact attentive and warmly engaged but is miscommunicating because of a motor system impairment. Similarly, suppose an adult says invitingly to a 3-year-old, "Come over here and play!" If the child has a motor system problem, she may wander here and there throughout the room before finally getting to the adult. Rather than getting impatient or giving up, the adult can maintain engagement by saying with words or gestures, "Oh, I see you coming closer!"

A therapist working with a child whose sensory and motor processing differences present special challenges will need to help the parents consider their expectations and fantasies about who their child is or should be. Sometimes, the parents' (or the therapist's) limitations in engaging are influenced by rigid expectations about a particular child. By becoming aware of and reconsidering such expectations, parents can free themselves to learn how their child actually experiences the world and to become more flexible in the ways in which they approach their child.

Floortime, Level 3: Two-Way Intentional Affective Signaling and Communication, and Level 4: Long Chains of Coregulated Emotional Signaling and Shared Social Problem Solving

As discussed in Chapter 2 ("The Functional Emotional Stages of Development"), two-way communication is essential for all learning; it is the basis for understanding causality and how the world is organized. It also provides the foundation for learning to differentiate between self and other, to control one's impulses, and to discern the intentions of other people. Two-way communication is the only process by which a child obtains feedback in response to her own behavior, thoughts, and feelings. Without such feedback, the child's inner world remains chaotic and fragmented.

To foster two-way communication during Floortime, one must meet the child on her own turf. There are only two rules: the child cannot hurt herself or anyone else, and she cannot break anything. The child is the director of the Floortime drama. Maintaining two-way communication with a child can be hard work. Adults sometimes fall into a pattern of merely watching the child play or standing apart and commenting on the child's actions without expecting a response. It is especially tempting to go this route when the child seems indifferent or actively ignores one's presence. The goal, however, is to foster two-way communication. It is therefore necessary in such cases to intrude oneself into the interaction. One starts modestly, by elaborating on whatever the child is doing. If she is playing with a car, one might form a garage with one's hands and try to elicit her help. If she ignores the garage, one might step up the intrusiveness by forming a roadblock in front of the car. The child is now forced to contend with the adult. If she pushes at the adult's hands, or makes a sound of irritation, she has built on the adult's gestures, thus beginning to open and close circles of communication. Note that this intervention follows the child's lead, staying with her preferred activity of playing with cars. The adult can then try to continue the interaction in a playful, non-threatening way, keeping in mind the child's individual comfort level with sounds, sights, and movement patterns. In this way, the adult gradually helps the child get used to interacting. As she begins to feel the novelty, pleasure, and mastery of interacting, she will likely begin to initiate more activities herself. This process works well for both very withdrawn children and very shy, cautious children.

When working with a child who is not using two-way communication and seems reluctant to do so, it is important initially to demand very little of him. One might put the garage in front of his car and ask, "Do you want me to take it away?" The child simply has to say "yes" or "no," or indicate the same by nodding, shaking his head, or pointing. Children who do not like to close circles will nonetheless often be willing to make a subtle gesture, such as a slight head nod or motion of the pinky finger, in response to the adult. The key is to help the child get started.

Even if he responds by pushing the adult away, this represents progress because if his word or gesture is intentional, two-way communication has begun.

Faced with a withdrawn or aloof child, many therapists make the mistake of merely commenting aloud on what the child is doing. If he is drinking water by himself, the therapist may say, "Oh, I see you like to drink water." This is a monologue, not two-way communication. Such verbalization is akin to parallel play. It may be useful at the beginning of therapy to get the child used to one's voice and to convey interest, but it does not provide an interactive experience and therefore does not foster differentiation between self and other, cause and effect.

Two-way communication should be approached in a manner that encourages the child's initiative and assertiveness. One of the biggest mistake parents, teachers, and therapists make is to try to control the action. The adult says a word and wants the child to mimic it. The adult shows the child a book and wants the child to look at it. An adult who is too successful at being the boss might foster a verbal and bright child, but this child will likely be overly compliant and passive as well.

If necessary, one can get an interaction going by a maneuver such as putting toys in front of the child, but then one must let the child discover how he wants to act, as opposed to acting for him. By way of example, a speech therapist described to one of us (S.G.) a child who would not take turns in a group setting. When the members of the group passed a ball around, this boy would keep the ball instead of passing it on to the next child. In an attempt to get communication going, the therapist would ask the child for the ball. If he refused, verbally or nonverbally, or simply held on to the ball, she continued asking him for it. What would happen if, after three days, the boy still held onto the ball? She said, "Well, I'd probably finally grab it from him and give it to the next person. He has to learn to take turns!"

What would the child learn from this experience? The two-way communication just described teaches him what can be done to him by someone more powerful, but it teaches him nothing about initiative. If the therapist intrudes and grabs the ball, the child's initiative is undermined, as is the goal of teaching him social communication and turn taking. In contrast, if one says, "Give me the ball," and the child says, "No" and one responds, "Oh, please?" and the child says, "No" and one says, "Give it here!" and the child says, "No way!" three circles of communication have been opened and closed, with the child in charge. Passing the ball should be considered only a vehicle for promoting interaction. It is always possible to get another ball and keep up the conversation with the recalcitrant child while the others pass the new ball. If the boy tries to take the new ball, the therapist could say "No" and block his path to it; as he gets frustrated and keeps trying to get the second ball, he may close 40 or 50 communication circles. Some of the best two-way communication occurs when a child is highly motivated.

Two-way communication can occur on many levels. The simplest of these involves physical touch. A child who feels a touch will often touch back. Even when very young babies hug and nuzzle, two-way communication often occurs: the baby positions herself, the parent shifts position in response to the baby's movement, the baby responds in turn, and so on. Touch can be used to very gently coax a withdrawn or frightened child into interaction. In working with one very withdrawn young boy, one of us (S.G.) tried placing a doll lightly on the child's leg. He pushed it off. A gentle game evolved, ever so slowly, of repeatedly putting the doll on his leg. After a few repetitions, he began anticipating the gestures and moving his leg away before the doll made contact. Sometimes the therapist would put the doll on his own leg, and the child would nod in approval.

In addition to touch, other senses may be used for simple gestural communication. A glance begets a glance. A sound begets a state of attentiveness and a sound in return. One person's shift in posture leads to a shift in the second person's posture, which leads to a further shift in the first person's posture. Clinicians often make the mistake of assuming that a child is interacting only when she is looking directly at the clinician. However, a vocal, tactile, or postural interaction may be occurring even while the child appears indifferent, aloof, or aimless. These subtle types of interaction often foreshadow more direct eye contact and other obvious signs of pleasure.

Simple patterns of two-way communication lead to more complex patterns. As a child gains experience in this mode of interaction, he opens and closes an increasingly large number of circles in a row. In addition, his individual gestures convey increasingly complex intentions. The toddler who points to his father's hat and then to his own head may be asking if he can put daddy's hat on. This sequence is more complex than simply vocalizing while pointing to the hat.

Distal communication, or communication across space, occurs from about 8 to 20 months of age onward. Distal communication can be fostered through Floortime. A child builds a tower of blocks and looks up at the adult a few feet away, who then claps his hands and says, "Wow! That's a tall tower!" When the child smiles and adds another block, the adult and child have closed a circle of communication across space. They may feel as though they are in each other's arms, although they are physically separate.

Floortime, Level 5: Creating Representations (or Ideas), and Level 6: Building Bridges Between Ideas: Logical Thinking

In many cases, a key goal of intervention is to help a child move from simply feeling emotions and discharging them in action to experiencing the *idea* of the emotion and expressing this through words or make-believe play. Many children brought to therapists for evaluation of aggressive behavior turn out to need help making this transition from action to what we sometimes call "emotional ideas."

During Floortime, one can help a child achieve this milestone by being available to interact with her in increasingly complex ways, especially in pretend play.

One needs to enter the child's world as an active play partner rather than simply observing and describing out loud what she is doing. For example, if a 4-year-old is playing with dolls and a tea set, a therapist or parent who comments, "You are feeding your doll so nicely," is not interacting. Such commentary does nothing to help the child amplify and differentiate ideas in the context of a relationship. Instead, the adult might ask the child to describe further why one doll got so mad at the other doll when the teacup was knocked over. Or the adult might enter the drama, speaking for one of the dolls: "I'm sorry I spilled the tea." At this point, the child might say, "Well, you are still being bad and you're getting spanked 6,000 times!" The adult then follows the child's theme: "Oh, please don't spank me!" "That's just the way it is—you have to get a spanking." As a general rule, one should try first to get two-way nonverbal or gestural interaction going with the child; this will make it easier to progress to interaction using words and pretend play.

This all sounds easy enough, and sometimes it is. Yet all too often, adults not only fall into parallel commentary but actively interfere with the child's use of emotional ideas. A parent playing "tea party" with a child might suddenly forget that this is just make-believe and say crossly, "Don't you dare bang that teacup, it's making too much noise," or "Don't hit that doll with the other one! You might break them." Not only will the child feel confused and undermined, but her creation of the imaginative drama will abruptly grind to a halt. The adult has suddenly forced the child into a more concrete way of thinking, in which the dolls' actions are regarded as real rather than as representations. A parent (or therapist or teacher) who cannot enter and maintain the make-believe mode may in this way derail a child's ability to use emotional ideas and to experiment with ways of picturing the world.

Even in reality-based conversations, it is possible to respond in ways that are too concrete and literal and thereby prevent a child from progressing developmentally. For example, suppose a child says, "I want to go outside right now!" Most of us have on at least some occasions found ourselves responding to such demands by saying, "No, you can't go outside now!" A power struggle ensues. The adult considers only the very literal message the child is conveying and assumes that a "yes" or "no" answer is required.

However, another kind of response is possible, one which gently pushes the child beyond concrete thinking toward the use of emotional ideas. Suppose, instead of granting or denying the child's request, the adult says, "You seem to think it has to be right now," or "Now? It has to be *right now*?" The adult focuses on the child's sense of urgency, which helps the child become aware of this emotion in himself. The emotion, rather than the action the child demanded, becomes the topic of discussion. The more the child and parent discuss or even argue about the child's urgency, the more likely both gestural and symbolic circles of communication are being opened and closed, giving the child an important learning experience fueled by his state of high motivation. Extended reasoning and arguing about his feelings and wishes will help him begin to picture these emotions and to label them. Most children who are involved in aggressive behavior or other kinds of behavioral discharge of emotion have parents who react in overly concrete ways in related areas of the child's life. If the parent can develop a less concrete, "Why now?" attitude toward the child's desires and demands and keep dialogues on these going longer, the child often starts doing better.

We can think of the use of ideas as developing in two stages: the concrete use of ideas to describe actions, and the truly abstract use of ideas to represent emotions. It is the abstraction that buys a child time to reason and be able to talk about an urge. The child can say, "I feel excited," without having to jump around or shout; she can say, "I'm mad at you," without having to punch or kick.

How does one help a child make this developmental leap when she seems to be locked into a behavior? It is necessary to help her make the transition in stages, as happens in normal development between about 16 and about 24 months. A verbal child who is unable to abstract emotions, label feelings, or express emotions through make-believe should be helped first to label her behaviors. An adult can (in addition to setting limits on the behavior) say to a 4-year-old who has been kicking and poking other children, "How do you feel when you do that?" The child may say, "I just like to kick them and poke them when they bother me," but may never say she is feeling angry. Instead of making the common mistake of saying, "You must feel angry," the adult could say, "What are the things you do when you feel like kicking?" and help the child label each behavior—kicking, poking, hitting, yelling, running around. The next question to ask is, "What do all these behaviors have in common?" The child may still not be aware of the anger inside, but she may say her muscles feel tense, she feels like exploding, or she feels like eating. It is important to help her describe her feelings in great detail, keeping in mind that these descriptions will often initially be of physical sensations. With a younger or less verbal child, the adult may need to start by describing the situation the child is in, such as being yelled at by another child, and describing what the child tends to do in the situation.

Obviously, such dialogues must take place repeatedly, over a long period of time, and be very interactive. The process requires a great deal of patience but is well worth the effort. By helping the child to describe behaviors associated with particular situations, the adult is helping the child create categories of behaviors. Categorization is one step closer to the abstraction of a feeling.

It is critical to help the child describe what occurs "inside the body" just before and during the behavior. Many children, and adults, who cannot abstract feelings can describe bodily sensations. "My chest feels tight," "My legs feel like they just have to move." As one teenager put it, "There was this pressure in my arm, and all of a sudden it was hitting people." Help the child describe each sensation as fully as possible. As he uses more detail, and as the interactive dialogue continues, his metaphors will likely become more vivid and more closely related to true emotions. "My muscles feel tense" may evolve to "they feel like a volcano about to blow up." As one empathically helps the child describe such physical states and categorize behaviors, he can gradually begin to connect a particular sensation with a general category of behavior. He will gradually begin to abstract and label that feeling we call "anger." This associative process is similar to the way children normally learn when they begin to identify feelings. As indicated earlier, it is critical not to label feelings for the child; this intellectualizes and, ironically, lengthens the learning process.

Once one has helped a child to use shared meanings—that is, to communicate abstracted feeling states or emotional ideas—the next step is to help her expand the depth and range of these feelings. Expanding the depth involves helping her make her pretend dramas more complex and nuanced. Two dolls get mad at each other, but the drama need not stop at this fact. What happens next? How mad is each character, and why? This process can also take place in verbal discussions. If the child says, "I'm hungry, I want some food," one should not just say "oh," "yes," or "no." Instead, one encourages the child to amplify the theme, to practice using emotional ideas. What would she most like to eat? When does she want it? What does it taste like? A child who complains of feeling angry at her friend should be asked to elaborate. What happened between the two friends, what does the angry feeling feel like, how angry does the child feel? One does not interrogate the child like a lawyer, of course, but verbally and gesturally invites the child to elaborate by staying empathic and interested.

Following the child's lead is not always easy, because one has to have some sense of where the child wants to go. Without leading the child, the adult has to be a half-step ahead. Open-ended questions, such as "What happened next?" are often helpful. Another useful technique is to make summarizing comments about the child's real-life story or pretend drama. "Let's see, the king and queen left their castle to hunt, then they got mad at each other and rode their horses into separate parts of the forest. I wonder what's going to happen next?" Such summaries help the child to feel understood and to take the story one step further.

Related to expanding the depth of feelings is expanding the range of feelings the child can experience and express. Some children play out only themes of compliance and cooperation. Their dolls or stuffed animals hug each other and talk sweetly but never get jealous, rambunctious, or angry. Another child may create scene after scene portraying fights and competition but avoid issues of love or separation entirely. The same techniques and style of interaction that help a child deepen his drama will help him broaden its range as well.

A therapist or other adult can best help a child broaden the drama by keeping an eye on both the forest and the trees. The "trees" are the details of the story: each way in which one horse is prettier than the other horse, each of ten different complaints one car has about another car. The "forest" is the overarching theme: each horse wants to be the prettiest, the cars are angry at each other. Through summarizing comments, the adult can articulate the theme by pulling together the disparate elements of the drama for the child. One should move back and forth between interactions that help the child amplify specific "trees" she is interested in and comments that help the child see the "forest" and expand its range. Another way to think of this process is that the adult moves back and forth between helping the child elaborate the story's content and conveying empathy with the feelings it portrays. One gets involved in the content for the purpose of finding opportunities to bring in the emotion or theme. Sometimes, however, children talk only about emotions and do not flesh out the story. If the child stays with statements like, "The purple horse is mad at the green horse, but she loves the pink horse," one focuses on helping the child amplify content: "What happened between the horses to make them feel that way?" As a child plays out a make-believe drama or relates real-life events, consider whether she is expressing mostly content and no feelings, or mostly feelings and no content. The goal is to help her flesh out both aspects of the drama.

The Floortime approaches we have described in this section will help a child not only to develop emotional ideas (level 5) but also to categorize and create logical connections between these ideas (level 6). As the adult helps the child open and close longer and longer chains of communication circles, amplify the elements of his real-life stories and pretend dramas, and move back and forth between content and emotional themes, the child is learning to define categories and to make increasingly complicated connections between meanings. He is learning to build logical bridges between his own different ideas, and between his ideas and the adult's.

To help a child begin the journey into categorizing, one coaches her to amplify both sides of any potential conflict. If she plays out a scene involving "good guys" and "bad guys," one can wonder aloud what makes the good guys good, what makes the bad guys bad. It can be particularly challenging to help a child amplify a drama centered on "evil" or "bad." She may create a chaotic series of scenes—a battle, followed by characters appearing to cooperate, followed by people getting hurt or dying, and so on. One may have to look very closely to find common themes or labels that can help her organize the diffuse content. One can encourage her to tell more about the particular details of the drama, then move to the "forest" by saying, "Okay, let's see if we can slow down for a second and figure out what's really going on here. I'm confused—I'm not sure who is fighting whom, and what's going on, and who's going to win, and why." The child may respond by clarifying, "Okay, these are the good guys, and these are the bad guys." In this way, the adult helps the child organize her ideas into categories and define how these categories are related.

For the child who becomes very fragmented and overwhelmed with the intense emotions and details of the moment, the best approach is not to focus further on details but to step back and help the child be aware of the overall theme of fragmentation. The most relevant categorization for this child may be the theme of chaos: "Everything is so confused, so wild."

To further the eventual categorization and connection of meanings, the therapist may have to help the child elaborate on meanings that are only hinted at and not put fully into the form of ideas. For example, a child may show teddy bears happily reading books to each other and also a wolf lurking in the shadows, but he may never develop a connection between these discrete elements. The therapist could say, "Gee, the bears seem so happy, and while there's an occasional wolf, they seem so safe and happy it's as if nothing bad ever happens to them." Such a comment may encourage the child to volunteer some information about the lurking danger.

At times, a child's drama may have a superficial quality; it lacks intensity. Perhaps she has dolls serve and empty tea cups repeatedly without much feeling. Again, one can comment in such a way that may open the door to more exploration of feelings: "Gee, it's so nice that they fill those nice tea cups over and over again." The child might say, "Oh, you think that's all they do? You should see what they do at night when everyone else is asleep." If, on the other hand, she says, "Yes, that's all they like to do, because they don't want to do anything else," one can simply pick up the thread: "Oh, why don't they like to do any other things?" By calling the child's attention to the possibility that she has a vested interest in shaping the drama in a certain way, one helps her build a bridge to other possibilities.

As we have seen in many of the examples considered so far, open-ended questions asking how, what, and why can be extremely useful. Bear in mind, however, that such questions can be misused to force on the child an interpretation beyond her capacity or inclination. For example, if a child has wolves attacking bears who are sitting around a fire reading, it may be tempting to ask, "Why do the wolves want to attack the nice bears? Is it that every time people are warm and close, something scary happens?" This kind of comment goes too far in suggesting to the child how the two themes are linked. Questions should be phrased in such a way as to enable the child to build her own bridges, not to establish a connection that the adult has in mind.

Adults will find it a challenge to stay with a child's pretend play or dialogue when its content is painful to them. When a child says, "I hate you!" or "You smell, I don't want to talk to you anymore," our gut reaction is to cut off the discussion: "Don't talk to me that way! You're being disrespectful." It is far more helpful, however, to remind oneself that the child is taking a chance by using words rather than behavior to express her feelings. One can then allow her to elaborate on the ways she hates the adult or feels the adult has been unfair. Then, particularly with a child of 3½ or older, one can raise questions as to whether there is any more to the story. In this way, one can see whether the child understands how her feelings of the moment fit into a larger context. At some point—if not immediately, then perhaps later the same day or tomorrow—the child may be able to reflect on the moment and see that her anger is only one aspect of her feelings toward the adult.

It is often extremely difficult for an adult to deal with a child in a state of intense emotion without undermining the child's use of emotional ideas. It takes hard work to tolerate the child's feelings and recognize that his expression of feeling in itself is positive as long as he is not hitting, breaking things, or using inappropriate language. (Although in therapy, using vivid or coarse language may be quite acceptable, using four-letter words at home or in public generally is not.) The goal is to help him continue to use ideas to describe his wishes and feelings, even when he is very upset. As an example, consider a young child upset because his father is away on a trip. During telephone calls home, the father can help his son put his feelings of sadness or anger into words and can also use words to help the child picture what his daddy is doing while he is away. The more that parents, therapists, and other caregivers can help a child represent intense affects, the more the stability, breadth, and depth of his representational system will be facilitated.

Bear in mind that every adult has his or her emotional Achilles' heel. No one of us is equally comfortable with every human theme. Themes that commonly trigger anxiety are sexuality, aggression, and intimacy. Experienced therapists are usually aware of their own Achilles' heels; that is what makes them experienced. Less experienced therapists, as well as parents and teachers, are more vulnerable to feeling bored, anxious, irritable, or controlling in response to the child's play or discussion. One should pay attention to such negative feelings and regard them as a clue that one's own anxieties or conflicts are being triggered by what the child is conveying.

One of the most important ways in which the therapist can assist parents or teachers is by helping these adults pay closer attention to their own reactions to the child's emotional ideas. The therapist reminds these adults that they are trying to help the child apply emotional ideas to a broad range of domains—separation, anger, and jealousy as well as intimacy, cooperation, and love. The therapist needs to point out to parents and teachers any general difficulty they may have in engaging the child on the level of emotional ideas, as well as their difficulties in tolerating particular emotions. These caregivers can be informed that it is normal to have strong reactions to some of what a child expresses and that no one can listen equally well to all of a child's ideas. One can, however, become more aware of one's emotional "hot buttons" and become more able to pause and reflect when these buttons are pushed instead of automatically jumping in with criticism, reassurance, or any other response that cuts off a child's expression of emotional ideas.

Floortime: A Six-Step Intervention Process

With children age 3 years or older who are fairly verbal, the intervention plan will in many cases call for Floortime to be employed as the core of a six-step intervention process. This process can be used to address a wide variety of challenges that children face, from handling aggression to building self-esteem.

Step 1: Establishing Floortime

Regardless of the problems, Step 1 is to establish a good baseline of Floortime between parents and child and between therapist and child if direct therapy is needed. By first using regular Floortime to solidify and deepen their relationship so that it incorporates the developmental levels of shared attention, engagement, and two-way communication using gestures and ideas, the adult and child lay the foundation for succeeding at the next steps, which are described later. For infants, toddlers, and preschoolers it is very important for parents to carry out these recommendations on a daily basis. The number of Floortime problem-solving and other interactions will be determined by the clinician and parents together. However, simply implementing the following suggestions during therapy sessions will also not be sufficient to support proper emotional growth and development because it is a child's daily experiences that are most essential.

Step 2: Problem-Solving Time

Problem-solving time is added after adult and child are regularly engaging well with one another in Floortime (depending on the child and adults involved, this may take anywhere from days to months). Problem-solving time is kept separate from Floortime and is an opportunity for adult and child to spend 15 or 20 minutes discussing problems, negotiating differences, and attempting to find solutions. Instead of following the child's lead, the adult is an equal partner with the child in creating the agenda. Whereas Floortime encourages pretend play and flights of fancy, problem-solving discussions are firmly grounded in reality. Their purpose is to help children learn to engage in logical communication and to anticipate and solve challenges they face.

The adult might use problem-solving time to bring up for discussion the fact that the child has been struggling with math homework, kicking other children on the playground, resisting going to bed on time, or appearing more melancholy and apathetic. One starts by bringing up the problem and asking an open-ended question: "Your teacher called and said that you hit three of your classmates during recess today. What happened?" It is important to listen to the child's perspective before giving one's own point of view. To be helpful, the discussion must be interactive, not a lecture. The child should be opening and closing circles of communication by building on the adult's comments with comments of her own. In this way, she gets practice in logical thinking, an essential foundation for the ability to solve problems. Although the examples we have just given apply to verbal children, even preverbal children can be engaged in problem solving. For example, a parent can use gestures to convey to a toddler that it is time to put away the toys or brush her teeth.

For various reasons, a child may be reluctant to enter into an orderly, reality-based dialogue. Children display a wide variety of ingenious avoidance tactics:

escaping into pretend play, answering the adult with "I don't know" or an unre-lated question ("What's for dinner?"), turning on the television, humming a tune, walking out of the room. It is important for the adult to persist in helping the child develop the problem-solving aspects of his personality. The child who says, "I don't remember," can be cued to recall the events of the day: "Well, usually during lunch period you sit beside Martha. Did you sit with her today, or with someone else?" If a child who is asked, "What did you do in school today?" responds by talking about how he's planning to fly to Mars on a spaceship, it is important to empathize with his escape route and the reasons for it: "It can be really hard to talk about school. It probably seems a lot more pleasant to think about traveling to outer space." Instead of pressuring him to disclose what took place at school, one en-gages him in discussing how hard it is to talk about school.

Keep in mind that many children converse more slowly than adults; they need an extra second or two or five to formulate a response. Especially with children who resist problem-solving discussions, it is tempting to slide into lecturing and miss opportunities to let the child take a more active role. For example, suppose a child wants to play with some of her classmates at recess but avoids approaching anyone, instead hanging back by herself and feeling lonely. Her father, feeling anx-ious about her evident unhappiness and desiring to help her, inquires why she will not ask anyone to play with her. When she says "I don't know," he launches into a lecture about how important it is to be assertive. "After all, what's the worst that can happen if someone doesn't want to play? It's hardly the end of the world!" His well-meaning pep talk does not, however, teach his daughter to be assertive, for he has given her no opportunity to speak for herself.

To really engage his daughter and help her practice assertiveness, the father could say, gently, "I guess it's hard to know the reasons," and then pause. If his daughter remained silent, he could say, "I'll bet you have good reasons for not talk-ing to each of the people you'd like to play with. Do you think it might help if we made a list? We could write down the names of each person, and then think about the reasons they might not want to play. What do you think?" Chances are, as the daughter considers the reasons she fears talking to each classmate, she will brighten up and become more talkative even though the "presenting problem" is not yet solved. She is now thinking about her difficulties rather than just avoiding them. She is having the experience of speaking and being listened to. Over time, she and her father may well figure out that certain classmates would feel less intimidating for her to approach.

Many of the recommendations already given for using Floortime to strengthen levels 5 and 6 also apply to problem-solving time. The process of helping a child gradually learn to describe his typical behaviors and then move toward abstracting feelings can take place during either Floortime or problem-solving time. When the child is cognitively able, it is extremely helpful to use problem-solving time to have him anticipate challenging situations and predict his likely reactions. "Do you think Sarah will try to take your toys again tomorrow? How will you feel when she does that? What do you think you will do?" When he has learned to make such predictions, one can begin having him consider other options. "What are some other things you could do?" By learning to picture and describe scenarios of events and feelings, the child is laying the foundations for better impulse control.

As part of problem-solving time, the adult should help the child observe how her specific behaviors are part of a larger pattern. As described in the discussion of Floortime, this involves helping to push her beyond concrete thinking toward emotional ideas. If a child is persistently whining for her parent to do something for her, such as put toys away, the parent could simply say "yes" or "no" but will accomplish more by saying something like, "How come I have to do it for you?" The child may thus be stimulated to consider this larger issue.

Problem solving is especially challenging for children with developmental delays. The next two sections provide examples of how to engage in problem-solving interactions with such children.

Reality-Based Dialogues With Developmentally Delayed Children

Parents, teachers, or therapists interacting with developmentally delayed children can easily miss opportunities to help these children increase the amount and complexity of their communication. Promoting such an increase is a primary goal of problem-solving time with these children.

For example, 3-year-old Sam can say few words and speaks only occasionally. Sometimes, he will point to the refrigerator to indicate that he is hungry. His mother's natural tendency is to say, for example, "Do you want some ice cream?" When he nods or says, "yes," she opens the freezer door and gets him what he wants, thereby closing a circle of communication with him.

Sam's mother could, however, push him to close six or seven circles by engaging in a different kind of dialogue that makes Sam work harder. When he points, she can ask, "What do you want?" If he looks as though he does not understand, she can mirror his expression by saying, "I don't know?" Sam will likely make an "I don't know" gesture with his hands. His mother can then offer a gradual approximation of what he wants, accompanied by multiple cuing of choices. "Do you want something to eat?" she can ask, simultaneously pointing to her mouth. If Sam nods and says "Yes," she can ask, "What?" If he looks blank, she can again mimic his "I don't know" and give him a few seconds to name the food he wants. If he cannot, she should list four or five choices. If he still looks blank, she can say something like, "Well, let me help," and then narrow the choices to three, showing him pictures of each food so he can point to what he wants. Once he has made a choice, she can say, "Do you want to open the refrigerator yourself?" while pointing to him and gesturing to the door. These interactive sequences are best attempted when the child is highly motivated. Keep in mind that combining gestures with one's words is the most effective way to facilitate the opening and closing of circles.

Reality-Based Interactions With Children With Pervasive Developmental Delays and Severe Receptive Language Impairments

Children who are nonverbal and only irregularly capable of intentional gestural communication present a particularly difficult challenge. Parents and clinicians often speak to these children in complicated sentences or abstractions that have no chance of being understood. In working with a child who is biting or repetitively opening and closing a door, a therapist might say, "Johnny is angry" or "Johnny likes opening and closing that door." As we have already noted, this kind of commentary is not interactive. Many severely delayed children have the language abilities of a normal baby of 6 or 7 months. Problem-solving work with such children begins with helping them achieve the level of purposeful two-way communication.

If a child is wandering aimlessly or banging her fists angrily on the floor, one can position oneself in such a way that she has no choice but to interact. If she is opening and closing a door, one might insert a finger in the door. If she indicates, with gestures or by grabbing the finger, "Get your finger out of the way!" the adult should point to the finger and look helpless. Such simple gestural interactions come close to the way one would interact with a normal 7- to 18-month-old. With a child who is having a tantrum, a parent can move in very gradually, using deep pressure on the child's back and a rhythmic, soothing tone of voice: "Let's calm down, it's okay, let's relax." Like a normal infant, the child will understand not the words but the tone. Even if she turns away, this is a response to the parent's communication, and the parent can respond in turn and thus keep the interaction going.

In working with language-delayed children, it is especially important to remain aware of one's vocal tone and rhythm. It is easy to fall into a pattern of singsong and baby talk that is nothing like the quality of normal conversation. As a therapist, one should help parents develop the habit of talking to their children in a normal tone and rhythm, using simple words and phrases while supporting these with lots of gestures.

Step 3: Identifying and Empathizing With the Child's Point of View

Step 3 is not a separate step but rather a principle that applies to both Floortime and problem-solving time—in fact, to almost any interaction with a child. This is the principle of empathizing with the child's goals. We often forget that no matter how inappropriate or egregious a child's behavior seems to us, children have good reasons for doing what they do. We need not agree with the reasons, but we do need to understand what they are. What is the child trying to accomplish? Each child's coping strategy is minimizing some emotional pain or meeting some emotional need.

Empathizing with a child's feelings, rather than criticizing them or trying to reassure them away, can be difficult. What loving parents would not want to save their child from painful feelings such as hurt and embarrassment? Often, this desire to protect children from pain leads parents to say things like, "Don't be silly, how could you feel that way? Of course your teacher likes you!" However, such responses seldom bring relief but instead leave the child feeling unheard and frustrated. They also tend to stop the discussion and thus to prevent adult and child from advancing to problem solving.

Instead, it is best to reflect back the child's feelings in a way that invites further elaboration: "It sounds like you feel really hurt and left out when your teacher calls on someone else." By communicating our acceptance and understanding of a child's feelings, we can better help the child to become aware of his own goals and to discover more constructive ways to reach them. If we can tolerate hearing the child elaborate on his own loneliness and fear of rejection, he will feel safe in sharing these feelings with us. A child who feels understood is more likely to join us in considering what situations trigger his bad feelings, how he typically behaves when he feels this way, what the results of his behavior usually are, and what other strategies might serve him better.

Step 4: Breaking the Challenge Into Small Pieces

Step 4 is based on the behavioral principle of shaping described earlier. Specific goals are broken down into component parts, and the child is helped to master one part at a time. With a child who is physically aggressive to others at school and at home, the intervention plan might focus first on helping her stop hurting people at school. If this goal seems too large and overwhelming for her to master, it could be broken down even further: first, stop in gym class. When the child is regularly using words instead of fists to express herself in gym, a second class period is added. If an entire gym class is too much to start with, the first challenge could be to stop hurting others for 10 minutes at a time. In short, the initial and incremental goals are made as small as necessary. This way, the child experiences a sense of competence and success early in the process and is less likely to get discouraged and give up.

Almost any problem or task, including sleeping problems, toilet training, and academic challenges, can be approached in this manner. For example, many children have difficulty learning math. Such children often turn out to have trouble picturing quantity. They do not intuitively sense that 10 is twice as big as 5, or 20 is twice as big as 10. A parent or teacher who tries to teach the child to memorize better will not succeed and will likely trigger feelings of failure in the child. Instead, the adult should start by joining the child in playing with blocks and have him make a stack of 5 blocks and a stack of 10 blocks. He can then compare what the two stacks look like. The second step is to engage the child in the same process without the blocks, by having him use his hands (and his imagination) to show what 10 and 5 look like. The third step is to begin with very easy numbers, such as $1+1=2$ and $2+2=4$, making sure that each time he can picture the quantities in his head.

Step 5: Setting Limits

Step 5 is the establishment of firm limits on misbehavior and avoidance. Often children will not want to practice whatever activities are decided on, even when tasks are broken down into small steps. Limits are essential to providing the structure and motivation for continued progress.

Ideally, limits and consequences for behavior should be decided on through negotiation and debate with the child during problem-solving time. In this way, one can make sure the child understands what the limits are, and she can participate in defining what sorts of sanctions are "fair." If adult and child cannot agree on these things, the adult will need to set reasonable limits and sanctions unilaterally. The child may not like it, but she will have benefited from participating in the problem-solving conversation nonetheless. Once limits have been agreed on or set, it is critical for caregivers to be firm in implementing them. Parents will have an easier time doing this calmly, without undue yelling, if the limits have been established in advance.

If a child is experiencing multiple challenges, it is important to set priorities rather than try to work on everything at once. Pick one or two problems to start with, advancing to others only when the child has experienced some success with the initial goals. Limits should be set on categories of behavior rather than specific behaviors. For example, a child is taught to "respect others' bodies and not hurt them" rather than simply to "stop hitting." In problem-solving discussions, the adult can help the child list the repertoire of behaviors that make up the category, "respecting others' bodies and not hurting them."

Parents should avoid setting limits in areas that are unimportant or that should really be under the child's control. Parents or teachers may feel tempted to limit behaviors they find annoying even when these behaviors are not truly problematic. For example, a child who jiggles his arms or tosses a tennis ball from hand to hand while he talks with an adult is not necessarily being disrespectful; on the contrary, these activities may be helping him focus on the discussion. There is no reason to limit or correct them.

Step 6: Balancing Limits and Floortime

An essential principle of limit setting is that whenever limits are increased, parents or other primary caregivers need to increase their Floortime with the child as well.

This helps maintain a warm, strong connection and ensures that the child continues to feel the parents' love and interest in her. It gives the child a time to express anger at the increased limits and helps the parent to empathize with her perspective. By helping to assuage any guilt the parent may feel about increasing limits, increasing Floortime helps parents maintain a firm stance when enforcing limits.

Summary

This chapter has outlined several principles of intervention based on the DIR model. In our review of traditional approaches to infant and child therapy, we attempted to define the strengths and limitations of these approaches. We briefly reviewed the features that make the DIR approach unique and distinguish it from the less comprehensive traditional therapies. We described Floortime, the core of DIR intervention, and its use as the foundation of a six-part intervention process applicable to a wide variety of emotional, behavioral, and learning challenges. Next in Chapter 5 ("Parent-Oriented Developmental Therapy"), we describe how to conduct DIR intervention with various types of children.

References

Ayres AJ: Tactile functions: their relation to hyperactive and perceptual motor behavior. Am J Occup Ther 18:6–11, 1964

Berrueta-Clement J, Barnett W, Schweinhart L, et al: Changed Lives: The Effects of the Perry Preschool Project on Youths Through Age 19. Monographs of the High/Scope Educational Research Foundation, No. 8. Ypsilanti, MI, High/Scope Press, 1984

Brazelton TB, Cramer B: The Earliest Relationship: Parents, Infants, and the Drama of Early Attachment. Reading, MA, Addison-Wesley, 1990

Escalona S: The Roots of Individuality. Chicago, IL, Aldine, 1968

Fraiberg S: Clinical Studies in Infant Mental Health: The First Year of Life. New York, Basic Books, 1980

Fraiberg SH, Adelson E, Shapiro V: Ghosts in the nursery: a psychoanalytic approach to the problems of impaired infant–mother relationships, in Selected Writings of Selma Fraiberg. Edited by Fraiberg L. Columbus, OH, Ohio State University Press, 1987, pp 100–136

Greenspan SI: A Consideration of Some Learning Variables in the Context of Psychoanalytic Theory: Toward a Psychoanalytic Learning Perspective. Psychological Issues, Monograph 33. New York, International Universities Press, 1975

Honig AS, Lally JR: Infant Caregiving: A Design for Training. Syracuse, NY, Syracuse University Press, 1981

Lally JR, Mangione PL, Honig AS: The Syracuse University Family Development Research Program: long-range impact of an early intervention with low-income children and their families, in Parent Education in Early Intervention: Emerging Directions in Theory, Research, and Practice. Edited by Powell DR. Norwood, NJ, Ablex, 1988, pp 79–104

Murphy LB: The Individual Child (Publication No. OCD 74–1032). Washington, DC, U.S. Department of Health, Education, and Welfare, 1974

Olds DL: Case studies of factors interfering with nurse home visitors' promotion of positive caregiving methods in high-risk families. Early Child Dev Care 16:149–166, 1984

Provence S: Infants and Parents: Clinical Case Reports. Clinical Infant Reports, No. 2. New York, International Universities Press, 1983

Ramey CT, Campbell FA: Preventive education for high-risk children: cognitive consequences of the Carolina Abecedarian Project. Am J Ment Defic 88:515–523, 1984

Ramey CT, Ramey SL: Early intervention and early experience. Am Psychol 58:109–120, 1998

Schweinhart LJ, Barnes HV, Weikart DP: Significant Benefits: The High/Scope Perry Preschool Study Through Age 27. Monographs of the High/Scope Educational Research Foundation, No. 10. Ypsilanti, MI, High/Scope Press, 1983

5

Parent-Oriented
Developmental Therapy

The results of a developmental, individual-differences, relationship-based (DIR) assessment of a child and family guide the clinician in determining whether to work primarily with the child, with both child and parents, or primarily with the parents. During the assessment interviews and the initial observation of parents and child playing together, the clinician may see evidence that the parents' own developmental lags, anxieties, or rigid views of their child prevent them from interacting in ways that help the child progress developmentally. In many such cases, the clinician will decide to work primarily or substantially with the parents.

General Principles of Parent-Oriented Therapy

As discussed in Chapter 4 ("Therapeutic Principles"), most DIR intervention plans begin with establishing a regular Floortime routine. Each parent should be encouraged to spend at least a half-hour or longer, depending on the challenges, each day in Floortime with the child. As the parents report back to the therapist about their successes and failures, the therapist coaches them and helps them gain insight into their responses to their child. In addition to discussing the parents' reports, the therapist can also observe and coach while the parents play with their child in session. With infants and children under 2½ years, it is often preferable to make such active observation and coaching a component of each session. With older children, the parents may need more sessions alone in order to speak freely as they explore their own feelings, conflicts, and family histories.

In their reports and in their interactions with their child and with the therapist, the parents will provide much evidence of how well they themselves have negotiated the developmental levels of shared attention; engagement; two-way gestural and problem-solving communication; symbolization; and organization, differentiation, and connection of meanings. As we have discussed in earlier chapters, parents may have global difficulties engaging their child at any of these levels, or they may have trouble handling a particular emotion or theme—anger, intimacy, competition—at one or more levels.

The therapist attempts to help the parents see where they have trouble relating to their child, to empathize with their fears and anxieties, and to help them understand how their own histories contribute to the ways in which they interact with the child. Perhaps, for example, a father complains that he starts daydreaming or reaches for a magazine whenever his son's play depicts characters acting angry or hostile. Perhaps the mother is also uncomfortable with aggression and fears that her son will "go out of control" if he has dolls or soldiers fighting. The therapist can help each parent explore what it is about anger or fighting that makes them so uncomfortable.

In sessions with parents and child together, the therapist must let the mother and father take separate turns in the play. In the role of coach, the therapist must be careful not to demoralize the parents by taking over or lecturing them on proper techniques of interaction. The therapist has to be available to the child without getting caught in the middle of the family's conflicts. For example, perhaps the mother mentioned above becomes so anxious when her son has the soldiers fight that she starts to call in "doctors." The therapist can wonder out loud, "Mom, you're bringing in the doctors, although there aren't any injuries yet. And [looking at the child] he hasn't even asked for help. He is still telling how angry everyone is." The mother may pause to watch what is going on. She may attempt to elaborate on the anger. If her anxiety again overtakes her and she resumes calling for the doctors—or, alternatively, tries to distract her son from the fighting drama by having "the three little pigs" arrive—the therapist can wonder out loud what it is about the fighting and anger that frightens her. She may be able to explore her anxieties with the therapist on the sidelines while her son plays, then return to the drama to try to follow the action from the child's perspective.

Whenever parents have difficulty with a particular emotion in their relationship with their child, it is important to explore how they handle that emotion in their relationship with each other. In the previous example, do the mother's and father's anxious responses to anger interfere with their own relationship? Does the father stop interacting with his wife when one or both of them are angry, and does the mother rush to appease her husband or distract him instead of confronting conflicts directly? Are the parents frustrated with each other because of these tendencies? How does their pattern affect the other children in the family?

The therapist works to help the parents not only to engage in daily Floortime sessions but also to institute a Floortime philosophy in all interactions with their child. The therapist also facilitates problem-solving discussions and effective limit-setting, as described in Chapter 4 ("Therapeutic Principles").

In cases in which a child's individual differences, such as oversensitivity to sound or touch or a tendency toward motor discharge, have made it difficult for the parents to engage her, parent consultation sessions can help the family understand the child's sensory or motor characteristics. The therapist can help the parents see their child more clearly, without distortions or projections.

To illustrate how a therapist can further a child's development by working with the parents, we now describe in detail two examples of parent-oriented therapy. In the first case, the child's problems lay in the early, presymbolic levels of attention, engagement, and two-way gestural communication. In the second, the child's problems lay mostly in the symbolic realm.

Case 1: Withdrawn Child, Withdrawn Parents: Helping Parents Engage

Danny, age 4 years, was very preoccupied with himself and uninvolved with other people. He was somewhat compulsive and ritualistic in his behavior, unable to represent feelings of yearning or dependency, and only occasionally—and barely—able to represent anger. He was referred for therapy because he was hitting other children at school. Danny was perceived as mechanical and aloof by both his mother and his teachers. He was very bright, able to do complicated math and language problems above his grade level.

During the first year of treatment, the therapist helped Danny establish two-way communication with his parents and others, initially through gestures, while helping the parents deepen their relationship with their son. After 1 year, Danny was able to abstract some of his feelings, particularly anger at other children who frustrated him or who would not play with him. He could assert his will and negotiate for what he wanted. He had more difficulty representing feelings of longing and need, but he began doing so intermittently. When his father was away on a trip, Danny would occasionally say that he missed him. On rare occasions, with a flirtatious glance, he would indicate he wanted to play a special game with his mother. He would sometimes talk about wanting a particular friend to come over and play.

As Danny became slightly warmer, he grew more flexible and was better liked by his peers and his own parents. His self-esteem improved enormously. Once a sense of better connectedness and two-way gestural communication was established, his school behavior improved, even before he began representing emotions. Once he became able to express his angry feelings symbolically, he stopped marching out of the room or having tantrums when frustrated. He gradually became more caring and empathic.

To facilitate his progress, Danny's parents had to work through their own anxieties and maladaptive coping strategies. Danny's mother described a pattern in which Danny was aloof or mechanical, and she responded by becoming depressed and withdrawing from him instead of reaching out to him. She worried that he was "disturbed" and interpreted every one of his behaviors as a sign of disturbance. She could see "no good" in him because of how he made her feel. Danny's father was very competitive and controlling; he had been "the king" in his own household as a child. He felt that "if my son wants me, he'll pursue me. I don't run after anyone." This attitude prevented him from initiating interactions with Danny.

As the parents worked with the therapist, they were able to understand where these feelings and attitudes originated. Danny's mother came to see how her feelings toward Danny were similar to those of her own mother, who had been aloof and depressed; as a result, she was able to reach out to Danny and to take pride in some of his qualities. Gradually, she drew him into a deeper relationship with her. As Danny's father became aware of his own fears of rejection, he too was able to woo his son. He found that he and Danny had much in common: intellectual pursuits and even a shared arrogance. Soon, there were two "kings" in the family. Danny's parents came to realize that even in their relationship with each other, they had been depressed, withdrawn, and competitively aloof. Slowly, they were able to strengthen and deepen their relationship.

After 2 years of work on the part of his parents, Danny was about halfway to where he needed to be. Progress was likely to continue, because a good foundation had been established. The most critical steps involved broadening and deepening the range of Danny's affect at the early, presymbolic levels. It is important never to skip the early steps, especially when the main problems are found there.

Case 2: Helping Parents Balance Their Empathic Range

Four-year-old Molly had a history of easily becoming upset, being negative and resistant, and having temper tantrums. Molly's mother felt so overwhelmed by her behavior that she would leave the scene whenever Molly became upset, yell at her, or punish her for being angry, demanding, and unwilling to calm down. Molly would respond by getting even more upset; she could literally cry for hours and then whine.

At the beginning of treatment, Molly hid behind her father's legs and insisted that he carry her into the therapist's office. She could be sweet, but she ignored the therapist. She impressed him as a very shy, yet warm and playful child who engaged well and interacted gesturally with her parents but could easily get overloaded and become very demanding. She was unable to process complex auditory input—that is, she could not answer "why" or "how" questions. She could engage in pretend play, but when she got anxious, she became aggressive and preoccupied with people being eaten or hurt. Her play became fragmented and disjointed. When frustrated with her parents, she dissolved in a crying fit, then continued to whine for a long time. The more impatient and angry her parents got, or the more they chose to ignore her, the more upset and disorganized Molly became, until she was throwing toys, crying, and screaming.

Molly's mother worked with the therapist on her own intolerance of Molly's moods and came to understand some of her conflicts about her daughter's behavior. After she had been practicing Floortime approaches for a month, she came in one day and said, "Molly's been doing great." She reported that she had been able to use an insight she had discussed at an earlier session:

> I finally realized that Molly feels unsure of herself. I couldn't face this fact before, because Molly was always my 'success story.' She would be the per-

son who would be better than my brother, which I couldn't be. We felt that she was so confident, because she'd been an early talker and had good motor skills. [Molly was a good runner, jumper, and dancer.] I also realized that, even though she was quite verbal in general, she did not find it easy to verbalize feelings, and she tends always to put feelings into behavior.... It's amazing what just being aware that your daughter can feel unsure of herself can do to your approach to her.

By way of example, Molly's mother went on:

We were in the middle of drawing, and for no apparent reason—after we had been getting along nicely for 15 or 20 minutes, and I was thoroughly enjoying the time—out of left field she started yelling and screaming and breaking the crayons and having a real tantrum. That's typical for her. Normally, I'd be enraged that she'd interfere with our nice play time together. This time, instead of yelling back at her and saying I won't stay in the same room, and leaving her, in which case she would probably have screamed for a good half-hour or more, I counted to 10 and thought to myself, there must be something here that she's feeling unsure of herself about. I stayed there and let her cry for a minute or two, and then just talked in a calm voice, asking her to let me know what was so upsetting to her. To my surprise (this has now happened many times), she said, "I messed up what I wanted to do."

The mother then asked, "Sweetheart, how did you mess up?" Molly showed her how she had drawn something that did not look quite like what she wanted it to look like, how the lines were "messed up." Her mother said, "This time I didn't exit; this time I didn't yell back, I actually felt bad for her. She crept into my lap and cried for a minute or two. I hugged her and then she said, 'I feel okay now.'" They were able to resume drawing and to enjoy the rest of their time together.

In another incident, Molly wanted to stay in the kitchen because her brother was there. Molly and her mother were on the verge of a power struggle, because her mother did not want both children in the kitchen arguing with one another. Instead of yelling at Molly or insisting she leave the room immediately, her mother accompanied her into the other room and asked her why she was insisting on staying in the kitchen. Molly replied, "I can't explain now, I can't get the words out to say what I want to." Her mother was patient and empathized with Molly's inability to find the words, because that seemed to frustrate her more than whatever she had actually wanted to talk about. Eventually, Molly was able to say that she thought her brother was going to get something to eat that she was not going to get, although she did not use the word "jealous." Her inability to express her reason for wanting to stay in the kitchen was what had been frustrating her and making her want to cry. As her mother empathized with her about how hard it is sometimes to say what one wants to say, Molly said, "Sometimes I feel my brain needs to be hit." Her mother's ability to empathize with her frustration enabled them to then discuss the situation and settle on a compromise: Molly and her brother each got to be in the kitchen with their mother part of the time.

As Molly's mother continued to engage her daughter with this approach, Molly was able to give up her pacifier, begin going to bed at a more reasonable hour, and become less finicky, angry, and belligerent during most of the day.

Implications for Working With Caregivers

Like Molly's mother, many parents have a perception of their child that makes it hard for them to empathize with a key part of the child's character. Molly's mother realized that despite Molly's apparent competence, she did feel vulnerable and unsure of herself at times. Seeing Molly's behavior in terms of uncertainty rather than as a willful act of belligerence was critical in turning around her daughter's behavior. Even more important, this mother's insight allowed her to empathize with the full range of her daughter's feelings during Floortime. If parents see their child in only one way, they cannot empathize with other aspects of her. It is as though one side of the child's character is cut off; because that part of her personality is never empathically mirrored by her parents, she never learns to put it into ideas or words, with the result that it is instead discharged in behavior. Instead of learning to think or say, "I feel frustrated with myself," or "I feel bad about messing up," the child discharges the feelings in tantrums or screaming fits.

No parent, however, is able to empathize with the full range of a child's feelings spontaneously or automatically, because all parents view their children through their own feelings and conflicts. A parent will be predisposed to favor one side of the child, such as her competence or her helplessness. As we have seen, the resulting empathic imbalance undermines the child's ability to represent fully her internal world. The therapist's goal is to help the parents increase their empathic range by helping them understand their own conflicts about one or another set of emotional themes. If the parents themselves tend to be concrete—that is, they have a global difficulty in representing feelings as ideas—the therapist will work to facilitate their representational access.

The long-term goal of this kind of work with parents is to help them understand their own fantasies and behavioral patterns so that they can become more flexible and adaptive in relating to their children. However, with parents who are not yet able to symbolize feelings, and thus cannot reflect on their own feelings and behavior, one can first work toward an important short-term goal: helping the parents meet the child's developmental needs in spite of their own perceptions and fantasies. For example, a very self-centered and impulsive mother was intrusive and overstimulating in her interactions with her infant son. We asked her what she wanted for him. "I want him to want me," she said. "How?" we asked. "To smile at me, hug, talk, and look at me." We also asked her what her long-term goals were: "What do you want him to be like as he grows up?" She answered, "Tough and strong, not to take shit from anyone." Although the mother was not yet aware of this, her long-term goal derived from her feeling, as a child, that she had to be tough and strong to cope with abuse by her father.

Using this mother's motivation to get her baby to meet her immediate needs ("to be hugged") and her long-term needs ("for him to be tough"), we worked with her on specific kinds of interactions. She thought poking her baby would get him to react to her and to be tough; we showed her "better" ways to get him to react: talking to him, handing him toys to see if he would hand them back, and so on. We talked about how she could make her baby "strong" by interacting with him in these new ways.

As this case illustrates, new interactive styles must be tied to the parent's needs and goals. These needs and goals may change over time if the parent can gradually learn to abstract ideas and, as a result, become more self-observing.

Conclusion

In this chapter, we have described how a therapist can help a child progress developmentally by working primarily or substantially with the child's parents. In determining an appropriate treatment plan, the evaluating clinician must consider which therapeutic strategy will best facilitate the child's ability to engage with her parents and others at all six developmental levels. Working with the parents alone; working in some sessions with parents alone and in some with parents and child; and conducting a combination of sessions with parents alone, parents and child together, and child alone can all be sound strategies. In cases in which the child's anxiety, negativism, or tendency to withdraw is severe and a parent's personality structure is very fragile, it may be essential to work directly with the child to enable her to take the lead in working out better interactions with her parents. However, most parents are available, and in many cases, the child can make progress without being seen alone very often.

A therapist faced with an extremely disorganized family can feel tempted to discount the family and work with the child alone, meeting with the parents only to offer support or specific advice. Many therapists give up on parents too readily. In most cases, one can work systematically with the parents as well as the child. Even in a very dysfunctional family, where one or both parents may have a severe character disorder or where the parents have serious marital conflicts, progress is still possible. The therapist may have to spend the first year simply getting consistent engagement and two-way communication established among family members. After these presymbolic capacities are firmly established, the child and parents have a strong foundation for gradually learning to symbolize feelings and to see the connections between them.

Many clinicians work with families whose problems are so numerous and so severe that the early goals must be to maintain contact with the family, foster a relationship, and stabilize critical parental and family functions such as the physical care, safety, and nurturing of the infant. The special challenges of working with multiproblem families were considered in some detail in an earlier work, *Infants in Multirisk Families* (Greenspan et al. 1987). We discuss these challenges in Chapter 10 ("Infants in Multirisk Families: A Model for Developmentally Based Preventive Intervention").

Reference

Greenspan SI, Wieder S, Lieberman A, et al: Infants in Multirisk Families: Case Studies in
    Preventive Intervention. Clinical Infant Reports, No. 3. New York, International Uni-
    versities Press, 1987

6

Clinical Strategies and Techniques for Different Types of Infants and Young Children

In the functional emotional developmental profile of any child, the evaluating clinician not only describes what the child is like but also offers explanations or hypotheses as to why the child is the way he is. By pinpointing the constitutional-maturational characteristics, family dynamics, and interactional patterns that contribute to the child's personality organization, the profile points the way toward interventions that will help the child make use of his unique qualities rather than allow them to become liabilities that make life more difficult for him. In the following sections, we describe several kinds of children, the factors that shape their experience of the world, and the styles of interaction that parents, teachers, and therapists can use to most effectively engage them and further their development.

Individual Differences and Floortime Procedures

In establishing procedures for Floortime and problem-solving time, it is essential to consider children's individual differences in sensory, language, and motor functioning.

Muscle Tone and Motor Planning Difficulties

Children who have difficulty with motor planning have a hard time doing rapid, alternating, sequential movements, such as quickly rotating their hands while slapping their thighs and then crossing over. They may have trouble putting together a six-step sequence of routine activities around the house, such as tying their shoes or putting things away in their proper place. Most people can, without really thinking about it, copy rapid, sequential movements demonstrated by another person. In contrast, for children who have motor planning difficulties, going from thought to action is not automatic but requires a great deal of effort.

For example, a child who appears to be clumsy may have a hard time copying his father's carpentry efforts or imitating complex activities demonstrated by a teacher, therapist, or parent during Floortime. He may be unable to follow along as other kids play "Simon Says." He may lack the fine motor skills and sequencing skills required to copy or construct complex designs.

Adults working with such children must respect the extra effort it takes for them to copy and sequence actions. Parents, teachers, and therapists can use Floortime and problem-solving time to provide these children with extra practice. Once a child can use ideas in a problem-solving mode, it is important for the adult to help her understand and adapt to the challenges she faces. As she exhibits her difficulties during Floortime and problem-solving time, the adult should empathize with her feelings of frustration. The adult should also point out that even though the child is gifted in using words or coming up with ideas, when she tries to make something out of her ideas—by cutting and pasting, drawing, or putting together pieces—doing so is hard for her. The child may say, with a look of amazement, "How did you know?" She may feel relieved that her problem is no longer her secret frustration but has now been named and described.

Elevating a child's difficulty to the level of conscious thought through problem solving enhances his sense of shared attention to a task and his sense of connectedness. Once his problem is identified, he can verbalize his full range of feelings about it, from anger and frustration to sadness and disappointment. He can become better able to use his strengths to tackle the challenge at hand. For example, if he is a good thinker and planner but has trouble implementing his ideas, he can learn to break tasks down into small steps. Having gained the insight that physical tasks take him a lot of thought and tire him out quickly, he can avoid overloading himself with too much motor activity in a brief period. He can learn to use his ideation or verbal ability to persist in a task by restating for himself what he needs to do, identifying each small piece of the task and taking one step at a time.

Such a child may also have slightly low muscle tone and may dislike feeling insecure in space. She may avoid going down slides or riding roller coasters. An adult working with her can help her understand that she likes to take care of her body and to be sure, in a very methodical, step-by-step way, how it is moving. Knowing this about herself will help her feel less embarrassed and defective when she notices that she is more cautious than many other children. She can even learn to take pride in her more careful and methodical approach.

Some children with motor planning problems associated with fine motor delays make a lot of seemingly peculiar movements. They may flap their arms or hold their bodies in odd ways. When they get excited, they may look very uncoordinated, with arms and legs moving in different directions. Sometimes, this kind of irregular movement is associated with other processing difficulties in the sensory and motor areas. It is easy for professionals to attribute such movements to nonspecific neurological illness or "organicity." However, everyone has some unevenness in maturation; some people show more than others do. Instead of generalizing from unusual movements to some vague notion of organicity, the professional should pinpoint the functional aspects of the maturational lag or dysfunction, whether it is in motor planning, auditory processing, visuospatial processing, or sensory reactivity. Children who have lags in more than one of these areas may look more "peculiar" than others in some of their mannerisms. Yet if the child is also an organized thinker, is comfortable being close to people and engaging with them, and has creative problem-solving abilities, the important elements of his personality may be well in place, and the apparent peculiarities limited to a mild lag in one or another area.

Word Retrieval Difficulties

Some children have what are called *word retrieval*, or *word finding*, problems. A child may be competent on the intake side, with no auditory processing (receptive language) difficulties, but still have a subtle expressive language impairment. Children with word retrieval difficulties have no problem articulating sounds but struggle to find the particular words they want to say. When one asks such a child what happened today at school, she may say, "Nothing," "Same old stuff," or "Can't remember," when in fact she has a good sense of what went on. She simply cannot access the words she needs to describe it, so she takes the easy way out. If asked by her teacher to describe a story the teacher has just read—or, in the fourth or fifth grade, to discuss the "theme" of a story—she may respond with vague generalities. She may simply say, "The book was good." This vagueness may not reflect poor conceptual abilities; some of these children are quite brilliant. However, if a child cannot easily find words, she may give up trying. She may have the abstracting ability to produce general answers but never provide details.

Children with word retrieval problems often need to be cued by the therapist, teacher, or parent to find the words to describe their experience. The adult should first empathize with the difficulty and frustration of not being able to remember. Helping the child become aware that recalling specifics is hard for him helps him begin to use his problem-solving ability—that is, his ability to use ideas and reflect on his difficulty. Second, the adult should provide cues to give the child reminders of how his day is usually sequenced.

For example, after empathically observing that it can be hard to remember what happened in school, the adult might say, "Maybe I can help. I know the first thing is free time, and often you like to play with Susie. Remember yesterday you told me she's mean to you sometimes." "Oh, yes," the child may respond. "She was mean again today. She took my truck away, and I was mad at her." The discussion is off and running. One may need to cue the child up for each part of the day: "Well, I know that after your free play, you usually do circle time. Did the teacher read a story, like she usually does? If she did, what was it about?" "I think she did, but I can't remember what it was about." "Well, I know often she reads to you about animals." "Oh, right, she read about a lion today." When engaging a child in this sort of dialogue, it is best to avoid getting into a power struggle by saying things like, "Why won't you tell me what you did today?"

Over time, an older child can learn to write down for herself the sequence of her day—math, English, free time—and to ask herself certain rhetorical questions that will provide the needed cues. It would be difficult for a child under 8 years to learn to cue herself, but older children, adolescents, and adults with word retrieval difficulties often learn to do this automatically.

Sensory Modulation Difficulties

A child who is overly sensitive to sensory stimuli is likely to find many experiences overwhelming and will naturally shy away from them. Because of the child's tendency to overreact to sensations, the barrier between his inner self and the outer world is not well developed. The child who is sensitive to touch, for example, will feel intruded on by a group and will want to find a corner where he can feel secure against two walls and only have to interact with one person whom he can see. He may react strongly to someone touching him on the back or bumping against him. He may dislike having his hair brushed. During Floortime, he may want to face the parent, teacher, or therapist and to always be able to anticipate what will happen next.

Alternatively, a child may be undersensitive to touch and therefore crave physical contact. He may like to roughhouse or go out of his way to bang against things. A cautious child who is easily overwhelmed by sound will not like loud noises or lots of talking, whereas a child who seeks out auditory stimulation may want the equivalent of a rock concert all the time and may try to create commotion.

One needs to recognize these differences to help each child identify how he is unique and learn to use his strengths in solving problems for himself. If one approaches the child's differences positively and empathically, the child can talk about situations he enjoys and those he finds frustrating. He comes to realize whether he likes loud noises. He discovers whether touch is something he needs to control and experience one step at a time or something he craves. This dialogue is a valuable part of problem solving that helps the child elevate his physical differences to the world of thought, idea, and judgment, enabling him to reflect on both his joys and his frustrations.

Furthermore, this self-knowledge allows the adult and child to collaboratively develop strategies that enable the child to achieve better control and modulation. For example, the child who is sensitive to touch can, with the help of her parents, teacher, or therapist, learn to anticipate situations where a lot of people will be present and determine how she wants to negotiate these situations. How can she become more comfortable during circle time? Perhaps she can position herself with her back to the wall. If a teenager is sensitive to sound, how can she better enjoy an upcoming rock concert? Perhaps she can wear earplugs. A child who knows what to expect, understands that her discomfort stems from a physical difference, and has a strategy ready will feel more at ease and more willing to participate in new experiences. Adults with comparable problems often find it very reassuring to review their history of being overly sensitive to touch or sound, such as the times they thought they were "going crazy" at big parties or felt suspicious of others' intentions. As they become aware of this trait and can anticipate situations when they will feel this way, the feelings no longer escalate to the point of feeling "crazy." The adult can say, "Gee, I'm getting overloaded. I'd better go to the powder room to relax or go outside to get a breath of fresh air." Children can learn to do the same things, and they find it extremely reassuring to know what to do.

Certain exercises help children who are extra-sensitive to touch to reorganize themselves. Squeezing their arms and legs and providing deep pressure or joint compression, such as in a skipping or hopping game or jumping on the bed, may be helpful. Large motor movement as well as firm pressure helps the touch-sensitive child to regain equilibrium. Knowing this about himself can give the child better control of his own body.

The child who is undersensitive to touch and craves sensation may easily lapse into socially inappropriate behavior, such as hitting other children, banging into things, breaking toys, and roughhousing too much. Understanding her craving may help such a child figure out appropriate ways to meet her needs. She can invent a game of "bear hug," so that she and her friends can hug one another. She can try to anticipate the activities she will enjoy during gym class and wait till then, rather than engaging in inappropriate behavior beforehand. At home, she can populate her playroom with big punching-bag balloon figures, which she can punch and jump on to get the sensations she craves.

The earlier that one identifies individual differences, the more that one can help a child find activities that give him a sense of mastery over his own body. For younger children who cannot yet use words in a sophisticated enough way to identify and anticipate difficult situations, the parent, teacher, or therapist should proceed on two fronts. The adult should collaborate with the child in identifying the kinds of experiences that he enjoys. In addition, the adult needs to create and structure difficult situations in such a way that they do not overwhelm the child but enable him to slowly gain control and confidence.

"Forest-Type" and "Tree-Type" Children

Optimally, one can be sensitive to detail and subtlety and at the same time understand how the details fit together into a larger pattern. Much of our emotional and intellectual life depends on the ability to blend these skills. Many individuals, however, are strong in one of these areas and relatively weak in the other. The "forest-type" person who can abstract and see overall patterns may have difficulty identifying the elements that make up a pattern. Such a person may try to figure out how she feels based on how she behaves: "I hit him, so therefore I must feel angry." A "tree-type" person who can perceive details knows that she feels angry, sad, happy, or excited but may have a harder time discerning the patterns that govern her emotions, such as "I feel angry when people reject me." A tree person may excel at empathizing with each character in a novel but have difficulty understanding the theme or overall plot. The forest person has a sense of the plot but may have trouble figuring out how each character feels. A tree person may handle simple arithmetic but have trouble with advanced math, like calculus, that depends on abstracting special patterns. The forest person may struggle with verbal skills and even arithmetic when she is young but do better with the more abstract academic tasks she faces when she is older.

An awareness of these differences helps an adult use both spontaneous Floortime and problem-solving discussions to provide a child with practice in the area in which she is weak. Suppose, for example, a tree child is playing out a drama with dolls. The dolls investigate secret passages in a haunted house. They are captured, escape, find someone who takes care of them, and are captured again. The drama is filled with rich detail: the child explains from moment to moment which character feels excited, which one feels scared, and so on. Day after day, the child plays out a drama involving excitement, fear, and security, all within 15 or 20 minutes. A parent or therapist who is aware of the difference between tree-type and forest-type children will recognize that despite this child's sensitivity, subtlety, and vivid use of language, she never describes the whole picture. Why are the characters exploring the house in the first place? Empathic comments can help the child consider the larger picture: "Let's see now. They were feeling excited, and they were feeling scared, and then they crawled along the secret tunnel. How does this all fit together? What are the explorers trying to do?" The child may then begin to create a larger structure or plot. At first, she will quickly return to the details, but after some practice, she may begin to develop a knack for thinking about the overall plot as well.

It can be surprising how seldom a tree-type child makes general statements. In a problem-oriented discussion, she may tell the adult lots of things that happened in school. One friend said this, another friend said that, one friend hurt her feelings, another friend played ball with her. The adult may get caught up in the child's excitement or fears without thinking to ask how the child would characterize her entire day. If a child is having difficulty with a friend who is very fickle—nice one day, mean the next, fun to play with one day, scary the next—one can, instead of getting lost in the details, ask the child, "Well, what would you say overall about Sam? How would you size him up?" If she can answer something like, "Well, he's really moody, but overall I guess I like him pretty well. I just wish he wouldn't change so much!" she is showing perspective and describing the larger pattern.

Helping a child learn to see the big picture can be very reassuring. To a person for whom a single detail seems like the only reality, emotions and interpersonal conflicts can feel overwhelming. As one verbal child put it, "When I'm mad, I think I will be that way forever." When such a child learns that his perceptions and feelings of the moment are part of a larger pattern, he realizes that they need not dominate his life. He can gradually feel integrated rather than fragmented. It is critical that the therapist guard against the temptation to get lost in detail along with the child. After all, one might think, it is my job to explore his anger or his sadness, right? Yet it is also the therapist's job to explore how different feelings fit together and how the child's tendency to feel fragmented or overloaded is itself an important feeling and an important pattern.

The child who has trouble attending to details or nuances, or the child who has difficulty discriminating among different sounds and words, faces a different challenge. Assume, for the moment, that the child also is gifted in seeing the forest and that this ability is supported by an unusually well developed visuospatial imagination. Such a child often describes his experiences in the broadest and most abstract way. When one of us (S.G.) asked one such child, "How was your day?" he replied, "My day was typical for a child my age." Asked about specific feelings, he responded, "What you would expect for a six-year-old." This apparently sophisticated and insightful answer was not matched, however, by an ability to fill in the details. When asked to describe his reactions in a particular situation, he had a hard time naming specific feelings or behaviors. He continued to speak in vague generalities. Nevertheless, he gave thoughtful answers, and he always seemed to be approximating some important truth. He did not respond with the same general principle to every question.

With patience, it was possible to help this child gradually fill in details. When he was asked about school, he first responded with generalities, but if the therapist then mentioned what children typically do first during the school day—hang up their coats, say "hi" to other children—he chimed in and said, "Oh, right—I did that." When led through the day with similar prompts, he gave more specifics. The therapist was helping him put the trees into the forest. When discussing feelings, the therapist similarly prompted him by speculating aloud about how some children might feel or behave in a similar situation. The child would sometimes disagree and volunteer that he thought a child might do or feel something different—or that he, in a similar situation, did something different. For every 10 words the therapist spoke, the child spoke 2 or 3, but he was clearly working hard and collaboratively.

The adult needs to progress from suggesting possibilities to finding ways for the child to suggest possibilities to herself. After many conversations in which one offers examples of how some children might feel or behave, one instead asks the child how *she* thinks others might feel or act. If she still cannot generate specifics, one needs to find a middle road—for example, drawing a picture of how some children feel and letting the child use this visual cue to stir her auditory-verbal memory. One might also mention to the child some friends she has previously spoken about who typify certain feelings and behaviors and wonder out loud if the child feels like any of them. In short, one finds ways to make the child do a little more of the work. Gradually, the adult must let the child do most of the work, until she can eventually fill in details on her own.

The forest-type person who has visuospatial strength often also has a weak auditory-verbal capacity. A particularly valuable exercise is to have him imagine the sound of someone who is mad or sad or frustrated. Having him play these sounds in his mind, and even mimic them, can help him dramatize the "trees" of his experience. The tree-type child, in contrast, often lacks a strong visuospatial capacity. A useful exercise is to have him visualize his feelings and experiences. He should be asked to picture a person at whom he is mad, a person he misses, or how his different feelings fit together.

Both tree-type and forest-type children can benefit greatly from early attention to their distinct processing styles. Because tree children often appear precocious in their verbal abilities, their parents and teachers tend to perceive them as very bright and to miss the fact that they need help constructing the forest. No one challenges them to develop the ability to think abstractly. As a result, they may earn stellar grades in elementary school but struggle more in high school, where abstract thinking is demanded. The forest-type child, who seems to use few words or have trouble recalling details, may be perceived by adults as "slow," or alternatively as a special breed of genius who has her head in the clouds. Adults who misperceive her as unintelligent will likely discourage her pursuit of knowledge and creativity, whereas those who see her as a genius will fail to challenge her to achieve a better balance between big-picture thinking and attention to detail. It can be extremely hard for parents and teachers to have the patience and make the effort required to help a forest-type child learn to identify the trees.

Occasionally, one encounters children who have difficulty with both detail-oriented and big-picture thinking. These children need practice in both modalities.

Shy Children: The Excessively Sensitive Child and the Withdrawn Child

Some shy children are extremely sensitive. They may be sensitive to the way someone looks at them, to the loudness or pitch of a voice, or to the way someone touches them. They may react strongly to being picked up and moved around in space.

The sensitive shy child is cautious, in part, because experiences involving sound, sight, or movement are often overwhelming. Such a child warms up to new people, situations, and physical surroundings very gradually. He needs to "go into the pool one toe at a time." Every teacher has encountered such children. When they enter a new classroom in the fall, they are extremely cautious and keep to themselves. In a couple of months, they may be moving into the group more, investigating more corners of the room, playing with more of the toys, and asking the teacher for help. Such a child seems to be saying, "I'm interested in you. I want to be part of the world, but I need to do it at my own pace." For this child, circle time, group time, and recess may be scarier than one-on-one play, talking to the teacher, or drawing alone at his desk.

In addition to inborn sensitivities, some of these shy children have parents who unwittingly intrude on and overwhelm them. For example, a father who believes only in rough-and-tumble play and constantly tries to "toughen up" his child can overstimulate and frighten the child, increasing the child's tendency to shyness and caution.

Another kind of shy child is not necessarily highly sensitive, but enjoys "marching to her own drummer." She has a hard time tuning in to others. She may, in fact, be *undersensitive* to sounds, words, touch, or visual stimuli. Such a child may appear withdrawn or unavailable. She seems to be focusing on her own inner voice, so that when someone starts talking to her, she only seems to be listening; it takes her a while to realize that anyone is talking to her. Then, when she says, "Would you repeat that?" the adult can easily become irritated and say, "But I've already told you!" In fact, one has not told her; one has been talking to her face, but not to her mind.

The withdrawn child needs someone to talk to her for a minute or two before she can begin listening. Unlike the first kind of shy child, she does not need time to warm up but instead requires a lot of wooing by adults and other children in order to engage. She may love relationships and love to be involved in group activities, but it does not come naturally to her to seek out experiences.

The two types of shy children need different kinds of help during Floortime and problem-solving time. In working with the oversensitive child, one needs to move slowly and in stages. The child will be able to tolerate the Floortime processes—shared attention and engagement, two-way gestural communication, communication with words and ideas, and building bridges between ideas—only in small doses at first. Gradually, one can help him to engage for longer periods of time at all these levels and to negotiate at each level a broadening range of themes, including those, such as assertiveness and aggression, that tend to be difficult for such children.

To respect the oversensitive child's need for caution—for example, in a classroom—a teacher may want to empathize with how new everything is and how scary new things can be. It is helpful to encourage the child to talk about how he experiences new situations, such as playing with the other children, doing a new kind of drawing, or listening to a new kind of music. As he shares his feelings, it is possible to gradually increase the number of experiences available to him. The teacher must break down into small steps the process of introducing the child to the group, to relationships, or to new academic exercises. The child needs to know that someone understands that he likes to take things slowly. He needs to be helped to feel that it does not make any difference how long it takes him to get where he is going; it is only important that he make progress. If a particular challenge, such as sitting in circle time, feels too hard, one should neither give up on it nor force the child to tackle it all at once. Instead, break the task into smaller steps. Perhaps the child can be in a little circle in a corner of the room with just one other child, then a second child, then a third child, then a fourth, until he feels comfortable enough to take his small group and merge it with the larger group. The same approach—being very supportive and empathic, keeping the stimulation at a level the child can tolerate, and breaking challenges down into small steps—applies to working with such a child one on one.

It is critical to help the sensitive child use his own action and initiative to master his environment. For example, if he indicates that the adult is sitting too close to him for comfort, the adult should try to get him either to indicate exactly where he wants the adult to sit or to move himself to a different position that suits him. The child who dislikes loud noise can learn to lower and raise the volume in various ways. By helping the child learn to take measures to increase his feeling of security, one supports him in becoming less passive and more assertive.

The withdrawn child who has a hard time tuning in to words or other stimuli requires a different approach. Because she is undersensitive to stimuli, she may not even notice someone who approaches her with a soft step and a gentle voice. To capture and sustain her attention, an adult must introduce new experiences with great enthusiasm and energy. Be very animated, talk in a loud voice, and vary the vocal pitch considerably. If the child's eyes brighten up, this is a sign of success. Initially, the adult may need to do 75% of the work to pull the child in. In a group, the adult can mobilize other children to play very exciting, high-energy games to keep the child interested and involved. A game that requires her and her peers to imitate each other may intrigue her, whereas drawing pictures side by side with another child may lead her to tune out, because she is not naturally inclined to look at the other child's drawings.

Many undersensitive children tend not to close circles of communication. A parent, therapist, or teacher may need to do a great deal of work to get gestural and verbal responses from the child and help the child close three or four circles in a row. Even when two-way communication has been established, the child may pull away repeatedly and return to her own play, as though she enjoys her own thoughts better than those of others. This appearance may be misleading. The child is comfortable with her own ideas and finds that figuring out what other people are saying is a lot of work. Keeping to herself feels easier, but not necessarily more interesting or exciting. As one painstakingly helps her open and close increasingly large numbers of circles, she becomes more and more interested in what one has to say, and more tuned in to the world around her.

Why do some children find it such a challenge to tune in to others? In many cases, the child has a problem with auditory processing, or receptive language. As a baby, he may have difficulty decoding the rhythm of people's vocal sounds. Whereas many 4-month-olds can understand a complicated rhythm, this child may understand only a simple, two-cadence rhythm; anything more complex confuses him. Later on, he has similar trouble understanding words. When one gives him three instructions: "Please pick up your coat, bring it over here, and hang it up," he remembers only the first one. After picking up his coat, he looks dumbfounded, as if to say, "What do you want me to do next?" This child has to work very hard to tune in to other people, because it is so hard for him to figure out their gestures and their words. He may be very creative and bright, but because he finds it so difficult to sequence other people's communications, he finds it easier to relax and listen only to himself. He needs to be convinced that the extra effort required to communicate with other people is worthwhile.

Certain caregiving patterns can intensify, or even create, a child's tendency toward self-absorption. Often, such children have parents who also tend to be self-absorbed and preoccupied. Perhaps the parents are sad, depressed, or worried about economic or family stresses. In some cases, the parents are overly cautious in approaching their child because they fear they will intrude on her. Whatever the reason, they do not work hard enough to engage her.

Whether one on one or in a group, whether in pretend play or reality-oriented conversation, it is critical to keep increasing the two-way nature of the child's communication. When he is playing out an elaborate fantasy, one must not stand passively by but rather become part of the drama. When the bad guys tromp the good guys, the adult can circle around, playing one of the bad guys, so that the child cannot ignore the maneuver and must make the good guys respond. If the child has the victorious good guys celebrate with an ice cream party, the adult can say, "I don't like ice cream," thus prodding the child to respond verbally.

At the level of logical thinking, this type of child easily gives up and retreats into her own world when challenged. When a situation calls for her to argue with her teacher or a classmate about why her way is better than theirs, she may instead simply say, "Okay," and proceed to daydream about having things her way. Instead of communicating or building bridges between her own and the other person's ideas, she may develop a wonderful Walter Mitty fantasy in which she tells the teacher she is going to take a nap or play outside rather than do whatever the teacher is asking. She will likely not discuss any of this fantasy with the adult, just as she did not present her arguments. If the adult tries to continue a reality-based conversation, asking, for example, "Why do you want to have it your way?" or "How are you going to do that?" the child may feel a bit confused. It is hard work for her to answer such questions, to think logically in the context of interactions with others. She can be logical only within her own thoughts and fantasies.

Adults should persist in pushing these children to use emotional ideas. If a child wants to stay outside, the adult can say, "Why don't you want to go inside? I know you're having a good time outside, but why won't you go in?" If the child says, "I don't know," the adult can respond, "I know you have good reasons." If the child still does not volunteer his reasons, the adult can patiently help him articulate them. "Well, how about telling me just one reason?" If he still won't respond, one might say, "Well, is one reason that you think it's a nice day, and children should be outside on a nice day?" At this point, the child might agree: "Yes, it's a wonderful day and children should be outside." Even though he has given one of the easiest possible answers, he has built on the adult's ideas, he is opening and closing circles, and he is beginning to get the idea of a logical, "lawyer-to-lawyer" conversation. In time, if the adult repeatedly engages him in this way, the child will begin generating and sharing imaginative new reasons and arguments: "Being inside is bad for you, because you don't get sunshine, and you need the sun to get vitamin D. Do you really want me to get sick from not getting enough vitamin D?"

In short, with the undersensitive, withdrawn child, one works to pull her out of her inner world. One captures her attention and helps her engage in increasingly long and complex interactions. Over time, these experiences can convince her that the world of interaction, although harder, is more rewarding than just marching to her own drummer.

The Quick-to-Anger Child

The child who easily becomes frustrated and angry presents a serious challenge to caregivers, particularly as a toddler. However, wonderful opportunities exist to help such children learn to use their considerable energy in constructive ways.

Some children who are quick to anger naturally tend to use their motor system to discharge energy. As a 3- or 4-month-old, such a child squawks loudly and moves around a lot when upset. As a 7- or 8-month-old, he may crawl and stand up well but may also love to be thrown up into the air and to bang into things. When he is angry, he is likely to bang the floor with his head or hands.

Such a child is often blessed with a high level of enthusiasm and exuberance. She may be outgoing, engage well with other people, and love new experiences. The world is her oyster, and she wants to take it all in. Naturally, when she is frustrated, she is not quiet about it. When she is interested in something she may be calm and attentive, but when uninterested she may become inattentive and active because she naturally tends make her needs known by using her motor system. Similarly, when frustrated and angry, she uses her muscles to change what she does not like. If a toy is not working, she wants to break it, not ask for help with gestures or words. If her parents are not doing what she wants, instead of whining to get their attention or convey her irritation, she will butt them with her head or push them.

What this active, physically aggressive child needs most is extra practice in two-way communication. By providing this practice when the child is a toddler, parents and teachers can save enormous amounts of energy and time when the child is older and needs to function in school. The first step, as described in Chapter 4 ("Therapeutic Principles"), is to use Floortime to establish a solid, nurturing relationship, with lots of shared attention and warm engagement. The aggressive child who does not seem to empathize with others is in particular need of warmth and engagement. He may, however, be fearful of closeness and avoid it. One needs to woo him gently and on his terms. If he is verbal, it is helpful to voice empathy with his fear, hurt, or other feelings underlying his avoidance of contact.

The second step is to make sure one is opening and closing many circles of communication in play and in other pleasurable interactions with the child. In this way, she learns that two-way communication can be enjoyable.

Next, one uses two-way communication to establish clear limits on the child's aggression or other problematic behavior. Keep in mind that the child may have trouble focusing on and comprehending vocal and physical signals. One should use very clear and vigorous gestures, like a police officer directing traffic. Suppose, for example, a toddler starts moving toward a forbidden electrical outlet. A typical parental reaction is to say, "No!" and pull the child away. An active, aggressive toddler, however, will run back to the outlet. When the parent again picks him up, he may throw a tantrum. The next day, the cycle repeats itself. The parent either becomes very adept at physical restraint or becomes exhausted from the constant battles, or both.

There is a better way to help the child learn limits. As soon as the toddler starts moving toward the outlet, get down on the floor in front of him, making very clear gestures, indicating "No" with head and arms while blocking the way. As he tries to get past, block his way even more while continuing to gesture with head and hands. Every time the child squawks and tries to get around the parent, the parent blocks the way and gestures "No." Every time the child responds with another squawk and movement he is closing a circle, and the circles are focused on the theme of limit-setting. The more circles are closed, the more the child is learning to understand and cope with limits as imposed by the parent's gestures, not just by physical restraint.

The parent must also learn to raise his or her voice. (This is often a greater challenge for mothers than it is for fathers, because women are so often socialized to be agreeable and pleasant rather than firm and assertive.) Vocal tone is an important gestural signal, as is facial expression. It is necessary to make one's facial expression very serious and to let one's voice get progressively louder. Parents for whom this does not come naturally can practice going from "1" to "10" in loudness and in seriousness of facial expression. This method is useful whether the child is moving toward an outlet, trying to grab something off the dinner table, starting to hit another child, or doing anything else she should not be doing. If, after a parent gets in front of her, gestures, and increases the intensity of seriousness, loudness, and animation from 1 to 10, the child is still trying to overwhelm any opposition, the parent may then need to use physical restraint. The experience of extended two-way communication, followed by physical intervention, will help the child learn to accept limits. When the child gets older and can use ideas, the parent can begin talking about the importance of "No-no" and the reasons she must follow the parent's directions at times. The child can express her frustration and anger in pretend play. When she is old enough to engage in logical communication, she will be able to present her point of view with great intensity. She may later become a fine trial lawyer who stomps and rages eloquently before the jury, just as she stomped and raged at her parents as a 4-year-old. If the parents have done their job well during the toddler years, the child will learn to accept their authority.

It can take practice to develop the art of progressively raising one's intensity. Some parents are reluctant to expend the energy needed to set firm limits early in an interaction. They may try extremely hard to be nice and agreeable. When the child approaches the wall outlet, his mother might say, in an even-toned voice, "Oh, come on James. Don't touch that. I said, don't. You aren't listening to me, I said don't touch that." The child smiles or giggles and continues toward the outlet. To raise one's voice to the midrange takes more energy and causes the parent discomfort. So she continues trying to be nice, nice, nice, all the while feeling more and more exasperated. Parents in this situation may get so frustrated that they go from 0 to 10 in an instant, exploding suddenly in anger and frightening the child, who had no warning. They may then feel guilty for their loss of control and try to make it up to the child by overindulging him. As a result, the child's environment is unpredictable and chaotic, veering wildly from extra-tolerant to explosive and back again. This pattern characterizes many families in which the children exhibit aggression and other problematic conduct. Instead, the parent needs to move in quickly. As soon as the child starts to challenge the parent's authority, the parent should see the situation as a learning opportunity: "Oh, good, he's challenging me again. Here's another chance to teach him about limits."

Two additional caregiving patterns can also intensify the aggressive behavior of a child who is very active and easily frustrated. Parents who believe in very concrete, law-and-order approaches to discipline may themselves be quick to act; the notions of pausing and reasoning before behaving and of putting feelings into words or gestures have no meaning for them. Such parents engage in frequent, intense power struggles with their child. Whereas a naturally cautious child might become fearful and passive with such intense, concrete parents, a physically active and assertive child may take a parent on and become increasingly aggressive. Another kind of parent engages primarily in intense, conflictual interactions with the child—perhaps because of marital tensions, family problems, or simply the parent's personality style—while failing to provide enough nurturing, soothing experiences. The child has no alternative but to conclude, "Love by irritation is better than no love at all. So I will irritate the heck out of you."

In many cases, the very active and aggressive child is also inattentive. This child may have a hard time processing auditory information, like the second type of shy child described in the previous section. She may find that tuning in to herself is easier than listening to other people. Another variety of active, aggressive child is not truly inattentive, though she may appear so; she tunes other people out not because she cannot comprehend what they say but because she prefers action to thought. Because she tends toward motor discharge, she acts on her environment rather than using ideas or thoughts, even up to the age of 4. Like the child with mild receptive language problems, she needs extra practice in using words instead of deeds. In pretend play, one can help her describe the characters' feelings; in problem-solving talks, one helps her describe her own feelings and use ideas. The goal is always the same: to help the child advance developmentally from simply acting to using more abstract forms of expression. When the child is young, one tries to help her move from aggressive behavior to gestural signaling of anger, frustration, and other feelings. Even the older child who is also working on using words needs a lot of help to become a better "gesturer"; she needs to learn to use gestures as warnings and as the beginnings of symbols. She needs to learn how to go from an intensity level of 1 to a level of 10 gradually, through the use of increasingly intense gestures, rather than instantly. As implied earlier, parents who can gradually escalate their intensity level will be better able to help their children do so than parents who switch suddenly from speaking softly to exploding.

Teachers and parents who deal with inattentive, aggressive children often feel capable of doing only one thing at a time. They get so busy setting limits that they forget to give the child extra practice in using ideas instead of actions. In fact, they are so happy when the child is quiet that they avoid initiating conversation or play with him. Without opportunities for engagement and two-way communication, however, the child cannot progress developmentally.

Parents and teachers should also keep in mind that the aggressive child may need more physical space than other kinds of children. Some children who are prone to motor discharge of aggression do much better when they have their own space with lots of room to play. In one day care center, children prone to aggression who had enormous amounts of space in each room did much better than they had done in more crowded settings. More space gives the child who is working out her own limits a little extra leeway.

Most quick-to-anger children are active, but a few are more like the oversensitive, cautious children described in the previous section. An oversensitive child can also have a short fuse and be prone to tantrums. For this child, one follows the same principles described for his more active counterpart. However, armed with the awareness that this child frightens easily, one wants to be much gentler and more gradual in communicating firmness and to provide extra practice in establishing limits. For this child especially, taking adequate time to develop the nurturing side of the relationship is critical.

With any aggressive child who is also verbal, articulate, and possessed of good problem-solving abilities, it is important to employ the entire six-step intervention process described in Chapter 4 ("Therapeutic Principles"). The child gets help in engaging; she experiences the adult's empathy for her goals; she is helped to determine ways to reach those goals without behaving aggressively; she is given the chance to collaborate in creating a step-by-step process leading to the curbing of aggression and the successful use of other ways to get her needs met; and she is given firm limits to motivate her. As limits are set, the adult also increases Floortime to ensure that the relationship is on solid ground. As the child collaborates in this process, she learns to anticipate situations in which she will experience aggressive feelings and to gain insight into her own pattern of escalation. Better anticipation and better self-awareness will enable her to implement new strategies to meet her needs.

The Inattentive and Distractible Child

Attention is an aspect of communication. By definition, the child who is inattentive does not open and close many circles of communication. The inattentive, distractible child needs a great deal of practice in this area during Floortime and problem-solving time. In order to help him open and close circles, one must pay attention to each sensory modality—vision, hearing, touch, smell—and assess whether that modality holds or undermines the child's attention. Loud noises or visually complex designs may distract him; soothing sounds, or vocal patterns that are not too complex, may help him focus. A certain type of lighting, not too bright or too dim, may help some children attend. Others love color or musical rhythms. One starts by providing the kind of sensory input that best enables the child to attend. Then, one gradually adds greater complexity and range of input, helping the child to open and close increasingly long chains of communication circles using vision, hearing, touch, and his own movement patterns.

Many children find it easier to be attentive when they are moving. The fidgety child who needs to walk around to focus should be helped to understand what kind of movement helps her attend better and to do it. If she understands her own motor system, she will collaborate in increasing her attentiveness if the adult respects the fact that she cannot necessarily be attentive in the way the adult would like, but she can be attentive in a way that is in keeping with her nature as an individual. As she becomes older and more able to use ideas, one can empathize with her inattentiveness and collaborate with her in determining ways to improve her ability to attend. If, at first, one meets the child 80% of the way to help her attend well enough to find the world interesting and satisfying, she will eventually find ways to adjust to most environments.

The child who is inattentive often has parents who think and act in a fragmented manner. The parents may be anxious, easily distracted, or trying to do so many things at once that their attention is spread thin. Such parents do not close their communication circles. Sometimes, due to marital conflicts, two parents have very different agendas for the child, causing the child to be pulled in different directions. Other parents constantly overexcite their children, causing them to experience chronic anxiety, which in turn can produce or exacerbate inattentiveness.

Many parents make a critical error in communicating with their inattentive children. They talk on and on, growing increasingly frustrated, without ever checking to see if they have the child's attention. One mother reported to her child's therapist how embarrassed she felt to be yelling at her daughter, "because I know she can't help being spacey." The mother would say repeatedly, "Come in for dinner" or "Do your homework now." The child would fail to respond, and the mother would end up screaming. The therapist asked, "When she doesn't respond, before you start yelling, do you walk over to her and see if she will look at you, and at least acknowledge what you've asked her to do?" When the mother said she did not, the therapist asked why. "That would feel too intrusive to me," the mother said. "But don't you think your daughter should at least look at you, when you talk to her?" The mother answered, "I know she loves me, it's just that she can't pay attention, because she's too distracted by what she's doing." The therapist: "I would bet that when the school principal talks to her, she looks at him!" The mother admitted that she had seen her daughter do just that. The therapist replied, "Well, it may be hard for her to look at you when she is busy doing something, but if her motivation is high enough, she'll probably pay attention to you. One of the problems is that you haven't helped her to become as motivated to pay attention to you as she is to pay attention to the principal." In intimate, loving relationships, people naturally tend to take each other for granted. A child who is easily distracted will be even more distracted in relating to people with whom he feels comfortable.

The mother asked, "You mean, I should just go over and say, 'Janie, can you look at me when I talk?' and repeat that till she looks at me?" The therapist: "Yes, and do it like a gentle top sergeant in the military: 'Hey, Jane! Whom do you think I'm talking to?'"

This case illustrates the important principle that a child who does not listen to an adult may have a primary auditory processing difficulty. The parent compounds the child's difficulty and creates opportunities for failure by speaking to the child without first getting his attention. If a child has not opened and closed even one circle of communication, it is unlikely one has his attention. Here is the advice we give to parents: First, position yourself in front of the child. Second, make sure the child is making eye contact with you. If not, raise your voice and say, "Hey! Why aren't you looking at me?" Keep raising your voice a bit each time until you get at least a fleeting glance. Shut off the television and eliminate other distractions. Once you have your child's attention, if he begins to tune out, stop and ask, "What just happened?" and find out why the child could not keep listening. The ensuing discussion will lead to the opening and closing of many circles, using both gestures and words, a process that will help the child work on the primary task of maintaining attention. If he decides not to focus, at least this is clearly a volitional, defiant act rather than true inattentiveness.

Recall that communication involves attending and engaging; establishing simple, two-way purposeful communication; and then establishing more complex two-way communication using gestures, symbols, and connections between symbols. These processes must all be in place before a parent gives a child specific instructions. It is important never to skip a step and to empathize with the child's tendency to look and listen to every passing stimulus.

The Clinging Child

The child who clings to an adult—usually a parent—drives the adult to attempt escape; the more the child senses the desire to escape, the more she clings. Instead of fleeing, the parent needs to forge a connection. He or she should set aside a half-hour of Floortime, at different times during the day, to engage the child without her asking. Floortime gives the parent an opportunity to initiate gestures signaling warmth and closeness, allowing the child to feel close without physically holding on. With children 2 years and older, one tries to use words signifying closeness. One can talk about dolls or bears hugging, or directly about the child's desire to hug. Sometimes, children's clinging reflects anger or frustration, and these feelings can be put into words as well. As the parent stops fleeing and proactively engages the child during Floortime sessions, he or she should also begin to set limits on the child's intrusiveness at other times. If the parent is on the phone and the child starts to interrupt and cling, it is time to be firm. The parent should use lots of gestures and eye contact to stay in touch with the child, while encouraging her to play nearby.

The Negative Child

The negative child poses a challenge to parents and other caregivers who attempt to engage him in Floortime. Negativism can take many forms. Perhaps the child will not play or converse with the adult but instead stubbornly sits and stares out a window or repetitively tosses a ball in the air. Perhaps he insists on very structured activities, such as playing a board game or having the adult read him a particular book over and over again. Adults faced with such responses often make the mistake of concluding, "I can't do Floortime with this child." They either give up or insist that the child get down on the floor and participate in pretend play or make up a story.

An adult who reacts this way is taking the concept of Floortime too literally. There is no such thing as a child not taking part in Floortime. Whatever the child is actually doing or saying—including sitting and staring fixedly at the ceiling—*is* the activity of Floortime. By definition, Floortime means simply that the adult is attentive, empathic, and ready to follow what the child wants to do. If, for example, a verbal child is sitting like a bump on a log and refuses to play, the adult can make an empathic comment: "It looks like you want to sit there staring out the window. There must be something interesting about that." If the child ignores the adult, the adult can sit next to her and mimic her behavior, saying, "Let's see what it feels like to do what you are doing." Because the child wants to sit and look, the adult can get in front of her and see if she will make eye contact. The adult can try making interesting or funny faces. If the child says, "Get out of here, you're blocking my view," she has at last responded. The adult can continue: "I didn't know I was blocking your view. What are you looking at?" The child may point at, but not say, what she is looking at, in which case the adult can follow up: "Oh, in that direction. You mean where the grove of trees is? I didn't realize that's what you were looking at." Adult and child are now involved in a gestural and verbal dialogue.

If the child persists in being negative—"I don't want you in front of me, I don't want to talk to you, just leave me alone!"—this is no impediment to continuing empathic two-way communication. "Oh, I understand now. You want me to leave you alone. Where should I go?" The child might say, "Anywhere. Just out of here," and the parent can reply, "Like where?" The slow pace of this dialogue will frustrate the child, who wants to get his message across more quickly, but the adult is successfully engaging him in Floortime. After 20 or 30 minutes, regardless of his negativism and indifference, the two will have opened and closed many circles, both gestural and verbal, and explored the child's main issue, his desire to be left alone. Eventually, the reason the child is so negative may emerge.

Along with taking the whole idea of Floortime too literally, adults sometimes take their children's comments too literally. The child says, "Leave me alone, get out of here," and the adult concludes, "If he doesn't want to play with me, I should leave him alone. That's the only way to be respectful and follow his lead." Remember that the point of Floortime is to *interact* with the child in ways that help her learn or strengthen the six core developmental capacities. One cannot be attentive and engage in two-way communication if one has left the room. If the child says, "Leave!" Floortime philosophy dictates that adult should communicate empathy with the child's wish but not actually do the deed. In another example, suppose a child engaged in pretend play says, "Now, I want you to bang your head against the wall." The adult, instead of taking the child's words literally, can make a distinction between reality and make believe—and between behavior and ideas—by merely pretending to bang his head.

When a child's words touch on an area that is anxiety-laden for a parent, the parent may take those words at face value. Parents who feel uneasy when their child is angry, for example, may take the child's "I hate you!" as a literal expression of truth. The parent may leave the room or respond with outrage: "How can you talk to me like that when I've done so many nice things for you today! I can't believe how ungrateful you are." Parents who fear they are "bad parents" if their children are not always feeling happy may feel driven to defend themselves against the children's specific complaints or criticisms. Yet a child's annoyance, resentment, feistiness, and dismissal of his parents are all part of his communications; they are feelings, not statements of fact. If the parents can see the child's statements in the spirit of Floortime, they can wonder out loud why he feels so angry at them or how they have disappointed him. The goal of Floortime is for the parents to stay engaged with him while helping him elaborate and abstract his negative feelings.

What about the child who wants to use Floortime only for structured games, like Monopoly or cards? The adult should enter into the game. Perhaps the child continually changes the rules to serve her desire to be the winner—that is, her underlying desire to be the boss or the champion, or to be invulnerable. Alternatively, the child may cast herself in the role of policewoman who keeps checking to ensure that everyone follows the actual rules. In either case, the child is giving her own meaning to the game; helping her abstract and explore this meaning is the point of Floortime. The adult should empathize with her wish to be the policewoman or to win at all costs by changing the rules. Instead of criticizing these maneuvers, the adult can express pride and pleasure in the way the child takes initiative. Each successive Floortime session may represent an act in a developing drama. Perhaps the child frequently changes both roles and rules; in this case, the overall pattern that emerges is one of vacillation.

Parents sometimes ask, "But if I allow him to make the rules during Floortime, how will he know when he's playing with his friends that he shouldn't change the rules?" The parent must help the child switch gears by making clear the difference between play sessions when he can set the rules and play sessions when he needs to follow the "real rules." For example, during a Floortime session (it need not be labeled "Floortime" for the child), the parent can comment, "Oh, I see we're going to be playing by your rules today." The child will likely indicate that he comprehends the statement. When the parent, the child, and a friend are playing Monopoly together and the child seeks to change the rules, the parent can calmly point out that with company, everyone needs to play by the actual rules of the game. The child will benefit by understanding what is expected in different contexts. Learning about context is one of childhood's most important lessons.

Parents need to feel secure about defining different contexts for their child. In this way, they help the child understand that in most instances, situations determine roles and behavior. Even though certain rules—such as not hurting other people—cut across all situations, most rules are at least somewhat dependent on context. One can wear a bathing suit to the beach but not to school. One uses certain kinds of words with friends but not with teachers. One eats in a different way at the dinner table than in the back yard. The children who function best socially are usually those who can understand and abstract rules from their contexts.

Summary

In this chapter, we have described several types of children and discussed the issues that parents, teachers, and therapists must keep in mind when working with each type. We described how to tailor Floortime procedures to children's individual differences in sensory, language, and motor functioning and how to help strengthen children's ability to perceive both forest and trees—that is, both the overall picture and the details of events and emotions. We described strategies for working with oversensitive, shy children; undersensitive, withdrawn children; quick-to-anger children; inattentive, distractible children; clinging children; and negative children. For each personality type, we described styles of interaction that tend to worsen the child's difficulties and recommended specific ways of interacting that make use of children's strengths and help them learn or improve capacities they have not sufficiently developed.

Many of the case examples we have given in this chapter and the previous one illustrate ways in which therapists, parents, or teachers can work directly with a child. In Part III, we describe the assessment and treatment of infants and children with particular disorders and further illustrate how the therapist and primary caregivers can work together to help the child.

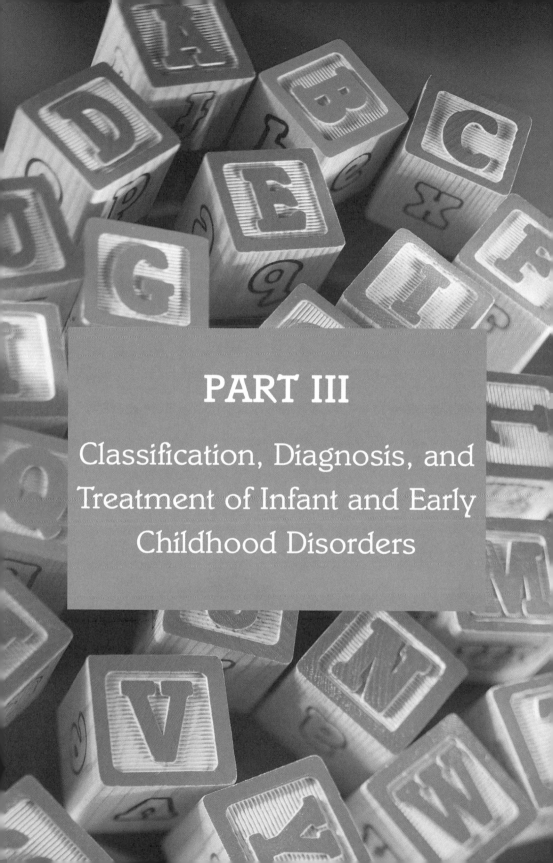

PART III

Classification, Diagnosis, and Treatment of Infant and Early Childhood Disorders

Introduction

The developmental biopsychosocial model presented in this volume provides a framework for classifying and treating different groups of infant and early childhood mental health and developmental disorders. Although each child must be described in terms of his or her unique developmental profile, it is often helpful to group patterns into broad categories to facilitate research, administrative record keeping, and the overall organization of clinical services. Such grouping also facilitates discussions that can improve comprehensive treatment programs.

Two organizations are now working to improve the classification of infant and early childhood mental health disorders. Several years ago, we had the honor of chairing the Diagnostic Classification Task Force for Zero To Three: National Center for Infants, Toddlers, and Families, resulting in publication of the *Diagnostic Classification of Mental Health and Developmental Disorders of Infancy and Early Childhood* (ZERO TO THREE Diagnostic Classification Task Force 1994). At present, there is an ongoing effort to revise the original classification framework. In addition, more recently we have initiated a Diagnostic Classification Task Force under the aegis of the Interdisciplinary Council for Developmental and Learning Disorders (ICDL) to further refine the diagnostic system for infancy and early childhood and expand it to consider developmental and learning disorders. ICDL has recently published its *Diagnostic Manual for Infancy and Early Childhood Mental Health Disorders, Developmental Disorders, Regulatory-Sensory Processing Disorders, Language Disorders, and Learning Challenges* (ICDL-DMIC; Interdisciplinary Council for Developmental and Learning Disorders 2005). The approach presented in the chapters that follow reflects this framework for conceptualizing infant and early childhood mental health disorders. In this book, however, we will not include the discussions on language disorders or learning disorders as they are beyond the scope of this work. The reader should refer to ICDL-DMIC for a full discussion of these disorders, as well as additional discussions of the disorders considered in this volume.

In this work, we consider three broad categories of disorders: interactive disorders, regulatory-sensory processing disorders (RSPD), and neurodevelopmental disorders of relating and communicating (NDRC). These three broad categories include the kinds of problems that are currently conceptualized within the diagnostic system that we helped develop at ZERO TO THREE as well as the classification system we have been developing with the ICDL. It also includes the types of problems currently conceptualized in DSM-IV-TR (American Psychiatric Association 2000).

Interactive disorders refer to challenges in which a primary contribution to the difficulty stems from the infant– or child–caregiver interaction patterns and related family and environmental patterns. *Regulatory-sensory processing disorders* are those challenges in which primary contributors are differences in the child's constitutional and maturational variations in terms of sensory over- or underreactivity, visuospatial or auditory processing, or motor planning or sequencing difficulties. *Neurodevelopmental disorders of relating and communicating* are developmental disorders, including autism spectrum disorders, in which there are significant difficulties with the fundamental capacity to relate, communicate, and think.

NDRC often include regulatory difficulties and interactive difficulties. If, however, basic relating, communicating, and thinking are disrupted, the problems would be classified under the NDRC category. RSPD may also involve interactive difficulties. However, if constitutional-maturational variations, as described earlier, are a significant contribution, the problems are classified in the RSPD category. Interactive disorders may involve constitutional and maturational variations as well as infant–caregiver interactions; however, in interactive disorders, the major contributor to the problems stems from the caregiver–child interaction and related family and environmental patterns.

In order to capture the unique qualities of each infant and young child and his or her family, it is essential to construct a developmental profile that captures these unique qualities. The profile, as we have discussed, will routinely include descriptions of the constitutional and maturational variations (regulatory profile), caregiver–infant or caregiver–child interaction patterns, relative mastery of each of the functional emotional developmental capacities, and family and environmental patterns. Therefore, the approach to classifying infant and early childhood disorders should always include, at a minimum, the following:

- The broad diagnostic category—interactive disorder, RSPD, or NDRC—and the specific type of disorder within the category
- The relative mastery of each of the functional emotional developmental capacities as described in Chapter 2 ("The Functional Emotional Stages of Development")
- The constitutional-maturational variations, in terms of sensory modulation (over- or underreactivity in each sensory modality), auditory processing, visuospatial processing, and motor planning and sequencing
- Characteristics of infant– or child–caregiver interaction patterns and family or environmental patterns

We recommend a multiaxial approach that characterizes the points made earlier. (Please note that the ICDL-DMIC includes additional axes, as well as more detailed discussions of this framework.)

TABLE III–1. Stages of functional emotional development

Functional emotional developmental level	Emotional, social, and intellectual capacities
Shared attention and regulation	Experiencing affective interest in sights, sounds, touch, movements, and other sensory experiences; modulating affects (i.e., calming down)
Engagement and relating	Experiencing pleasurable affects and growing feelings of intimacy in the context of primary relationships
Two-way intentional affective signaling and communication	Using a range of affects in back-and-forth affective signaling to convey intentions (i.e., reading and responding to affective signals)
Long chains of coregulated emotional signaling and shared social problem solving	Organizing affective interactions into action or behavioral patterns to express wishes and needs and to solve problems (e.g., showing someone what one wants with a pattern of actions rather than words or pictures) *Fragmented level:* Little islands of intentional problem-solving behavior *Polarized level:* Organized patterns of behavior expressing only one or another feeling state (e.g., organized aggression and impulsivity; organized clinging, needy, dependent behavior; or organized fearful patterns) *Integrated level:* Different emotional patterns—dependency, assertiveness, pleasure—organized into integrated, problem-solving affective interactions (e.g., flirting, seeking closeness, and then getting help to find a needed object)
Creating representations (or ideas)	Using words and actions together (ideas are acted out in action, but words are also used to signify the action) Using somatic or physical words to convey feeling states ("My muscles are exploding," "Head is aching") Putting desires or feelings into actions (e.g., hugging, hitting, biting) Using action words instead of actions to convey intent ("Hit you!") Conveying feelings as real rather than as signals ("I'm mad," "Hungry," or "Need a hug" as compared with "I feel mad," "I feel hungry," or "I feel like I need a hug"). In the first instance, the feeling state demands action and is very close to action; in the second, it is more a signal for something going on inside that leads to a consideration of many possible thoughts and actions. Expressing global feeling states ("I feel awful," "I feel OK," etc.) Expressing polarized feeling states (feelings tend to be characterized as all good or all bad)

TABLE III–1.   Stages of functional emotional development *(continued)*

Functional emotional developmental level	Emotional, social, and intellectual capacities
Building bridges between ideas: logical thinking	Expressing differentiated feelings (gradually there are more and more subtle descriptions of feeling states, such as loneliness, sadness, annoyance, anger, delight, and happiness) Creating connections between differentiated feeling states ("I feel angry when you are mad at me")

- **Axis I will contain the primary diagnosis** as described in the next three chapters.
- **Axis II will reflect the functional emotional developmental levels** mastered and the degree to which they have been mastered. See Chapter 2 ("The Functional Emotional Stages of Development") for a description of each functional emotional development level and Chapter 3 ("Assessment") for a description of how these levels are observed during the clinical consultation. For each level, it should be noted whether that level is

    a. fully mastered in an age-expected manner
    b. constricted (partially mastered in that selected emotional themes or areas of sensory and motor processing are not operational at that level) or
    c. not present or evidences a deficit (level is not at all reached).

    Table III–1 outlines the functional emotional developmental capacities.

- **Axis III describes the regulatory profile of the child.** As described in Chapter 8 ("Assessment and Treatment of Infants and Young Children With Regulatory-Sensory Processing Disorders"), a number of constitutional-maturational differences affect the way in which infants and young children respond to and comprehend sensory experiences and plan actions. The different observed patterns described in Chapter 8 exist on a continuum from relatively normal variations to disorders. Disorders occur when the variation or individual differences are sufficiently severe to interfere with age-expected emotional, social, cognitive, or learning capacities. The clinician should indicate in this axis the presence or absence of regulatory differences in the categories described in Chapter 8. It should be noted, however, that if the primary diagnosis is a regulatory disorder, these patterns will already be described and this axis need not be addressed again. To summarize the range of these regulatory differences, the clinician may use the following demarcations to indicate the degree to which the pattern represents normal variations versus severe impairments:

    a. Not present
    b. Present, but within a range of normal variation

TABLE III–2. Multiaxial approach

Axis I	Axis II	Axis III	Axis IV	Axis V
Primary diagnosis	Functional emotional developmental capacity	Regulatory profile	Caregiver, family, and environmental patterns	Other medical or neurological diagnoses
Interactive disorders Anxiety disorder Developmental anxiety disorder Disorder of emotional range and stability Disruptive behavior and oppositional disorder Depression Mood dysregulation-bipolar patterns Attentional disorder Prolonged grief reaction Reactive attachment disorder Traumatic stress disorder Adjustment disorder Gender identity disorder Elective mutism Sleep, eating, and elimination disorders **Regulatory-sensory processing disorders** *Type I:* Sensory modulation challenges *Type II:* Sensory discrimination challenges *Type III:* Sensory-based motor challenges	Shared attention and regulation Engagement and relating Two-way intentional, affective signaling and communication Long chains of coregulated emotional signaling and shared social problem solving Creating symbols or ideas Building bridges between ideas; logical thinking **Rate each capacity as—** Age-expected With constrictions Not present (deficit)	*Type I:* Sensory modulation challenges *Type II:* Sensory discrimination challenges *Type III:* Sensory-based motor challenges **Rate these capacities as—** Not present Present, but within a range of normal variation Mild to moderate impairments (e.g., makes it difficult for the child to get dressed or remain calm in noisy settings)	**Rate these patterns as—** Fully supporting the child's age-expected functional capacities Evidencing minor interferences such as difficulty in engaging a child in the specific area of emotional functioning while supporting others (e.g., family conflicts over aggression) Moderate interferences such as when caregiver or family patterns are unable to support whole domains of functioning such as assertiveness or autonomy	

TABLE III-2. Multiaxial approach (continued)

Axis I	Axis II	Axis III	Axis IV	Axis V
Primary diagnosis	Functional emotional developmental capacity	Regulatory profile	Caregiver, family, and environmental patterns	Other medical or neurological diagnoses
Neurodevelopmental disorders of relating and communicating *Type I:* Early symbolic, with constrictions *Type II:* Purposeful problem solving, with constrictions *Type III:* Intermittently engaged and purposeful *Type IV:* Aimless and unpurposeful		Severe impairments (makes it difficult for the child to engage in relationships, form basic patterns of communication, or learn to think)	Major impairments such as when caregivers or family patterns undermine the fundamental foundation of healthy functioning such as the capacity for intimacy and relating	

    c. Mild to moderate impairment (e.g., makes it difficult for the child to get dressed or remain calm in noisy settings)

    d. Severe impairments (makes it difficult for the child to engage in relationships, form basic patterns of communication, or learn to think)

- **Axis IV characterizes caregiver family and environmental patterns.** These are obviously complex dynamic patterns that can only be captured with a detailed narrative. However, for the purpose of this axis, it should be noted whether the caregiver family and environmental patterns are supporting or undermining the child's functioning. Therefore, caregiver family and environmental patterns may be characterized in terms of

    a. fully supporting the child's age-expected functional capacities

    b. evidencing minor interferences such as difficulty in engaging a child in the specific area of emotional functioning while supporting others (e.g., family conflicts over aggression)

    c. moderate interferences such as when caregiver or family patterns are unable to support whole domains of functioning such as assertiveness or autonomy

    d. major impairments such as when caregivers or family patterns undermine the fundamental foundation of healthy functioning, such as the capacity for intimacy and relating.

- **Axis V describes other medical or neurological diagnoses.**

    Table III–2 summarizes this multiaxial approach. A full description with illustrations of this multiaxial approach can be found in the ICDL-DMIC. Although the multiaxial approach summarizes the child's functioning, it does not replace the narrative developmental formulation that describes in more detail each of the factors outlined in these axes.

    In the following chapters, each broad group of disorders is described and a comprehensive developmental approach to the treatment of each disorder is elaborated.

References

American Psychiatric Association: Diagnostic and Statistical Manual of Mental Disorders, 4th Edition, Text Revision. Washington, DC, American Psychiatric Association, 2000

Interdisciplinary Council on Developmental and Learning Disorders Diagnostic Manual for Infancy and Early Childhood Workgroups: Interdisciplinary Council on Developmental and Learning Disorders Diagnostic Manual for Infancy and Early Childhood Mental Health Disorders, Developmental Disorders, Regulatory-Sensory Processing Disorders, Language Disorders, and Learning Challenges. Bethesda, MD, Interdisciplinary Council on Developmental and Learning Disorders, 2005

ZERO TO THREE Diagnostic Classification Task Force: Diagnostic Classification of Mental Health and Developmental Disorders of Infancy and Early Childhood. Arlington, VA, ZERO TO THREE: National Center for Clinical Infant Programs, 1994

7

Assessment and Treatment
of Infants and Young Children
With Interactive Disorders

Interactive disorders are characterized by the way a child perceives and experiences his emotional world and/or by a particular maladaptive child–caregiver interaction pattern (Greenspan 1992). The caregiver's personality, fantasies, and intentions; the child's emerging organization of experience; and the way these come together through child–caregiver interactions are important components of the basis for understanding the nature of the child's difficulty and for devising an effective intervention plan. As with all infant and early childhood disorders, it is important to consider the contributions not only of child–caregiver interactions but also of the child's regulatory-sensory processing profile and family and environmental stress factors.

Infants and young children with interactive disorders tend to have their primary challenges with child–caregiver, family, or environmental patterns rather than their regulatory-sensory processing profile. Although each child has a unique regulatory-sensory processing profile, constitutional-maturational variations are not a major contributing factor in interactive disorders, as they are in the category of regulatory-sensory processing disorders, which we describe in the next chapter.

Many symptoms can arise from disorders of interaction. Regardless of the symptom, however, the goal of treatment is not only to alleviate it, but also to

131

facilitate the child's progress toward an age-appropriate developmental level and toward an age-appropriate degree of stability and range of thematic experience.

Symptoms that can reflect an interactive disorder include anxiety, fears, behavior control problems, and sleeping and eating difficulties. The same symptoms can be reflective of any number of challenges. This is understandable in light of the limited number of behaviors or limited expression of feelings of which infants and young children are capable. This category also includes transient situational reactions, such as a child's response to his mother's return to work. It also includes certain reactions to trauma in which the response does not involve multiple aspects of development.[1]

Primary interactive disorders include the following, which we examine in this chapter's subsequent sections:

- Anxiety disorders
- Developmental anxiety disorder
- Disorder of emotional range and stability
- Disruptive behavior and oppositional disorder
- Depression
- Mood dysregulation-bipolar patterns
- Attentional disorders
- Prolonged grief reaction
- Reactive attachment disorder
- Traumatic stress disorder
- Adjustment disorders
- Gender identity disorder
- Elective mutism
- Sleep disorders
- Eating disorders
- Elimination disorders

Discussion and Illustration of Interactive Disorders

Consider a withdrawn 4-year-old who never formed relationships well. As a baby, she tended to disengage, particularly when confronted with anger or other intense feelings; her parents never knew quite how to woo her back. Under the pressure of

---

[1]For a fuller description of this diagnostic category, please see Interdisciplinary Council on Developmental and Learning Disorders: *Interdisciplinary Council on Developmental and Learning Disorders Diagnostic Manual for Infancy and Early Childhood* (ICDL-DMIC). Bethesda, MD, Interdisciplinary Council on Developmental and Learning Disorders, 2005 (www.icdl.com).

competition from other children, she becomes angry and withdraws. Another 4-year-old, in contrast, engaged well from infancy, learned two-way gestural communication, and learned to symbolize his emotions; however, he has difficulty clearly distinguishing between aggressive feelings and warm, loving feelings. Whenever he feels aggressive, he becomes frightened and anticipates that others will reject him; he copes with these feelings by becoming aloof and withdrawn. The behavior or presenting patterns of these two children may appear identical, but the underlying interactive disorders that give rise to their difficulties are very different.

The first child displays an aloof, cautious manner upon entering the evaluating clinician's playroom. She may not warm up at all, or may warm up only very slowly. Whenever the situation does not feel quite right to her, or the play or conversation suggests any emotion, she withdraws anew. The clinician has the strong impression that this child never mastered the very early developmental task of engagement and intimacy. Once treatment begins, this understanding guides the therapist not to wait passively for the child to begin talking about her feelings; hanging back would simply replay the child's early experiences of disengagement. Instead, the therapist tries to empathize with the child's uncertainty about how to be close and tries to explore associated fears.

When the second child comes into the playroom, he will likely be warm and engaged, use interactive gestures, and play out themes such as aggression and love, showing that he can represent emotional experience. However, the clinician begins to see that he confuses aggressive and loving themes in his play, and that as these themes become increasingly merged and chaotic, the child cuts his play off at a critical point. This child clearly negotiated the interaction patterns of early development well, but had difficulty negotiating complex symbolized feelings in the context of an ongoing relationship. The therapist needs to discover what it is about the child's key relationships that prevented him from learning that aggressive and loving feelings can be part of the same relationship.

It is important to highlight that multiple observations of interactions with the child are critical, including those with the evaluator. These observations are especially important when symbolic play representing the child's experience was not observed during the prior interactions and can then be elicited by the evaluator for those children capable of dynamic play.

Anxiety Disorders

Infants and young children may evidence persistent levels of anxiety and fear that impede age-expected ranges of emotions and functioning. Anxiety can take the form of specific fears or verbalized worries, obsessions or preoccupations, excessive tantrums, distress and agitation, and avoidance behaviors. The primary source of the anxiety, however, may not always be clear.

Presenting Pattern

Depending on the age of the child, the expression of anxiety takes different forms. Infants and very young children who cannot yet communicate or elaborate verbally show anxiety of a more generalized nature in which symptoms—such as excessive fearfulness, tantrums, agitation, avoidance, panic reactions, and worries—are in evidence on a persistent basis, even when the child is not threatened by separation from a primary caregiver. The older child may talk about his fears but not respond to reassurances, or he may have a freeze, fight, or flight reaction. In some cases, children may even have counterphobic reactions where they do just what they are afraid of to alleviate the anxiety they cannot control and to "get it over with." The child is clearly distressed and fearful and cannot carry on usual routines and activities without significant disruptions during the day or night.

We also observe, even in very young infants (3–4 months of age), hypervigilant behavior. The child appears frightened, overly reactive, and overly focused, as though there were imminent danger. Infants who are abused may show this reaction quite early in their development, although it can manifest itself at any time.

Most typically, anxiety will be manifested in a moderate level of apprehensiveness and fear in relationship to many age-expected experiences, such as playing with peers, going into a new social setting, attending a birthday party, performing in school, or trying new foods. These behaviors may be accompanied by whining, crying, withdrawal, and refusal. Not infrequently, difficulties with sleeping or eating, and in older children, difficulties with toilet training and comfortable patterns of elimination, can arise from the child's anxiety even when they are not the source of the anxiety. It should be noted, however, that difficulties with sleeping, eating, toilet training, and elimination can also be related to regulatory-sensory processing disorders, depending on whether the primary contributing factors lie in infant–caregiver interactions or constitutional-maturational variations.

We can see an interactive disorder when the child's anxieties and fears are related to the primary caregiver(s) not sufficiently providing regulating, comforting relationship patterns. For example, the caregiver may be unable to use various strategies, such as helping the child anticipate what might be anxiety-producing through problem-solving conversations, practice in pretend play, preparing the child for what will occur, and planning strategies to use to help the child become less anxious. The caregiver may not be able to soothe, negotiate, and reassure the child sufficiently if the anxiety increases.

Often, the caregiver is also anxious and distressed. The caregiver's anxiety may stem, in part, from anticipating the child's anxiety and feeling ill equipped to help or feeling annoyed or overly worried. The caregiver may also be bringing his or her own anxieties to the situation at hand—such as a social inhibition or a specific phobia, such as a fear of dogs—or be overidentifying with the child who reminds the caregiver of similar experiences in his or her own childhood. In either case, the interaction between the child and caregiver increases the anxiety and distress.

Developmental Pathway

A particular type of infant–caregiver interaction combined with a particular regulatory-sensory processing profile (within the normative range of individual differences, but not at the level of a disorder) often results in a child's evidencing excessive anxiety. Individuals prone to anxiety tend to be overresponsive to sensations like sound and touch and to experience and express affect intensely. In a child at risk for anxiety patterns, the caregiver does not shut down but instead overreacts to the child's emotional communications. As a consequence, the child feels overwhelmed and dysregulated. Instead of experiencing a loss or rupture in the relationship (as the depressed child might), the anxious child constantly feels overwhelmed and experiences dysphoric or unpleasant affects associated with being overwhelmed.

For example, when a toddler shows strong emotions, such as crying to be held or fed, the caregiver reacts as though this routine communication were a major catastrophe. The caregiver may vocalize loudly, speed up the affective rhythm of interaction, and intrude into the child's physical space by quickly picking him up before he gestures his wishes.

Developmental Anxiety Disorder

Development itself can induce significant anxiety in some children who have difficulty negotiating the expected emotional milestones and making developmental transitions. As development launches children into new experiences and uncharted emotional territory, some apprehension or mild anxiety is expected with emerging emotional awareness, until the child begins to feel safe and later develops regulating interactions around emotional understanding of his or her experience. For example, recognizing a stranger and realizing this person is not someone that he or she knows reflects this awareness. With repeated interactions, which are sensitive and responsive to the infant, he or she begins to experience the new person as safe and enjoyable, and is able to adapt. Similarly, as the infant or toddler recognizes the experience of separation, sensitive caregiver interactions help the child adapt and make use of additional solutions, such as a transition object (a teddy bear or blanket) to feel secure.

As the child continues to develop, other emerging emotional experiences may challenge her sense of security and competence. For example, fears of bodily injury, what is real or not (monsters or ghosts), aggression, and related worries may emerge. With supportive interactions, the child develops an understanding of these experiences through regulating interactions, conversations, and symbolic play. She learns to take charge of her own security through words and play, using good judgment and seeking support when needed.

In some cases, however, the anxiety is very intense and highly disruptive. For example, the child may be extremely fearful of separation from his primary caregiver and venturing out into new situations. Overt behaviors include desperate clinging, crying, and tantrums. In addition, the child may be overly anxious even anticipating the separation. He may not function as usual, even when separation is not involved, and avoid expectably interesting age-appropriate experiences with toys, peers, or new physical settings. In other cases, anxiety persists way beyond the developmental stage and may generalize to other fears as well.

As with other interactive disorders, the child's individual differences and/or the caregiver's experience may underlie the anxiety. Multiple dynamics can contribute to the intensity of the anxiety or prolong it. Caregivers who find it difficult to provide adequate support to their child to master new developmental tasks may have or have had similar anxieties themselves.

The child may be at risk or vulnerable due to other health matters in the past. The caregiver may have conflicts or fears related to the child growing up, or is reminded of her own separation challenges in the past as well. In some cases, the child's anxiety masks other problems related to the parental relationship or other environmental stressors. The child may sense some threat or danger related to the caregiver and want to stay with her. Or, the child may be more overresponsive to the unexpected impact of touch and sounds in a new busy environment and become anxious without the security of a protective caregiver nearby.

Whereas stranger and separation anxieties are very familiar, other developmental anxieties are identified less frequently. For example, the toddler becomes aware her body can get hurt, usually after she has mastered some motor autonomy in being able to walk, run, and climb. This awareness is not yet discriminated, in that the child does not yet "know" if it is a big deal or little deal as each bodily insult may be experienced as a potential catastrophe with attendant kisses and band-aids for the boo-boos. With developmental maturation and adequate sensory-motor capacities, these concerns typically resolve within the next year or two, as seen when the child seeks help if really hurt, takes appropriate risks during physical activities, and copes with doctor visits or medical procedures. When the expected developmental anxiety does not resolve, and the child continues to be excessively anxious, avoids physical risks, tends to panic, and is fearful of bodily injury, even in the absence of experiencing real injury or trauma, we often see a developmental anxiety disorder.

Caregiver interactions play a critical role here as well. On the one hand, if caregivers are also anxious about bodily injury because of their own experiences, trauma, or fears, they may find it hard to provide the reassurance and supportive experiences their children need to master body competence. On the other hand, if they are embarrassed or ashamed of their child's fears or timidity, they may transmit these feelings or even shame their children. These interactions can exacerbate the child's anxiety and need to be carefully examined to understand the caregiver's experiences.

As development moves forward, additional emotional milestones can generate anxiety, including negative affects such as jealousy, competition, fighting, retaliation, and other forms of aggression. As children become aware of these affects, they may always insist on being only the "good guy," only claim positive feelings, deny negative motives and feelings, have frightening dreams, and avoid conflict or competition lest they lose. Anxiety is often palpable as the child shows alarm, fear, impulsivity, and even panic in the face of threats related to aggression. The child may even become aggressive toward others.

Typically, these heightened emotions are accompanied by the development of symbolic solutions as the child begins the process of differentiating reality and fantasy. When children begin to report dreams and worries about ghosts and monsters, they are beginning to imagine the first symbols of danger and vulnerability. Those who can imagine these symbols can counter their fears with symbolic solutions. They can imagine the use of magical power (e.g., that of wands, wizards, and witches); employ symbolic play with action figures; or dress up in a drama to fight back and outwit their or their playmates' imagined enemy. Some children become the enemy or bad guy just to be sure they are in charge of the danger. Eventually, children can explore both the good guy and bad guy sides and abstract the reasons for their fighting. These symbolic experiences lay the foundation for higher level abstract thinking and personal standards.

When the child is not prepared to deal with the broader range of affects, anxiety can increase significantly. This is indicated when the child keeps safe by avoiding all negative emotions, protesting vehemently, getting angry, or throwing objects if approached with these themes by other children. The anxiety can escalate into panic as the child experiences himself in danger, can drive the child into avoidance of experiences that make him uncomfortable, or can even trigger regressions as the child tries to escape into the safety of dependency. Other children move into these new emotions more slowly, may temper their anxiety through overreliance on magical solutions, may attempt to control the environment, and are unable to move forward into logical reasoning and building the boundary between reality and fantasy.

As with the other developmentally based anxieties, caregiver interactions can have a crucial impact on the child's emotional development. Here, too, the caregiver's comfort or discomfort with certain emotions can support or impede the child. If the caregiver is only loving when the child is "good" and rejecting of anger, jealousy, meanness, and aggression, the child may not get the support to experience the full range of emotions safely and learn that both positive and negative feelings can be part of relationships. If the child does not have the opportunity and encouragement to experiment and practice with feelings in safe symbolic ways, the developmental process can be derailed.

Presenting Pattern

Children with developmental anxieties present with similar patterns as children with other anxieties and trauma reactions. Some children cling, cry, lash out, hit, bite, or throw tantrums, often in panic proportions. Others may just appear very apprehensive and subdued, if not alarmed, and withdraw from their usual interests and refuse activities. The verbal child may protest or express more worries and fears, show mood shifts, and avoid or withdraw from anxiety-inducing situations. In some cases, the child is afraid to go to sleep or wakes up frequently, reporting frightening dreams or nightmares, or is unable to report feelings but perhaps appears sweaty or anxious. Eating can also be disrupted, with changes in appetite and food choices or even difficulty holding down food. All children with this challenge evidence more intense or prolonged reactions than expected at developmental crossroads and are not readily soothed or reassured.

The anxiety can also be readily transmitted back and forth from child to caregiver and caregiver to child. In some cases, the child's development may have been proceeding smoothly until the anxiety becomes obvious. In others, it is preceded by struggles to master earlier developmental transitions. The anxiety may also be a very intense but transient experience as the child is actually trying to move forward developmentally, and his anxious, disorganized, and even regressive behavior can be the step taken backward before moving forward.

Developmental Pathway

The child may not have adequate symbolic capacities to comprehend emerging emotions, or the child may not be employing these capacities effectively to deal with the expanding range of emotions that development inevitably presents. Developmental anxiety can result from 1) individual differences in the child that contribute to greater vulnerability in negotiating the steps of emotional development and 2) caregiver–child interactions around these developmental steps. The caregiver may not realize the emotional developmental tasks at hand and why they may be challenging the child. Caregivers may not be sufficiently aware of how their past emotional experiences influence their present caregiving and may have unresolved conflicts or fears that intrude into the child's emotional experience.

A number of regulatory-sensory processing vulnerabilities can also contribute to the excessive anxiety evidenced around developmental challenges. These include overresponsiveness in auditory, tactile, or vestibular-proprioceptive capacities; poor visuospatial processing; and motor planning problems. Any one or all of these can make navigating new emotional territory more challenging, especially as expectations increase for the child to interpret and respond to the environment appropriately and not to be derailed by unexpected sensory intrusions.

Disorder of Emotional Range and Stability

Infants and young children tend to show a gradual increase in their emotional range and stability as they develop from early infancy into the preschool years. For example, a 2- to 3-month-old infant tends to shift emotional states rapidly and to evidence a few global emotions, such as joy, delight, distress, rage, and so forth. In contrast, a 16-month-old toddler may evidence warmth and security, pleasure and delight, curiosity, excitement, caution, fear, annoyance, assertiveness, rage, sadness, and so forth. The adaptive toddler, however, experiences and expresses these emotions in a relatively stable manner in relationship to expectable experiences; for example, showing happiness and pleasure when mommy or daddy comes to the door, with a big smile and a readiness to get down on the floor and play. Anger and frustration may predominate when a favorite toy is put back on the shelf because it is bedtime.

Although difficulties with age-expected emotional range and stability may be subtle and less obvious than states of anxiety, these kinds of difficulties can have long-term consequences and are important to recognize. The child's capacity to experience the full range and stability of age-expected emotions is an important foundation of his future social and intellectual development.

To determine if a child has difficulty with age-appropriate emotional range and stability, a clinician must have a roadmap of expected emotional development in infants and young children, observed in their relationships and interactions with family and friends, as well as in pretend play themes. This developmental roadmap starts with emotions related to dependency, pleasure, security, separation, disappointment, bodily competence, injury, surprise, joy, and satisfaction. More negative emotions emerge as the child encounters the reality around him in relation to others and may feel anger, jealousy, sibling rivalry, competition, aggression, and a wish for control and power over others. These "negative" emotions can challenge the caregiver–child interactions if the relationship does not embrace the full range of human feelings. As the child masters reality testing and reaches higher emotional developmental levels, emotions expand to friendship, loyalty, justice, and morality.

While the rudiments of most emotions are present from infancy, emotions become further differentiated as the child develops in the first 5 years of life. In these first years, the child becomes able to describe more complex feelings and the reasons for these feelings, which include ambivalence and conflicting emotions. A 2-year-old may bop his baby sister and then hug and kiss her. At 3, he may pout and grab her toy. At 4 years, he may protest verbally that mommy never spends time with him and that the baby always comes first, but he also acknowledges his love for the baby. Between ages 5 and 6, he may be protective and helpful but can also talk about his jealousy.

It is the lack of differentiation, range, and stability of emotions that characterizes a disorder of emotional range and stability. In contrast to children with developmental anxieties, these children present with constrictions and a very narrow range of affects or interests without the full-blown intensity of anxiety reactions.

Presenting Pattern

Many infants and toddlers do not evidence the increasing range and stability of emotions just described. As toddlers and preschoolers, they may persist in evidencing only a few global emotional states, such as joy and rage, depending on the circumstances. The lack of stability may be seen in rapid fluctuations from one emotional state to another or in variations in the intensity of the same set of emotions, with little or no capacity to tolerate frustration in an age-expectable manner resulting in disrupted functioning. Or they may even confuse or reverse emotions inappropriately. Questions about feelings are hard for them to answer; the connections among thoughts, feelings, and behaviors are fleeting; and little reflection is available. Interests tend to be limited as the child selects and focuses on just a few areas, such as construction, vehicles, or transformer toys, and seems uninterested in the emotional drama that could accompany these ideas. Play with other children may also be affected as the child has fewer emotionally based ideas and is less interested in the symbolic play of others.

Developmental Pathway

Sensory underresponsivity and low muscle tone, a mixed pattern of underresponsivity and overresponsivity, or overresponsivity to sensations alone can contribute to this disorder. These patterns of responsivity make emotional regulation more difficult; clearly, sensory modulation challenges can make it harder to negotiate the functional emotional developmental capacities in a stable, regulated manner and vice versa. The key contribution, however, is from caregiver–child interaction patterns that do not optimally foster a broad range of feelings at each functional emotional developmental level. As an example of the contributions of both sensory processing and interaction patterns, the child may be underresponsive to his own bodily sensations of emotion (e.g., not feeling the tightening of his muscles as he gets angry, the scowls in his face as he gets frustrated with a task, or the pit in his stomach as he becomes fearful). When this underresponsivity is coupled with interactions that also avoid the safe expression of the full range of emotions or with interactions in which only certain emotions are acceptable, the child has fewer opportunities to explore and navigate his emotional world. Parents may deny the child's feelings (e.g., "Don't feel mad, and don't feel sad"; "There is nothing to be afraid of!"; or "You always have to be nice"). Other parents are conflicted about recognizing or expressing their own emotions and avoid the same in their children, sharing only "happy" times. Thus, the child may learn to accommodate the parents' comfort level.

Disruptive Behavior and Oppositional Disorder

Disruptive behaviors are a common challenge in infancy and early childhood. As the toddler begins to walk, problems with impulse control often first emerge. For example, a toddler may hit, bite, or scratch instead of using interactive gestures and emotional signals to convey intentions. During the preschool years, children may display a combination of attentional and disruptive behavior challenges. The preschooler may evidence a high activity level; show poor frustration tolerance; react to frustration with pushing, hitting, or throwing objects or being oppositional; and rapidly shift from one activity to another. Often, when assessing the child's relative mastery of functional emotional developmental capacities, we observe that although the child has some mastery of each level, he shows constrictions at each level. These constrictions can especially impede self-regulation and social problem-solving where disruptive behavior derails symbolic solutions using language, negotiations, and pretend play to express needs and feelings, resolve conflicts, be flexible, and delay gratification.

In addition, when the child behaves disruptively, we often observe a caregiver interaction pattern characterized by a lack of regulating and limit setting in response to the infant's signals. The caregiver may read and respond to the infant's signal of pleasure and joy or fear with a variety of appropriate reciprocal gestures (smiles beget smiles, fear begets comfort, and so forth), but when the same toddler begins to show annoyance and anger, the caregiver may evidence, often due to momentary anxiety, a lack of response or an exaggerated response. Sometimes caregivers appear almost stone-faced at the moment of truth as the child is getting increasingly angry and beginning to get ready to push or bite. Other times, the caregiver may move in too quickly in an overly punitive manner. Not infrequently, one caregiver "freezes" while the other is overly punitive. The result is that the child does not receive sensitive reciprocal regulating and limit-setting responses.

In some cases, disruptive behavior can be extreme, with even young children acting very aggressively. They might hurt others, set fires, destroy property, or torture animals with little remorse. They may become aggressive in a caregiving environment that is overly punitive or unavailable and be relatively unable to successfully master the organizational levels dealing with engagement, empathy, coregulated emotional signaling, and limit setting. If the immediate environment doesn't provide warmth and nurturing, as well as firm, consistent limits, or if limits are imposed abusively, the tendency toward seeking sensation can take on an enraged quality, with indiscriminate, aggressive acting out[2] (Lewis 1992; Yeager and Lewis 2000).

Developmental Pathway

The pathways include the way the child reacts to and comprehends different sensations and plans actions (an expression of his or her biological patterns), the ways in which his or her caregiving environment interacts with these individual differences, and the levels or stages of emotional and intellectual organization that are negotiated through these interactions.

For example, infants and toddlers who are underresponsive to touch and sound are often physically very active and sensory seeking or craving sensation. These children often become aggressive in a caregiving environment that is overly punitive or unavailable. They are relatively unable to successfully master the organizational levels dealing with engagement, empathy, coregulated emotional signaling, and limit setting.

Although an overresponsive pattern is related to a very different underlying processing challenge than underresponsivity, it also can manifest with aggressive behavior. Children who are overresponsive to sensations such as touch and sound may easily become overloaded in noisy or busy environments, such as a preschool or a shopping mall. A sudden, unexpected touch from another child can easily be misperceived as hostile or aggressive by the tactilely overresponsive child. He may then push or hit as a response. Infants and toddlers who are sensory overresponsive to sensations such as touch and sound likely become aggressive if the caregiving environment is too intrusive or overwhelming.

Depression

In healthy development, infants and young children gradually expand their capacities for emotional expression and for experiencing a wide range of feelings. This gradually expanding capacity is part of the infant–caregiver relationship pattern. Adaptive interactive patterns enable infants to successfully negotiate each of the functional emotional developmental capacities, and thereby experience, by the time they are toddlers, a large range of emotions from joy, pleasure, and enthusiasm to transient sadness and fear. They are also able to enjoy assertiveness and exploration, as well as a growing curiosity.

---

[2]Among children deprived of nurturing affection in the early years of life, including those in institutional care, two tendencies have been observed. One group of children became withdrawn, depressed, or apathetic. Some stopped developing physically, failed to gain weight, and even became quite ill and did not survive. Those in the other group sought out sensation, becoming aggressive, promiscuous, and indifferent to others, relating to them only to fill their own concrete needs (Spitz 1945). In another study, researchers found a higher-than-expected degree of subtle difficulties in the functioning of the nervous system among antisocial children and adults, with problems in perception, information processing, and motor functioning (Bowlby 1944).

Presenting Pattern

Infants and young children can begin showing a consistent mood pattern rather than the range of emotional states expected for their age and developmental stage. For example, some toddlers and preschoolers display a persistently sad or depressed affect. They may indicate that they are sad or well up with tears when asked about feelings or even seeing someone else feeling sad or crying. They appear to show little pleasure or interest in their usually enjoyable activities and do not initiate "fun" activities. Sometimes they may have difficulty showing or verbalizing expectable feelings of sadness in situations that would ordinarily elicit sad feelings or insist they are "happy" even as they cry or look very sad. As they become symbolic, they may play out and talk about depressive themes. Preschoolers may, for example, enact in play and/or verbalize persistent feelings of being "bad," and slightly older children may talk about wishing they were not alive or present themes of dying in their play (when it is not part of a bereavement or trauma situation).

Infants and young children may also evidence persistent agitation and irritability, with nothing pleasing them; or in contrast, they may move very little, show little energy, and turn down activities they may have once enjoyed. Other children have sleep or eating difficulties (with weight loss or gains), which are common symptoms related to various sources of stress.

The severity of the mood disorder may be reflected in the intensity of just a few of the behaviors described above, or in the increasing number of challenges, the longer the child feels depressed. Infant–caregiver interaction patterns often play a major role in the child's difficulties in regulating mood. The child may experience the loss of love or support when the parent cannot accept his or her full range of behavior and feelings. For example, the parent may be very loving in response to compliance and being good, but pull away when the child is angry or aggressive. The parent may not be able to respond to the child when the parent's own conflicts are triggered and thus becomes ambivalent or unpredictable to the child.

The depression becomes apparent over time when the child experiences some loss or conflict with others and is unable to rely on an internalized, nurturing image to soothe and comfort. Such difficulties can, if left unaddressed, persist into adulthood.

Developmental Pathway

Sensory overresponsiveness, stronger verbal processing capacities, and weaker visuospatial processing capacities characterize the pattern we have observed in many individuals prone to depression. In a child at risk for depressive patterns, the caregiver tends to shut down when the child's affect is becoming intense (i.e., the caregiver finds it hard to maintain a pattern of coregulated affective interaction at these moments of heightened affect). The child experiences a loss or rupture in the relationship, sometimes only for a few seconds. This very brief sense of loss becomes associated with strong affect. As expectations are formed, due to better pattern construction, the child expects loss and/or emptiness when he has strong feelings. As the child becomes more symbolic, this pattern can be experienced in terms of images of loss and, later on, "I must have caused the loss by being bad or angry or demanding." Instead of an internal security blanket of warm, soothing, comforting images and expectations, the child experiences loss and sadness.

Mood Dysregulation: A Unique Type of Interactive and Mixed Regulatory-Sensory Processing Disorder Characterized by Bipolar Patterns

In recent years, there has been growing interest in early identification and treatment of bipolar-type mood dysregulation in children (Carlson and Weintraub 1993; Cytryn and McKnew 1974; Egland et al. 1987; Geller et al. 2001; Lish et al. 1994; Radke-Yarrow et al. 1992). In children, manic or hypomanic states often cause aggressive behavior or agitation rather than the frantic, grandiose thinking commonly seen in adults. Diagnosing bipolar patterns in children is therefore difficult (Harrington et al. 1991; Strober et al. 1988). We do not have a clear understanding of the antecedent variables leading to bipolar disorder in children, although a host of neuropsychological vulnerabilities or deficits have been suggested, including problems in the areas of language, motor development, perception, executive functioning, and social functioning (Castillo et al. 2000; Sigurdsson et al. 1999). Furthermore, a comprehensive intervention program that addresses family interactions and educational issues, as well as biochemical treatments, has not been formulated.

Presenting Pattern and Developmental Pathway

We propose a novel hypothesis: bipolar patterns in children can be understood as arising from a unique configuration of antecedents involving sensory processing and motor functioning, early child–caregiver interaction patterns, and early states of personality organization. Specifically, we suggest that children at risk for developing bipolar-type mood dysregulation share the following characteristics (Greenspan and Glovinsky 2002):

1. An unusual processing pattern in which overresponsivity to sound, touch, or both coexists with a craving of sensory stimulation, particularly movement (most overresponsive children are more fearful and cautious). Sensory craving is usually associated with high activity and aggressive, agitated, or impulsive behavior. Therefore, when overloaded with stimuli, children with this unusual

combination of processing differences cannot self-regulate by withdrawing, as a cautious child might. Instead, they become agitated, aggressive, and impulsive, thereby overloading themselves even more.

2. An early pattern of interaction, continuing into childhood, characterized by a lack of fully coregulated reciprocal affective exchanges. In particular, caregivers are unable to interact with the infant or child in ways that help her upregulate and downregulate her moods to modulate states of despondency and agitation.

3. A personality organization in which the fifth and sixth functional emotional levels of development have not been mastered. Emotions either are not addressed at the symbolic level, instead remaining at the level of behavior or somatic experience, or are represented as global, polarized affect states rather than in integrated form.

Attentional Disorders

Infants and young children may evidence challenges in sustaining attention. Attentional disorders are one of the most complicated mental health disorders. Although certain shared symptoms, such as inattentiveness, characterize a large number of children who receive this diagnosis, there may be many different patterns (i.e., many different pathways) leading to these symptoms, and many different reasons for inattentiveness. A comprehensive approach to understanding attentional problems needs to address the different and combined processing patterns as well as the different developmental organizations and interactive patterns of infants and young children.

Here, we focus on challenges with attention that stem primarily from interactive difficulties and the developmental pathways that contribute to these challenges. Attention needs to be given to the relevant developmental tasks at hand to explore whether developmental anxieties (fears), the environment, or social challenges in the environment may be disrupting the child's attention and can be addressed or modified.

In both the interactive and regulatory-sensory processing attention problems, the same developmental pathways are involved, and interactions can be more challenging. Based on a complete profile, the clinician can determine which developmental pathway is contributing to the symptom choice.

Presenting Pattern

Variations in attention can be expected in early development. Difficulties sustaining attention can be observed as early as 2 to 4 months when the infant becomes more capable of turning and focusing to look and listen and coo responsively. By 8 to 12 months, the infant may attend only fleetingly, rather than in the sustained manner needed for two-way interactions, such as peek-a-boo, pat-a-cake, or enjoying a shape sorter with another person. In the second year of life, the toddler might just move from toy to toy and appear highly distracted even when playing with an object of choice. Later, the young child may always be on the move, always changing topics, unable to stick with a conversation or a game. Another pattern involves spurts or intermittent stop-and-go interactions. Or the child may be too self-absorbed or overfocused on special interests and finds it hard to shift his attention to others, even when called.

Variations in attention can also be related to the functions at hand so that young children may be attentive to books, videos, or other forms of entertainment—but less attentive when expected to attend and participate more actively to what others choose or where they have less interest and less interaction available, as in circle time. Often, the tolerance or expectations of the environment affect perceptions of the problem (e.g., when a child plays alone for long periods, it might be considered an asset rather than a pattern signaling possible self-absorption; changing activities every few minutes at preschool or at home may be considered necessary because assumed attention is very short in young children). Despite all these variations, attention difficulties are readily identified, and determining the primary contributions based on the child's individual profile is the next step.

Developmental Pathway

Motor and regulatory-sensory processing patterns and child–caregiver and family interactive patterns (and often combinations of both) can be significant contributors to attentional challenges. First, consider interactive patterns.

As in anxiety and depression, we have observed a pattern of reciprocal affective interchanges characteristic of attentional difficulties. Typically, coregulated reciprocal affective interactions with caregivers are established from about 9 to 24 months. When we observe an infant–caregiver interaction pattern characterized by short bursts of back-and-forth communication or signaling, rather than long chains of back-and-forth communication, a problem is evident. Some caregivers respond to the child's short bursts of interaction by becoming fragmented with the child. They jump from one thing to another with him rather than trying to sustain a long chain of interaction. They also frequently give up entirely and let the child play alone.

Other caregivers attempt to overcontrol the child, which can lead the child to be rigid. Such a child seems to focus but not with true, shared attention. No real back-and-forth problem solving occurs. Overcontrol also mobilizes catastrophic affects that can lead to even shorter interactions. The child's constitutional-maturational variations as well as the caregiver's characteristics contribute to this type of interactive pattern. In addition, the caregiver's attentional capacities should be explored.

The absence of consistent opportunities for communication and interaction with adults can lead children to become more self-absorbed or preoccupied with their own interests and seemingly inattentive to others. The critical factor, how-ever, is that these children can be readily wooed into interaction and focus when engaged in a wide range of conditions (e.g., in quiet environments, in the class, in a small group).

In some cases, what appears as poor attention may be related to anxiety and avoidance patterns, and other interactive disorders should be considered. Chaotic families or very self-absorbed ones can certainly contribute to a disorder, and one may also see symptoms of anxiety and/or depression in children in such settings.

In most cases, when regulation, interaction, and engagement are available, poor attention usually relates to regulatory-sensory processing disorders or neu-rodevelopmental disorders described in the next chapters.

In considering the interactive patterns of children with attentional problems, two reasons appear for the short bursts of interaction: 1) each child brings unique biological patterns into the interaction; and 2) interactions stem from these bio-logical patterns or intensify them, as described above. Now let's look at the regu-latory-sensory processing differences that may contribute to the developmental pathways of attentional problems.

As a group, children with attentional problems tend to have one or a number of processing difficulties, most frequently with motor planning and sequencing. Six regulatory-sensory processing and modulation patterns, as well as some com-binations, are associated with problems with attention. These are described below:

1. *Motor planning and sequencing.* It is hard for children with attentional problems to engage in long action sequences (i.e., a number of actions in a row). In their spontaneous play, they'll tend to do two actions in a row, such as take the car and put it into the house. They do not complete eight or ten actions in a row, such as take the car, put it in the house, then take it out of the house and go to the pretend schoolhouse, then go to the store, etc. We see children who, even as toddlers, can sequence four or more actions in a row (e.g., moving trucks differ-ent places) and children who can do only one or two sequences.

    When a child has biologically based motor planning and sequencing chal-lenges and perhaps other processing challenges as well, it's harder for him to engage in long chains of back-and-forth interaction. If he's a one- or two-step action sequencer, the adult interacting with him must work with him much harder to sustain an interaction than with a child who ordinarily is a four- or five-step action sequencer. When older, children with motor planning prob-lems may have a hard time with such basic skills as learning to tie their shoes, learning a complicated sequence of dance steps, mastering the steps involved in new sports, and in following directions that involve motor performance. Therefore, motor-based schoolwork can be very challenging.

    These children also can have difficulty with a range of basic academic and so-cial tasks that often are associated with a lack of attentiveness. For example, they are inattentive and have difficulty complying with a range of school activities, including such basics as standing in line, marching in an orderly way to the library or lunchroom, organizing their backpacks with the proper homework assignments, carrying out the steps in doing the homework, and returning the homework the next day. Children with this challenge may understand all the concepts involved in the homework, but they may receive a low grade because they either don't take the homework home or don't hand it in the next day. Because of their difficulty with sequencing, they may also have difficulty handling complex social interactions, as with negotiating different relationships in a party or on a soccer field. In addition, sequencing ideas in an essay or an oral argument may also be problematic.

2. *Underresponsivity to basic sensations.* These children often have challenges in registering basic sensations, such as touch and sound. Therefore, they tend to retreat into their own fantasies. A typical 4-year-old with this pattern would be described by his parents as tuning out all the time and engaging in pretend play on his own. His teacher would describe him as tuning out as well, and that she has to work very hard to get and maintain his attention.

3. *Sensory seeking.* These children may be underresponsive to sensations such as touch and sound, as the group above. However, sensory-seeking children tend to be physically active and seek out sensory input, sometimes to compensate for their underresponsivity. They tend to differ from the previous group in some important ways: they are often underresponsive to the sensation of movement and, therefore, crave it, which tends to contribute to their activity levels; they are *less* likely to have low muscle tone, which the previous group often evidences; and their muscle tone contributes to their ability to seek out sensation, in contrast to the previous group, who would tire quickly from too much activity.

    The sensory-seeking group also tends to have difficulty with registering sensory input and, therefore, these children are often inattentive when someone is trying to talk with them or challenge them to focus on an academic task. Because they also tend to seek sensations, however, they frequently fidget, touch everything nearby, and attempt to create loud noises and movement for themselves and others. Therefore, they often evidence high activity levels and move rapidly from object to object. They may also, in their zest for new sensations, evidence a great deal of risk taking and aggression. The aggression can become especially prominent if there are insufficient nurturing interactions, insufficient limit setting, and practice in creative (imaginative) thinking and reflective problem-solving.

4. *Overresponsivity to sensation.* Children with this pattern tend to overrespond to basic sensations, such as touch and sound. In a noisy classroom, they tend to be distracted easily by the sounds around them, such as another child chewing or the sound of the boiler or air conditioner or a noise outside. Rather than

retreating into their own fantasy worlds and having a hard time registering sensations, these children register too many sensations and jump from one thing to another. They have a hard time sustaining their attention. They may also evidence some reactive aggression and impulsivity when they are overloaded with sensation. In this group, it is often the sensory overload, rather than a fundamental difficulty with anger, that is associated with this type of behavior.

5. *Auditory-verbal processing challenges.* Children with this pattern evidence inattentiveness secondary to processing or comprehending auditory, verbal experiences (i.e., language). They may show difficulties with following directions, understanding the sequence or steps in solving a problem, or their ability to comply or carry out any number of social or academic tasks. Their confusion and lack of sustained direction often lead to, or appear to be, inattentiveness.

6. *Visuospatial processing challenges.* This pattern relates to difficulties in processing or comprehending visuospatial experiences. Visuospatial experiences involve understanding spatial relationships, such as where the park is in relationship to one's own house; how the different rooms in a new house are laid out or how to find a hidden object; or, at a more advanced level, how to picture different visual designs from different angles, such as figuring out the mirror image of a pattern of blocks.

   Advanced concepts in mathematics and science also depend a great deal on visuospatial thinking, as does the more general ability to "see the forest for the trees." Children who have difficulties with visuospatial processing often have a hard time understanding the larger patterns within which they are operating and, therefore, can easily get "lost in the trees." They may be quite gifted verbally and have excellent verbal memories, but nonetheless, have difficulties with complex patterns that require a great deal of sequencing or difficulties with the ability to put all the pieces together into a larger whole. Such children can easily evidence distractibility and inattentiveness when the tasks are oriented toward big-picture thinking or require the manipulation of objects or concepts in spatial contexts.

7. *Combinations and severity.* Many children evidence combinations of the above underlying processing difficulties. The more severe the interactive patterns and the processing differences described earlier, often the greater the attentional difficulties.[3]

---

[3]It is important to note that neuropsychological and educational batteries do not always test for all these processing challenges. For example, they do not test for over- or underresponsivity to sensations such as touch and sound. They do, however, pick up auditory-verbal processing challenges and certain types of sequencing challenges.

Prolonged Grief Reaction

The loss of a parent or primary caregiver is so profound it always requires clinical attention.

Presenting Pattern

Reactions can take many forms and may progress over time. Most often, when infants and young children experience the loss of a primary caregiver, they evidence an initial grief reaction characterized by the child searching and protesting the caregiver's absence. The child may also withdraw, become more passive and self-absorbed, and avoid expected or pleasurable activities. Fear, anxiety, and agitation following the loss may give way to despondency and self-absorption, depending on the length of the loss. In other cases, the child may hardly seem to be reacting, especially if he or she takes on the role of comforting or distracting the other grieving family members by entertaining or becoming more demanding of the caregiver and insisting they be cared for.

Reactions can also take the form of increased separation anxiety. Some children cannot tolerate separation from the remaining caregiver and are very clingy. Some express their anger and aggression at the remaining parent who is still there, with or without the idealization of the missing parent. In some cases, children appear to carry on in one environment but not another, such as at preschool or daycare versus at home. Many evidence sleep and eating disruptions, weight loss, and/or weight gains; become ill; have a variety of somatic complaints; show reduced frustration tolerance; exhibit regressions in recently mastered developmental tasks, such as toileting and dressing; or show other ways of feeling helpless. The persistence and/or multiplicity of these symptoms move expected grief reactions to the level of a disorder.

Comprehending the permanence of the loss is developmental in nature, but it is important not to underestimate the impact of the loss on infants and toddlers or children with significant developmental delays. These infants and children may have many of the reactions described above, which other caregivers may not always link to the loss and grief or don't expect the child to remember. It is not unusual for the verbal child to express an expectation of the parent's return or to imagine the parent is living elsewhere and that they will be able to reunite at some point. Similarly, some children show marked distress at reminders of their missing caregiver, whereas others seek reminders that are positive reflections of their experiences and they want nothing changed or moved.

Whatever the reaction of the child to the loss of a parent or primary caregiver and however they try to comprehend its meaning, it is important to help the child, given the overwhelming significance of the loss and the child's limited resources to understand the reason or the finality of the loss. The age of the child and the emerging developmental profile of the child determines, in part, how long a period of loss is necessary for a prolonged grief reaction or disorder to be considered.[4] An important factor is the availability of a nurturing substitute caregiver who provides extra security and emotional warmth, the opportunity to express feelings, and, in preschoolers, the opportunity to play out emerging worries and fears as well as feelings of loss. Such a caregiver can be especially helpful in enabling the child to cope with grief.

Developmental Pathway

Disruption of the child's functioning is likely to take the form of any vulnerability in the child's constitutional-maturational patterns before the loss. Children who are overresponsive may become more irritable and fussy, with increased reactivity to the environment. Underresponsive children may become more withdrawn and self-absorbed and less responsive to attempts to arouse and engage them. Many children have mixed patterns and may show many fluctuations in unpredictable ways—sad and withdrawn one hour and frustrated and aggressive the next. If regulation was fragile to begin with, more difficulties are to be expected. But even when the child's functioning is good, some short- or long-term dysregulation can be expected.

Reactive Attachment Disorder

Forming an attachment or, more broadly, an emotionally trusting relationship, is a well-established critical dimension of healthy emotional development. We can observe, however, many compromises in forming or sustaining healthy relationship patterns.

Presenting Pattern

Attachment problems include a wide range of challenges in infants and young children, including those who are not able to engage in any type of intimacy; do not seek or respond to comfort; and may be very despondent, withdrawn, or self-absorbed, or diffusely aggressive, impersonal, or promiscuous in their relation-

---

[4]Bowlby described and the Robertsons filmed very young children evidencing such a grief reaction when separated from their primary caregivers during a hospitalization. (These famous films are available at the New York University film library (Bowlby and Robertson 1953).

ships. Other infants and young children show more subtle variations in degrees and qualities of intimacy, empathy, and the capacities for negotiating and sustaining relationships.

When extreme, disruptions in early attachment patterns can be associated with compromises in the child's growth and weight gain (failure to thrive), as well as with language, cognitive, and social difficulties. The most severe versions of these reactions are seen in children who grow up in orphanages that do not provide sufficient nurturing care and in children who experience extensive neglect or abuse within their families. If attachment problems have significantly disrupted the fundamental capacities of relating, communicating, and thinking, the child may appear to have a neurodevelopmental disorder of relating and communicating, such as autism, with little capacity for shared attention, social reciprocity, or social problem solving, and require the same type of treatment program as children with derailed development.

In many cases, however, attachment and relationship problems in infancy and early childhood are not extreme. There are many subtle variations in which the early relationship lacks emotional depth, range, and optimal levels of trust and security. In looking at the more subtle attachment and relationship problems of infants and young children, the clinician should employ a framework that considers the implications of infant–caregiver relationships in light of the infant's capacity to successfully master each of the functional emotional developmental capacities. The attachment relationship needs to be viewed from the perspective of the full range and stability of age-expected feelings and progression through each of the functional emotional developmental capacities. These levels may be difficult to negotiate with parents who have often experienced severe deprivation themselves, as seen in multiproblem families, and who are then unable to form intimate attachments with their own infants. The interactions may also be embedded with anxiety, despair, or ambivalence, and other compromises in the parent's experience or current relationships.

The clinician also needs to consider the contributions of the child's regulatory-sensory processing profile. For example, infants who are very responsive to sensations such as touch and sound may evidence far more insecurity in their early relationship patterns than other infants. Alternately, challenges in forming relationships can lead to challenges in sensory modulation, sensory processing, and motor planning, all of which can appear to have a biological origin, even when they are secondary to interactive challenges. Infants who are born with very competent nervous systems, including good muscle tone and abilities to focus, attend, and respond to visual and auditory sensations, can lose these competencies during the first 2 to 3 months of life if their environments are either very chaotic or nonnurturing (Greenspan et al. 1987). Infants can develop low muscle tone, underresponsivity to touch and sound, difficulties in auditory and visuospatial processing, sensory hypersensitivity, and patterns of avoidance (in the more chaotic, overstimulating environments). Even when these patterns are secondary to interactive difficulties, infants with a reactive attachment disorder may be indistinguishable from infants who are born with these processing challenges, such as infants with extreme regulatory or neurodevelopmental difficulties in relating and communicating.

Developmental Pathway

Two major pathways and their variations need to be considered. One pathway includes the interaction between the environment and the child. When the environment is neglectful, abusive, or otherwise stressful, it may not provide the nurturing interactions necessary to form relationships that can support each functional developmental level. In some cases, the environmental stress may be related to external factors such as poverty, family disruption, or illness. In other cases, the parent may not have the personal emotional and relationship capacities to help the child form a secure relationship and maintain it.

The other major pathway involves understanding the child's unique individual profile and the contribution of the child's challenges. For example, the infant may be more sensory over- or underresponsive or have challenges in the way he or she processes auditory and visuospatial information and plans motor actions. These variations can challenge the parent's competency and derail the development of a secure and trusting relationship as the infant and parent struggle to regulate and enjoy their interactions.

Traumatic Stress Disorder

The term *traumatic stress disorder*, rather than posttraumatic stress disorder, is used because infants and young children often respond to severe trauma or stress immediately. The reaction may then continue, depending on factors discussed below.

Presenting Pattern

Infants and young children may be exposed to a range of traumatic stresses that can disrupt their emotional, social, language, and intellectual development. Children experiencing or witnessing serious unexpected events that threaten them or others, such as accidents, animal attacks, fires, war, natural disasters, or overwhelmingly frightening interpersonal events such as abuse or a parent being killed, are some examples.

Such children may experience a disruption in a number of basic capacities. Most common are disruptions in sleep, eating, elimination, attention, impulse control, and mood patterns. Physiological disruption is common and reflects the enormous impact of the traumatic stress on the young child's autonomic functions and regulation of basic states such startle responses, increased heart rate, heavy breathing, shaking, or sweating. Other children become sick and needy. The child may also find it difficult to focus and may be so on guard, anxious, or avoidant that they are unable to participate in and enjoy typical routines or social activities.

New fears not present before the trauma may also emerge as the child becomes more worried about other things and displaces fears of recurrence of the traumatic event. These fears may be accompanied by nightmares. Other children ask continuous questions about the event, repeating questions they already know the answer to. Children who play symbolically may reenact the trauma in their play over and over again, unable to change the story.

Whenever a known single event or series of discrete events are associated with an immediate or delayed disruption in the child's age-expected range of emotional and social or related language and cognitive capacities, a traumatic stress disorder becomes a likelihood. The child's reactions may be tempered by the parent's ability to help the child feel safe again as quickly as possible, but reactions may surface later on as well. Ongoing mastery of the functional emotional developmental capacities may be disrupted in relationship to the traumatic event. For example, regarding shared attention and regulation, the child's difficulties with concentration and/or overvigilance may make it challenging for him to attend and engage because of the insecurity following the trauma. Engagement may be disrupted as the child may either feel distrustful or angry for the failure to protect him or becomes more clingy, frightened, or sad. The child may also become less communicative and helpless, unable to sustain the longer back-and-forth problem-solving interactions he had before. If he is able to play symbolically, the child may reenact some form of the trauma as the victim or the perpetrator, or he may become avoidant and constricted, unable to use symbolic play or language to deal with his feelings. Reality testing can get derailed as the child resorts to denial, confuses what is real or not real, or regresses to magical thinking.

Developmental Pathway

The child's basic regulatory and developmental patterns often interact with the stress. Infants and toddlers who are underresponsive to touch and sound—who are also sensory seeking or craving sensation and are physically very active—often become aggressive and/or antisocial following the trauma, especially if they also suddenly lose the caregiver's protective security provided through engagement, empathy, coregulated emotional signaling, and limit setting. Children who are underresponsive but not sensory-seeking may shut down further and appear more lethargic or depressed and difficult to arouse.

Children who are overresponsive to sensations such as touch and sound may easily become hypervigilant or overloaded. The sensory overresponsive child is also likely to describe fear, panic, and being overwhelmed. Even a sudden, unexpected touch from another child can easily be misperceived as threatening or aggressive. He may then push or hit when others become too intrusive or overwhelming. Caregiver–child interaction patterns that are soothing and regulating foster initiative and social responsiveness, and the elaboration of emotions and ideas in play and words often help children deal with stress. Where these patterns are compromised, stress can be more difficult.

Adjustment Disorders

Infants and young children, like older children and adults, will evidence temporary challenges in response to expectable situations that they have difficulty adapting or adjusting to. Experiences such as a change of caregiver, starting school, conflicts with peers, temporary illness of a parent, birth of a sibling, parents' separation and divorce, or moving from one house to another may trigger an adjustment reaction. What is unique, however, about the infant's or young child's adjustment reaction are the types of behaviors and interactions that vary from their prior adaptation.

Presenting Pattern

In addition to easy-to-observe temporary shifts in sleeping, eating, minor regressions in language and behavior, mood shifts, poor frustration tolerance, increased anxiety or fears, oppositional behaviors, or impulse control patterns, one must also look for subtle changes in the child's ongoing mastery of each of the functional emotional developmental capacities. Does the child who was fully engaged withdraw even a little? Does the child begin to object to going to preschool or leaving the house? Does symbolic play get restricted to earthquakes or battles?

Developmental Pathway

Adjustment reactions can have a number of different developmental pathways related to the child's unique processing profile and prior adaptation. A temporary disruption can relate to the most recently mastered developmental task, such as separation or toilet training. A child–caregiver interaction pattern characterized by a caregiver overresponding to a child's expectable feelings can be associated with a tendency to become fearful with a temporary challenge. A regression can occur in the area where the child struggled in the past, such as falling asleep related to overresponsiveness to sound or difficulties self-calming. The underresponsive child might withdraw or become more self-absorbed. Symptoms can also relate to the processing system that is less developed; for example, not listening or following directions (weaker auditory processing) or losing and not finding favorite toys (weaker visuospatial processing). It is often possible to understand the family dynamic or sensory-based reasons for the adjustment reaction by examining the child's earlier adaptations and profile.

Gender Identity Disorder

In infants and young children, gender is beginning to form. One can see gender-specific behaviors throughout infancy and early childhood. These become more pronounced in the latter part of the second year and into the third and fourth years of life. Children's difficulties with their own biological gender are most frequently identified when a preschooler insists on dressing up as the opposite gender, not simply as part of playful exploration and experimentation but as a persistent pattern. In play, there may be a strong preference for opposite-gender roles, dolls, and so on. There may also be a strong preference for opposite-gender playmates, as well as for activities associated with the opposite gender. Verbal preschool children may express a clear dislike for their own anatomy and a wish to change their genitals. This reaction can be particularly strong and associated with a great deal of anxiety as the preschool child becomes more aware of the anatomical differences between boys and girls. The patterns of preference for the opposite gender and dislike of or anger at one's own gender can begin in early childhood. If not addressed, these patterns can persist and intensify as the child develops. They can emerge at older ages as well.

Often, there may be unique constitutional-maturational variations as well as caregiver–child interactions and family patterns contributing to a child's gender identity difficulties, for example, parental conflicts or a parent's wish for a child of the opposite sex. Underlying concerns with separation from the primary caregiver, conflicts over aggression and assertiveness, conflicts identifying with the same-gendered parent, or the absence of a positive relationship may contribute to the child's difficulties (Coates et al. 1991).

Developmental Pathway

These children tend to be more overresponsive to sound, light, and touch, as well as more challenged by difficulties with sensory modulation, motor planning and sequencing, and visuospatial processing. This combination, coupled with caregiver conflicts and the developmental tasks at hand, may undermine the security and physical and emotional competence of the child who then seeks change of gender. Because gender conflicts also emerge at the time the child is expected to expand emotional range and become more able to experience increasingly negative emotions such as anger, jealousy, retaliation, and fears of aggression, the child may seek to avoid or flee from his or her own gender, which may mask the anxieties related to these feelings.

Elective Mutism

Elective mutism refers to a continuing difficulty in talking in social situations, coupled with an ability to comprehend language and to speak in other settings, such as at home. This pattern is reported to be found in less than 1% of children, but it is nonetheless challenging for parents, educators, and the child.

Presenting Pattern

Children with elective mutism tend to be anxious and are often very reactive to new environments or changes in environments, especially ones with lots of people, noise, and so forth, where sounds and movements can be surprising and unpredictable. The inability to speak is often associated with a subjective state of overwhelming fear and vigilance. Often the child attempts to retreat in a selective manner. In play or conversation with a child with elective mutism, one often observes content related to fear, worry, and danger. One may also see patterns of avoidance (e.g., in seemingly safe nonemotional scenes, such as tea parties). Relationships are often characterized by an anxious dependent pattern with a reluctance to take initiative and be assertive. Although the child appears most anxious and becomes selectively mute and overvigilant in selected settings, constrictions of the functional emotional developmental capacities are evident even where the child is comfortable speaking. Unresolved developmental anxieties related to fears of body damage, aggression, and other negative emotions are evident with constricted capacities to symbolize and express feelings safely in play or conversation. Although related to anxiety disorders, the highly specific symptom of elective mutism warrants a separate disorder.

Developmental Pathway

The somatic state is one of tension and anxiety and, as indicated earlier, overreactivity to sensation. The child with elective mutism is also described in the section on regulatory-sensory processing disorders. Often, early infant–caregiver interaction patterns do not optimally support the child's initiative and self-regulation. Overanxious caregiver response patterns, dysregulating ones, or those that undermine initiative may be seen.

Sleep, Eating, and Elimination Disorders

Difficulties with sleeping or eating, and in older children, difficulties with toilet training and comfortable patterns of elimination, are very common in infancy and early childhood. In some cases, they initially appear to be the only challenge the child experiences. Often, these difficulties arise in response to various interactive challenges, including trauma; anxiety; and adjustment reactions to transitions, illness, and psychosocial stress. The expression of the symptoms is often determined by the underlying sensory-motor vulnerability in combination with the developmental anxiety and/or interactive patterns. Difficulties with sleeping, eating, toilet training, and elimination can also be related to regulatory-sensory processing disorders.

The contributing factors may lie in infant–caregiver interactions or constitutional-maturational variations. The child's developmental profile always reflects the relative contributions of constitutional-maturational variations, child–caregiver interactions, and family and environmental factors.

Sleep Disorders

Establishing sleep-wake cycles is one of the first tasks of infancy, and most children establish sleep-wake routines within the first few months or year of life. Many factors may contribute to challenges. Disruptions in sleep patterns can naturally occur with illness, changes in location, transitions in development, and other stress, but these patterns usually get re-established with the resumption of security and soothing relationships. In some cases, healthy sleep routines were not established early on, with inconsistent times or settings for sleep or when infants do not learn to fall asleep on their own and are accustomed to being held, fed, or lain in physical proximity to the parent. Some infants rely on nursing or sucking a bottle to initiate sleep. Parents do not always learn other techniques for helping the child to become calm and fall asleep independently. Other infants do not change their patterns even after maturation appears to have resolved fussy and irritable periods during infancy, and sleep rhythms still do not get established. In still other cases, the environment is too chaotic to sustain routines and security, and disorganized sleep patterns result.

Another factor to consider pertains to the family culture. Complaints of a sleep disorder can be subject to the perceptions and feelings of caregivers who may have varying tolerance for irregular or disrupted sleep patterns or have similar patterns themselves. In other cases, parents come from cultures where sleeping with a child is acceptable or desired, and all children share this experience. What presents as a sleep disturbance for one parent, therefore, may not be for another.

Because sleep disorders are such a common pathway for conveying distress, they can signify any of the primary interactive disorders described earlier, or they can be rooted in constitutionally based regulatory-sensory processing disorders associated with other regulatory challenges described below.

Presenting Pattern

Infants and young children may have difficulty settling into sleep when they first go to bed, or they wake up and cannot fall asleep again on their own. Some of these infants may even wake frequently throughout the night and are restless and sensitive sleepers. Others may be hard to arouse and sleep too much. Sleep disruption can also occur when the child awakens from a scary dream or nightmare as she becomes more symbolic and is not sure what is real or not.

It is often the interactions between caregivers and children that become the determining factor of a sleep disorder. Relationships are often characterized by neediness, negativism, and impulsivity, with different parts of this pattern dominating in different children and families. Some parents are puzzled and feel very inadequate when they hear that their child can fall asleep with others but not with them. Other parents blame each other for not being able to get the baby to sleep, and marital conflict may also fuel the maintenance of the sleep disorder.

Developmental Pathway

Infant–caregiver interactive patterns combine with underlying sensory and motor patterns, including overresponsivity and/or underresponsivity related to poor arousal as contributing factors. Particular infant–caregiver interaction patterns to look for include overresponding to the infant's cues and undermining initiative; difficulty creating rhythmic, soothing interactions; insufficient interactive opportunities during the waking hours; and intrusive, frightening interactions.

Eating Disorders

Eating disorders, like sleep disorders, can be symptomatic of many of the interactive disorders as well as of a regulatory disorder with sensory hypersensitivities and oral motor difficulties (described below in the "Developmental Pathway" section). When related to an interactive pattern, eating disorders may reflect the residual anxiety of unresolved biological problems, such as gastrointestinal difficulties, reflux, or other illnesses with resulting anxiety and lack of pleasure around eating.

It is often the interactions between caregivers and children that become the determining factor of an eating disorder. For example, eating can become an overly relied-on source of comfort and self-soothing in the absence of appropriate nurturance. Refusal can become an expression of fear, anger, or rejection in the absence of symbolic expression.

Presenting Pattern

The eating disorder may involve poor or irregular intake, food refusal, vomiting, and restricted or insatiable eating. Because eating is so essential for survival, it is not a challenge that can be overlooked for long. Because the health and weight of the baby is often seen as a reflection of "good" parenting, the eating disorder can become an enormous source of worry, stress, and inadequacy to the caregiver. The interaction between the child and caregiver can result in vacillations between neediness, negativism, and anxiety, with different patterns dominating in different children and families. Even simple feeding challenges can undermine the confidence of the infant and caregiver when coincidental with family disruptions, transitions, or difficult resuming or establishing more organized eating patterns. In other cases, the absence of routine and timely family eating patterns or eating disorders in the caregivers themselves can derail the development of healthy eating patterns.

Developmental Pathway

Two pathways are involved. The infant's underlying sensory-motor vulnerability can include both hypersensitivities to food textures, tastes, and smells and under-reactivity to tastes and smells that reduce the awareness and enjoyment of eating. In addition, infants may have reduced muscle tone and oral motor difficulties that make feeding or eating challenging (e.g., difficulties getting food off the spoon, moving food to be chewed and swallowed, lip closure). An eating disorder can develop when these sensory-motor vulnerabilities combine with infant–caregiver interactive patterns related to conflict, anxiety, and fear.

Elimination Disorders

Elimination disorders include functional encopresis and enuresis. In a primary elimination disorder, expected urinary or bowel control has not been reached beyond the variations of developmental expectations. In a secondary elimination disorder, this control has been reached but is subsequently lost. In both types of elimination disorders, as well as in children who withhold their stool or urine, the child often experiences a range of affective states. Fear, shame, and embarrassment over the "accident" are readily observed. However, at a deeper subjective level, the child often feels unsure about his or her body. There is a pervasive sense of insecurity about bodily functioning with significant anxiety over "not being in control" of unexpected urges. Some children defend against the bodily signals to eliminate and may hide or deny their bodily needs. These children may compensate by trying to "control" everyone else. They may experience the demands of their body as coming too unpredictably and then become anxious. Some children are not sufficiently aware that they need to go until it is "too late;" or they have poor sensory registration of their bodies' signals coupled with reduced muscle tone, leaving them confused and embarrassed.

For others, mastery of toileting implies overly high expectations to be a "big boy!" Or, persistent wishes to still be the "baby." These conflicts may be the child's or the parent's, and usually become intertwined as caregiver and child struggle with fears of loss and separation, changes in alliances, (e.g., babies belong to mom but big boys go to daddy!), fears of incompetence, or other conflicts.

The child's mental content in play and conversation tends to mirror the affective patterns described above. Play themes are often characterized by avoidance of strong affect, explosive bursts of affective content, and vacillations between the two. The child often verbalizes a wish to "do better" and please his caregivers, coupled with negativism and intermittent impulsivity. In the content of the child's play, one sees shame, embarrassment, avoidance, impulsivity, and fragmentation. An examination of functional developmental capacities can help identify the constrictions contributing to these problems and the specific dynamic formulation that may be relevant.

Developmental Pathway

Underlying sensory-motor vulnerabilities combined with interactive challenges contribute to elimination difficulties. For example, the child may have low muscle tone and poor motor planning, as well as sensory underresponsivity. This combination makes it difficult to sense and then execute motor control over basic bodily functions. Others may be too sensitive to or fearful of the flushing. Some limit their toileting to a specific bathroom in their home or cannot orient themselves visually and spatially in unfamiliar settings. But somatic states also tend to express the particular types of affects and physical challenges that the child is evidencing (e.g., discomfort). For some children, withholding can become a way to express anger or retaliation in the absence of a more symbolic use of words or play to communicate their feelings. Relationships are often characterized by vacillations between neediness, negativism, and impulsivity, with different parts of this pattern dominating in different children and families.

Therapeutic Implications

It is important to help the child deal with his sense of uncertainty and insecurity so that he can arrive at a realistic picture of how the body functions. It is also important to help the child work through fears of anger or assertiveness, as well as help the caregiver and family (as a whole) provide an emotional climate that supports both security and initiative. Often, caregiver–child interaction patterns are compromised in terms of fostering assertiveness and initiative in a secure and regulated manner, at both the level of affective gestures and symbols. Sensory and motor processing can be supported to facilitate the child's sense of competence in his body through related and other sensory-motor and visuospatial activities. It is important to help parents manage their feelings regarding these basic body functions, to define what these functions mean to the parents and how they feel, and to find what allows the parents to implement an effective approach to support the child. The more supportive and empathetic the family and the better it can help the child embark on a constructive intervention approach, the more likely that the family relationship patterns will be characterized by comfort, security, and shared pleasure.

Principles of Intervention

This first step in the therapeutic process involves a detailed understanding of the presenting problems in the context of the developmental, individual-differences, relationship-based (DIR) model. In cases in which a thorough DIR assessment of a child and family reveals that the child's presenting symptoms and developmental lags stem primarily from some difficulty in interaction patterns, the evaluating clinician must consider the interaction patterns characteristic of each of the six developmental levels and determine which patterns have been negotiated successfully and which are absent or constricted.

For example, consider a withdrawn 4-year-old who never formed relationships well. As a baby, she tended to disengage, particularly when confronted with anger or other intense feelings; her parents never knew quite how to woo her back. Under the pressure of competition from other children, she becomes angry and withdraws. Another 4-year-old, in contrast, engaged well from infancy, learned two-way gestural communication, and learned to symbolize his emotions; however, he has difficulty clearly distinguishing between aggressive feelings and warm, loving feelings. Whenever he feels aggressive, he becomes frightened and anticipates that others will reject him; he copes with these feelings by becoming aloof and withdrawn. The behavior or "presenting problems" of these two children may appear identical, but the underlying interactive disorders that give rise to their difficulties are very different.

The first child will display an aloof, cautious manner upon entering the evaluating clinician's playroom. She may not warm up at all or may warm up only very slowly. Whenever the situation does not feel quite right to her, or the play or conversation suggests any emotion, she will withdraw anew. The clinician will have the strong impression that this child never mastered the very early developmental task of engagement and intimacy. Once treatment begins, this understanding will guide the therapist not to wait passively for the child to begin talking about her feelings; hanging back would simply replay the child's early experiences of disengagement. Instead, the therapist will try to empathize with the child's uncertainty about how to be close and will try to explore associated fears.

When the second child comes into the playroom, he will likely be warm and engaged, use interactive gestures, and play out themes such as aggression and love, showing that he can represent emotional experience. However, the clinician will begin to see that he confuses aggressive and loving themes in his play and that as these themes become increasingly merged and chaotic, the child cuts his play off at a critical point. This child clearly negotiated the interaction patterns of early development well but had difficulty negotiating complex symbolized feelings in the context of an ongoing relationship. The therapist will need to discover what it is about the child's key relationships that prevented him from learning that aggressive and loving feelings can be part of the same relationship.

As discussed earlier, many symptoms can arise from disorders of interaction. Regardless of the symptom, the goal of treatment will be not only to alleviate it but also to facilitate the child's progress toward an age-appropriate developmental level and toward an age-appropriate degree of stability and range of thematic experience at that level. The six-step intervention process described in Chapter 4 ("Therapeutic Principles"), beginning with the establishment of regular Floortime between parents and child to build a consistent, warm relationship and two-way communication, can be used to great effect to help families heal disorders of interaction. Because we have already described this process in detail, we focus now on specific challenges that can confound families (and therapists) if they are not addressed.

Recall that once Floortime is well established, a problem-solving approach is added to help the child learn or strengthen cause-and-effect thinking and anticipate situations, feelings, and alternative behaviors. This challenges the parents to anticipate their child's functioning in problematic situations and to help their child learn to anticipate as well. When the parents feel overwhelmed by a particular symptom, however, their ability to anticipate calmly and to think in an organized way about their child's functioning can become severely compromised. For example, a child who experiences a great deal of separation anxiety may become so demanding that his parents, feeling beleaguered and desperate, may begin thinking too concretely, focusing only on the here and now. Their goal becomes "to keep him quiet and settled so we can have a moment to ourselves." If he is having a difficult time separating in the mornings to go to preschool, the parents fear to bring up the subject at other times during the day, "because then he'll think about it and get upset."

Parents who take this approach cannot help their child anticipate and plan. Instead, they must shift to a problem-solving mode. In the comfort of his own house, in the warm security of an intimate exchange with his mother or father, the child may indeed be able to picture how he will feel at school the next day and how he will likely behave when he gets that feeling. Simple prediction—without the expectation of change—is the first achievement. Once the child can clearly predict his likely feelings and responses, he and his parents may be able to design a strategy to ease his anxiety. Perhaps they can plan for mother or father to be at school with him the whole time the first day, the whole time minus a half hour the second day, minus an hour the third day, and so on. Even if these negotiations do not hold up under the pressure of the next day, the ability to anticipate the feelings and likely behaviors associated with the difficult situation, together with some available alternative behaviors, can only prove helpful. In order to make the required shift in approach, however, parents who have become overwhelmed and concrete must first be helped to identify and verbalize the feelings that have left them so paralyzed. A therapist working with the family needs to help the parents verbalize and explore their anger, resentment, and fear that their child "will never grow up, and will always be a burden on us."

The third step, empathizing with the child's perspective, also presents a serious challenge in situations in which interaction patterns underlie the child's symptoms. When a child is exhibiting serious fears, anxieties, or behavior control problems, it is almost tautological that whatever the natural history of the problem has been, once it becomes a dominant force in the family's life, the ability to take the child's perspective is absent. Parents who cannot empathize with their child cannot help her see what goals and basic assumptions are motivating her actions and reactions.

In situations such as these, it usually turns out that one or more of the child's emotional themes—dependency longings, anger, vulnerability, curiosity, sexual excitement—are not being engaged by certain family members. As we have discussed, a theme can be ignored at the level of engagement, two-way gestural communication, representational or symbolic elaboration, or representational differentiation. If a theme is ignored at several levels or at all of them, its contribution to a particular symptom will play an important role in the maintenance of that symptom and in the potential correction of it.

For example, an intense, energetic 3-year-old boy clearly enjoyed competition. His parents, however, denied and avoided aggressive, competitive themes and felt strongly that sharing and cooperation were the most important values in life. Whenever the child wanted to compete with his father at the behavioral level, by horsing around and jumping on his father's stomach or wrestling, his father would quickly discourage this "aggressive" behavior and try to engage his son is a more structured activity. When the boy came home from preschool and told his mother that another child had been mean to him, his mother could not tolerate hearing about his anger or his desire to hit the other child back. As a result, she could not empathize with his feelings or allow the opening and closing of "circles of communication" about his school experience. Before he could get many words out, she would interrupt with advice and wishful thinking: "Just ignore him…maybe he is really nice." Both parents would habitually withdraw from their son whenever he seemed angry with them. This family was clearly unable to effectively address the themes of anger and competitiveness at the levels of engagement, two-way behavioral interaction, the symbolization of feelings, and the differentiation and connection of feelings. However, the parents were able to engage their son at these levels in situations involving feelings of dependency or curiosity. They had no trouble understanding how much he loved his mother or father, exchanging hugs and kisses, or listening to their son describe how much he missed them when they were away at work.

The parents brought their son for an evaluation because he had frequent nightmares filled with monsters that were burning down his house. He felt very worried about his parents being hurt. When the clinician first saw the child, heard his history from his parents, and observed their interaction, he sensed that the child was quite angry with his parents. It was not surprising that he was constantly having his house burned down in his dreams. Later on, after treatment had progressed, the child was able to verbalize how frustrated and angry he was, especially about having situations that he found difficult at school not only ignored by his parents but reinterpreted to him all the time. Once the clinician was able to help the parents engage, interact, and symbolize with their child the competitive and aggressive aspects of life, the boy's symptoms receded. A critical step in enabling the parents to empathize with their son was exploring with them why they found these themes so frightening. Themes that a parent has difficulty tolerating generally hold some specific, often distorted meaning for the parent related to his or her own history. For example, in the clinician's work with this boy's parents, it emerged that the father had had a hyperactive sibling. His son's horseplay and other physical expressions of competitiveness triggered the father's fear that, if allowed to engage in such activities, his son would become "too aggressive" as his brother had been. The father was helped to verbalize his feelings about his brother and to separate these feelings from the reality of his son's need to engage in normal, healthy competitive activities.

In this case, the parents needed to tolerate certain feelings and themes and to engage their child in these areas. Sometimes, however, it is the child who has greater difficulty with a feeling or theme. Step 4 in the intervention process, breaking a challenge down into small steps, can be used to help such a child to gradually approach feelings that have been warded off and to organize these feelings at an age-appropriate level. For example, a child who is fearful of her needs and longings may vacillate between excessive clinging and aggression. In addition to helping her control her behavior (a project that also needs to be broken down into small steps), parents and therapist can help her play out and verbalize her feelings, especially those of frustration when her needs are not met. This process cannot occur all at once. It may begin with a reference to a doll or even a pet fish or hamster. Perhaps the child will have the doll or pet play out these feelings as well. Ten steps later, she may talk about the frustration felt by some other child; by the twentieth step, she may be able to talk about such feelings in relation to herself.

In interactive disorders, as well as in other developmental difficulties, conflicts can be very important. Behind most anxieties, fears, or behavior-control problems lies a conflict between the greedy, tyrannical, or aggressive side of the child and the fearful or worried side. Children will always do better with their fears if they feel secure that their greedy or aggressive side cannot get out of control. They need to know that they can rely on their parents to assist them by maintaining some structure. This is where step 5, limit setting, becomes critical. The structure should be neither overly punitive nor overly permissive, and it should be created in collaboration with the child, particularly the child who is verbal.

To illustrate why limits are important in interactive, family-based problems, consider the child who is excessively fearful about playing with other children and joining in activities at school. Such a child may also have nightmares. He wants to stay with his mother all the time, refuses to go to preschool, and refuses to let his father carry him. He insists that he should be able to push and hit his baby sister because "she scares me when she takes my toys." This is the child some clinicians refer to as "the fearful tyrant." The mother feels anxiously overprotective, and she is afraid that if she is punitive, her son will only get more fearful: "How can I punish him for pushing his sister, when he's already so scared? He'll only have more nightmares." In such a situation, it is critical to establish some structure by setting limits in a few areas at once: first, on hitting and pushing his sister; second, on his avoidance of challenging activities like going to preschool, interacting with his father, and letting his father carry him; and third, on his demands that his mother be at his beck and call. If the first four steps in the intervention process—engagement through Floortime, problem-solving discussions, empathizing with the child's point of view, and setting up small steps in areas that the child finds challenging—are instituted effectively, one can introduce additional structure, bolstered by incentives and sanctions, to motivate the child to move from one step to another in tackling each challenge. For example, this child should face a sanction every time he hits or pushes his sister. The argument that punishment scares him will not hold up, because the parents will feel secure that their Floortime and availability to the child are supportive and reassuring enough to help him cope with the sanctions. Furthermore, by consistently following through on sanctions, the parents will communicate to their son that they will prevent his aggression from getting out of control; this will decrease, not increase, the child's fear. In problem-solving discussions, the parents will help him anticipate difficult feelings and consider alternative ways of coping with each situation; the parents can thus assure themselves that their child usually has fair warning of challenges he will face.

The child should also be given incentives not to avoid school altogether. At first, he may need to attend part time and have his mother with him. Each step needs to be negotiated with firmness. In addition, the child should spend part of each day with his father, whether he wants to or not. The father should use Floortime strategies to try to make the experience fun, but he should not demand that his son demonstrate pleasure. Nor should he take an overly concrete approach by leaving the room every time his son says, "Get out of here, Daddy!" Instead, he needs to keep the interaction going, as described in earlier chapters. A flirtatious, and at times playfully provocative, parent can succeed in wooing the child into a relationship. Meanwhile, the mother should become slower to acquiesce in every one of the child's demands. As structure is established in all these areas, the child will feel more confident that the greedy, tyrannical side of his nature cannot get out of control. At the same time, through Floortime and problem-solving time, he has the chance to explore and verbalize the other side, his feelings of fear and worry.

As described in Chapter 4 ("Therapeutic Principles"), every time structure and limits must be intensified, it is crucial to increase Floortime proportionally.

The goal is to foster a balance of structure and limits with support for higher-level, more elaborative communication.

In this chapter, we have highlighted issues involved in treating children whose symptoms and developmental lags stem primarily from disturbances in the interaction among family members. (The case studies of Danny and Molly in Chapter 5, "Parent-Oriented Developmental Therapy," provide further examples of the treatment of interactive difficulties. Recall that Danny's parents needed to learn to relate to him in a warmer, more engaged manner, whereas Molly's mother needed to recognize that her daughter felt inadequate at times and to tolerate her daughter's expressions of insecurity without fleeing or punishing her.) As discussed in the next two chapters, however, even in situations where a child has a primary regulatory disturbance or a disturbance of relating and communicating, family interaction patterns can exacerbate the child's difficulties, and helping family members interact in new ways can help the child achieve her potential. All parents have their own histories and conflicts, and these will influence how they perceive and relate to their children.

Case Illustrations

Sammy

The parents of 19-month-old Sammy brought him to me (S.G.) because he was "hitting and biting mother and being defiant." Apparently, he did this less with father and the babysitter, and mother was worried that Sammy was "mad" at her. In addition, he was waking up once or twice at night, and only sleeping for 7 or 8 hours.

Although ambivalent about having children, as soon as Sammy was born, mother "fell in love with him." Her feelings for him were so strong that she was "always worried about undermining his confidence or denying him anything emotionally."

The pregnancy and delivery were unremarkable, and Sammy was born a healthy 8 pounds, 6 ounces. As an infant, he was alert and able to look and listen and calm himself easily. His motor development was on schedule; he was sitting up by 5 months, crawling by 7 months, and walking by 11 months. He had good fine motor skills and could pick up Cheerios by 8 months and hold a pencil and make scribbles by 15 months. His language development was also on schedule, with lots of vocalizations toward the end of his first year and a few words by the beginning of his second year.

Mother described Sammy as warm and happy. He had smiled by 4 months and interacted with her intentionally by 7 or 8 months, using gestures and playing peek-a-boo–type games. As a toddler, he had started some more complex interactions, mother thought, but had obviously not developed fully in this area. Mother also admitted that there were "lots of problems" in her marriage and that she and her husband stayed together out of "inertia."

I watched mother and son interact. Sammy was very exploratory, looking in every corner and closet of the room. He had good attention and focus but not much follow-through as he examined each item, such as the telephone. He spent 10 or 15 seconds on one object, then went on to the next. However, he was very engaged with mother; circles were opened and closed with gestures and even with vocalizations. For example, when exploring the telephone, he said "phone," and gestured to mother as if he wanted to dial it. "He wants a real phone, to make a real call," mother said to me. She shook her head, no-no, and he nodded, yes-yes at her, and pointed again to the phone, while babbling. Not only were they engaged with and focused on each other, but they could exchange information two ways, with each one building on the other. Then there was a small battle over the phone: mother gestured for Sammy to stop playing with the buttons and he refused. Mother's tentativeness was obvious; her voice did not increase in degrees of assertiveness, nor did her facial or motor gestures emphasize a desire for him to stop. Instead, she got whiny and helpless, with a very anxious, tentative voice. Feeling like he could do what he wanted, Sammy did not stop until mother physically restrained him. He clearly was not getting the range of gestural feedback he needed for his exploratory nature.

Although Sammy seemed to have shared attention, engagement, and the exchange of simple gestures as part of two-way communication, he did not sustain complex gestures with mother. He closed a few circles in a row, but not 10 to 30 circles in sequence as part of a complex, preverbal drama. Although his affect was pleasant and warm, it did not show the range that his brightness indicated he might be capable of. He looked serious, pleased, and annoyed but did not show deep joy or anger.

Playing with me, Sammy roamed around the room (as he had done at first with mother), but closed fewer gestural circles. He moved away while making eye contact with me and babbled when I asked him what he was doing or looking at. He preferred to play by himself than play with me, but he used me for help; for example, he pointed at me when he could not reach inside the doll house to get a car, so I reached in and got it out for him. He nodded, and enjoyed playing with the car, but did not get involved with me again.

He played with mother again, and I watched to see if he could elaborate a more complex dialogue by opening and closing circles. Unfortunately, mother got impatient and overcontrolling with him instead of waiting for him to build on her responses. When she asked something like "What next?" or made an equivalent gesture and he did not respond immediately, mother would move in with several more issues. She did not give him time to build on her initial prompting.

In our second meeting, mother and Sammy were again very engaged and connected. Their vocalizations and facial and motor gestures indicated shared attention and a sense of relatedness. There seemed to be increased depth to their sense of pleasure and engagement and a greater range of affect. Their evident progress was in part related to my suggestion, after the first session, that mother begin Floortime with Sammy.

They had some dialogue about whether Sammy wanted to draw with a pencil. Through head nods, vocalizations, and pointing, with many circles closed in a row, they negotiated which pencil he would use and how he would hold it, and he showed a nice grasp of the pencil. He also took the initiative and related to me more this time, exchanging and throwing a ball with me. Then he said, "Mom" and the word "ball," indicating that he wanted to throw the ball to her. Gesturing pleasurably, he threw the ball to her and she threw it back. He smiled and said "ball" again, pointing to mother and throwing the ball back to her. I waved to him to throw it to me, and he looked at me and made a "no" gesture. He said

"Mom" again, throwing it to her. I asked if he would hand me the pencil, and he said "no" again and handed it to mother.

After a short break, I encouraged them to try some pretend play. Mother took a puppet and made it bite Sammy's leg. He turned away, and mother said, "See, he doesn't like me to play with him in this way." She seemed unaware that her main theme was somewhat intrusive and aggressive. Later on, after they had done some drawing together, Sammy threw her the ball, smiling nicely and saying "ball" again. Mother looked at me and said, "He just threw me the ball to get me out of his hair." I responded, "Maybe that's the game he wants to play—'Get out of my hair.'" Mother replied, "Great. 'Get out of my hair.' So I'll leave him alone." I said, "Sometimes, even 'Get out of my hair' and rejection can be part of a playful interaction, not to be taken literally." She asked, "When should I take him literally?" I pointed out that this was a key question for her, and she said that she had a hard time knowing the difference between when Sammy was doing something in play and when he felt strongly about it. Consequently, she did not know when she should take his behavior literally or with a grain of salt.

We had discovered an important dynamic: mother was taking her 20-month-old son literally and having her feelings hurt, because the question of "literalness" was often around rejection or separation or mother not feeling worthwhile. At the beginning of the session, mother had admitted, "I almost didn't come back this session. I felt very self-conscious about your watching my play. I felt so unnatural. I am a good play partner." Her fear that I would think otherwise seemed related to the issue of "literalness."

In the third session, father came in for the first time and said, "I want Sammy to be assertive and experiment with taking risks. I'm afraid if we curb his aggression too much, we will inhibit him." However, father was concerned that Sammy had bitten and gouged people in the face. "I think what he does is abnormal," he admitted. "He even bashes his own head on the floor sometimes." Still, he did not want Sammy to be a "wimp." Mother added, "And I don't want to hit him or give him mixed signals by modeling my hitting." To which father replied, "We disagree on how to handle him."

Father described himself as compulsive, sloppy, slow, and methodical. After many years in the federal government, he now worked as a commercial real estate broker. Mother came across as chronically depressed; she seemed to feel overwhelmed and fragmented and responded to the emotions of the moment, as opposed to father, who tended to shut out any emotions.

Mother felt they had lost their communication and connection and confessed that she was thinking of "leaving the marriage." Father too felt the need for "renewal" and said that he knew what mother wanted. He complained about a lack of sexual intimacy, while she complained that he did not communicate with her. She also had no interest in his "methodical" way of thinking, and he found it hard to empathize with her emotionality. They elaborated on their backgrounds, saying that early in their marriage, they had empathized with each other more than at present. After Sammy's birth, however, they lost their appreciation for each other's style of thinking and did not know how to regain it. They spent almost no time together to rekindle their early feelings; they never went out on the weekends, and once they got Sammy to bed at night, each went his or her own way.

It became clear that their difficulty understanding each other was mirrored in their problems with understanding Sammy's behavior. Mother could not understand Sammy's motivation or how to interpret his gestures and speech. When he said, "Get away," should she take it literally, or see it as part of an interaction? Father had trouble understanding Sammy's emotions but not his basic messages. He wanted to know how to empathize with Sammy's desire to be angry sometimes while recognizing his need for limits. This was confusing to a man who liked things laid out logically.

"Why can't Sammy learn to stop behaving so aggressively?" mother asked. "Why does he feel that just because he's mad he needs to hit or bite?" I wondered aloud if Sammy's idea that a feeling leads immediately to an action was paralleled by the way mother sometimes interpreted things literally. When she asked what I meant, I pointed out that she had said that when he gestured for her to leave the room, she sometimes felt compelled to do it—in other words, to immediately respond to his intention with a behavior. This was exactly what Sammy did—take an intention and immediately put it into behavior. If mother responded physically every time he had an intention or a wish, she was confirming a literal and concrete way of relating to the world.

I elaborated—over the course of many sessions—that at this stage in life, Sammy was learning how to move from a literal, behavioral orientation to the world of emotional ideas, where he could contemplate wishes and intentions without needing to put them into behavior. If his intention could exist as a thought or wish, he could begin to delay and reason about it and consider many different behaviors, from make-believe elaboration of the wish, to inhibiting the wish, to finding a substitute way of satisfying it or even relinquishing the wish. However, if mother remained concrete, she would not help him learn to elevate a wish to the level of ideas. I went back to when they were playing together and he gestured to her to "bug off." If she could empathize with gestures and a few simple words like "Mommy away" and have a dialogue about him wanting mommy to go away, Sammy could begin to separate the word from the deed. She could acknowledge his desire, while at the same time continuing to engage him empathetically. If he continued to point at her to leave, she could empathize with how much he wanted her to leave. She could even become quiet for a few seconds, showing some respect for his wish, but remain in the room with him and engaged. She could then try to play out the drama with dolls or gesture around it and see how it would develop. In other words, Sammy pointing at her to leave would only be the first step in the drama.

In this session, we also discussed the need for mother and father to empathize with each other's way of communicating. They agreed to begin their own version of "Floortime" together—at least a half-hour together each night plus one evening a weekend. They could not even begin to work out their difficulties, which perhaps involved deep-seated emotions and conflicts, without some sense of shared attention and engagement. As they tried to understand each other, we could look at the hurdles they ran into.

We also talked about a half-hour of Floortime each evening with Sammy, focused on opening and closing circles and encouraging his gestural and preideational patterns to be as elaborate as possible. He tended to be a little bit fragmented and could use help in stringing together circles into a more elaborate drama, whether it was just a gestural drama around drawing or a presymbolic drama with cars moving, or perhaps even some early representational or symbolic play. I emphasized the need for father to spend Floortime with Sammy, because it was clear that Sammy and mother had a very intimate relationship but that it was being acted out with power struggles and anger.

We also talked about how to create and define limits. First was using lots of gestural interchanges around limits, with mother varying her voice pitch and facial gestures before using physical restraint and then using varying degrees of physical restraint. I suggested that father do the same thing. Sammy was not getting much emotional or gestural preverbal feedback to his challenging behavior, because mother was anxious and afraid of somehow depriving him (in part as a reaction to her original wish not to have him). Meanwhile, father's affect was isolated and he did not want Sammy to be a wimp. They were both too ambivalent about setting limits for him. The second component was a limit-setting approach that would not let Sammy's behavior get to the point where they blew up at him in frustration but would move in gradually and very firmly. Clearly, Sammy perceived mother's tentativeness and felt that he was in charge with her; mother would have to become firmer, and father would have to become firmer and much more involved.

I also suggested elimination diets to see if these would facilitate better behavioral control and a better sleeping pattern for Sammy. The different food groups to be tested included dairy products, additives such as preservatives and dyes, sugars, caffeine and chocolate, peanuts and nuts, salicylate-containing fruit, and wheat products. Each food would be eliminated for 10 days, and then reintroduced for 2 or 3 days to see if Sammy's behavior or symptoms were affected.

Finally, we discussed a bedtime ritual that would give Sammy a lot of cuddling time with mother and father as well as the opportunity to play quietly in bed. During this time they could facilitate closing circles, gestural interaction, and perhaps some early symbolic play. Once this pattern was in place, they would gradually encourage Sammy to put himself back to sleep in the evenings: letting him cry for increasing periods of time, looking in to make sure he was safe, and weaning him from their going in to him in the middle of the night.

The parents became aware of their issues around concreteness, both with Sammy and with each other. Mother took Sammy literally, not realizing that he needed to be understood in terms of his wishes without those wishes necessarily being granted or translated into behavior. Sammy was learning that wishes and behavior were the same, which inhibited his moving from the behavioral and gestural level to the ideational and representational level. Meanwhile, father needed to address his own sense of confusion—which he dealt with through avoidance and isolation of affect—and realize that Sammy needed to be assertive but also to have limits.

Over the next three sessions, we expanded these themes in terms of family patterns. More complex gestures and early symbolic play started to emerge in Sammy's Floortime at home and in the office. Father became more involved, and Sammy played out aggressive themes, such as car crashing, with him. With mother, Sammy still chose themes of "leave me alone"; often, while drawing, he would turn his back to her, then flirt with her and bring her in, and then mildly reject her. Mother recognized his desire to be left alone. "He doesn't want me," she said. Yet when she stayed in there, empathizing with words like "Mommy away," and then looked sad for a second, Sammy giggled and would pull her back in, often with a gesture such as touching her nose or handing her a crayon to draw with him.

Mother and father experimented with a gradual approach to limits, being firmer but also giving lots of gestural interaction when Sammy was about to throw a tantrum or bite or kick someone. They could recognize the expression on his face that usually preceded this behavior, and whenever he had that look in his eye—the beginning of a pattern in which he would usually touch another child on the head and then start to pinch—they would raise their voices, point their finger at him, and say "no-no." Then they would motion for him to come to them (he resisted doing this at first, but after being physically restrained several times, he began responding to their gestures), and they would say, "Sammy—hit yes or hit no?" Sammy would giggle and say, "No hit." This pattern resulted in Sammy gradually hitting, biting, and poking less and less frequently.

The elimination diet showed that Sammy had a slight sensitivity to salicylate-containing fruits as well as caffeine and chocolate. He was also mildly sensitive to eating a lot of dairy products in one day. With dietary refinements, plus the new play and interaction patterns, he began sleeping through the night. His concentration was also slightly improved, although this was fairly good to begin with.

The work with this family continued in short-term treatment for about eight sessions (with one session every 4–8 weeks) to consolidate the gains they had made. Although Sammy's behavior continued to improve, the parents' marital relationship moved much more slowly. They began spending a little more time together, and mother showed a more pleasant affect in father's presence, but how well they could work things out remained to be seen. Most importantly, however, Sammy made nice progress and emerged as a confident, outgoing, warm, and—most of the time—respectful child.

In this case, we observed an approach to working with a child who was having difficulty learning to regulate his impulses and control his behavior. The capacity to learn impulse control and regulation ordinarily occurs between 16 and 24 months of age, and having an opportunity to work with a child as this important capacity is forming is a unique opportunity to favorably influence development. Such a case is a dramatic illustration of the importance of infant and early childhood mental health. It is clearly much more difficult to help a child master patterns of aggressive behavior once they become more firmly established.

In working with Sammy, we saw the relative contributions to his challenging pattern. As indicated, a critical element was the caregiver–toddler interaction at the level of gestures. These interactions were not providing Sammy with the type of affective signal-reading experience that he needed in order to learn what was appropriate and what was not appropriate behavior. It is important to emphasize that children's first lessons in impulse control emerge way before words are ever used to a significant degree. Interactive emotional gestures communicated with voice tone, facial expression, and motor actions enable a child to learn how to regulate his own emotions and behaviors. Helping a family master this critical capacity, however, requires—as this case so well illustrates—work with each parent and his or her personality, the family relationship pattern, and the way in which these play out in the moment-to-moment and day-to-day interactions with the child.

In Sammy's case, exploring his sensitivities to certain food groups was also an important factor. Although the research on food sensitivities and behavior is at present not definitive (some studies suggest food sensitivity can contribute and other studies suggest it only contributes in rare instances), it is important to recognize that each child can be observed in his own right. It is particularly important to do this in areas where research is not definitive. My own clinical experience is that children have very different thresholds and that select children are very reactive to their physical environment. The best way of determining this food sensitivity is to conduct an elimination diet in a very systematic manner, as we would with a rash of unknown etiology. The family history can also be helpful. Environmental sensitivities, however, are often only one component of a complex pattern. The key is to organize a comprehensive approach.

In Sammy's case, the emphasis is on the interaction patterns between Sammy and his caregivers. As we were able to improve these and, in particular, the affective signaling dealing with regulation and limit setting as well as constructive forms of assertiveness, we were able to help Sammy make significant progress. In terms of our classification approach, Sammy's pattern comes closest to what we have described as disruptive behavior disorder. In very young children such as Sammy, however, such disruptive behavior challenges need to be thought of as dynamic processes very open to change.

Sammy and his family continue to do well with periodic reevaluations. As with all families, however, there is a tendency at times of stress to lapse into old patterns. Periodic reevaluations, even after the treatment program has been completed, is an excellent way to monitor progress and provide additional help, as needed, during a child's formative stages of development.

Jamie

When Jamie's parents brought him in to me (S.G.), mother talked about her history of depression. She was currently in psychotherapy, but she was still chronically depressed. She was worried about how to relate to her 4-month-old son, saying, "He doesn't look at me; he cries whenever I touch him or hold him." There was either "something wrong with him or something wrong with me," she said. She explained that he never looked or smiled at her and cried whenever she approached him or looked at him.

In contrast, she said, her husband related a little better; Jamie would relax and not cry with him, although there was still no pleasure or enthusiasm. There was also a nanny at home, a 21-year-old from the Midwest, with whom Jamie related better; he gave her occasional faint pleasurable looks and even a "smile or two."

I watched mother and baby interact and was struck by how stiffly she held him. She seemed anxious and worried and had almost no facial expression. She vocalized in a depressive monotone, with a few utterances such as, "Baby, baby look," followed by pauses of 3 or 4 seconds, and then another monotone utterance. She had no movement (in terms of rocking) and very little orienting of her body posture to Jamie's. Also, when she did talk to him, she spoke in a whisper as well as a monotone. Jamie looked past mother with an indifferent, flat, vague stare; there were no looks, smiles, frowns, or motor gestures. After about 10 minutes, he became irritable and began crying and twisting.

Father was more relaxed holding Jamie; he picked him up and walked around, first with the baby on his shoulder and then trying some roughhousing, like quickly moving Jamie up and down and to the sides. Yet he also talked in a relative monotone with little facial expression. Jamie looked a bit at father but had few smiles; he vacillated between looking at father and looking around the room.

As I held and played with the baby, he started off by looking around me, not at me: he glanced to the left, right, up, and down with a fairly vacant look. As I vocalized, saying his name and how cute he was, I tried to use lots of facial animation and very slow variations in pitch at rhythm and was able to elicit a little smile and then another one and another one. It took about 5 minutes to get these three little smiles and 5 seconds of focused interest.

When, as I tried to keep his attention, my facial expression became too animated or my voice pitch went up with enthusiasm or my rhythm became very fast, Jamie cried. I also noted that when I left his field of vision, putting my head to the left or right to see if he would turn, he began to cry, as though uncomfortable with the change. I tried speaking slightly louder to his parents as I held him, and he again started to whimper and cry. However, he did seem to enjoy brisk up and down movement and doing little sit-ups in my lap.

The pregnancy and delivery were unremarkable, and Jamie was born healthy at 8 pounds, 2 ounces and with 9/9 Apgar scores. He seemed to have good motor control and to be both alert and calm. He responded to sights, sounds, movement, and touch in the first few days and weeks after birth. Yet by the second month, mother noticed that he was not as responsive as he had been as a newborn to her looks or father's looks or their vocalizations. "He's learned to hate me," she said.

Mother's chronic depression began in late adolescence. In spite of this, she had been able to finish college and graduate school. Now in her late 30s, she was an accountant who worked 8–12 hours a day.

Father was also a busy accountant. He presented himself as a rigid, controlled person who liked things done in an orderly fashion on his schedule. He showed little interest in emotions and was "frustrated" that Jamie was "hard to warm up." He was angry at his wife, whom he viewed as "deficient in her mothering abilities," but was willing to talk about how to improve these abilities. Although recognizing that she worked, he wanted her to be a "better mother" and was very angry at her for "not being a good mother" and, by implication, not a good wife. He alluded to many instances in which she had disappointed him, without going into detail. He was closed about his own background, claiming it was "not terribly important."

By the end of the session, it was clear that Jamie and his family needed intensive work; at 4 months of age, he was already not fully engaging with or attending to the human world, although he could be drawn in with some work and skill. Even more worrisome was his parents' interactive pattern. Mother seemed completely unable to be flexible in trying to engage him and help him attend, and father seemed somewhat disinterested, except for his rough-and-tumble–type playing, which was effective to a limited degree. I suggested that they return in a few days with their nanny for a follow-up meeting, so I could determine how to involve her in a program that would help both the baby and the family.

At the next session, I observed the nanny interacting with Jamie. She had more warmth and relatedness than either parent and clearly had an emotional interest in the baby. She held him gently about 6–8 inches away from her face and made little facial expressions and sounds at him. Her approach was conventional—talking and making sounds. (She reported that she was the oldest of five and had used this approach when babysitting for her siblings.) She was able to catch Jamie's attention fleetingly, as I had, and he gave her a faint look and smile, but only for a second or two; there were no robust, warm smiles or focused looks lasting any period of time. She confirmed that it was hard to get him to look at her or show pleasure. She might try getting him to look at pictures in a book, but he showed only a brief interest. When she tried to play with him and he was less responsive than she expected, she would get discouraged after a minute or two and just let him "do his own thing" as she cleaned the house.

The nanny described her father as rather bossy and her mother as warm but nervous and controlling. She hoped to be a mother someday herself and was using this job to get from the Midwest to the East, where she hoped to find another kind of job in a year or two.

I worked with Jamie again and confirmed my impression that he was sensitive to high-pitched and loud noises and overly animated facial expressions; he tended to focus in for a second or two, then look at other things, then tune in again. He gave only the faintest smiles. However, his muscle tone and beginning motor planning capacities seemed fine. It was hard to assess his auditory or visuospatial processing because his looks were so brief, and it was impossible to tell whether he responded better to simple or complex rhythms. As in the first meeting, he responded well to robust movements in space—up and down and side to side.

We formulated a plan: the parents would work with a colleague of mine on infant–parent interaction patterns. I explained that this would help Jamie learn to attend and enjoy interacting with people more. We reviewed the factors contributing to his difficulty negotiating the early stage of shared attention and engagement. There were his individual constitutional and maturational differences, including his sensitivity to loud and high-pitched sounds and to complex visual input such as extremely animated facial expressions. In addition, there were the family patterns, such as mother's depression and feelings of hopelessness and helplessness in regard to Jamie. She acknowledged that it was hard for her to relax and try the things she knew she should try in order to engage him. Father did not acknowledge his own patterns but saw mother's limitations and recognized that a parent/family component and an interactive component were contributing factors. On mother's side there was a history of depression but no history of thought disorders or other severe pathology. Father indicated no history on his side.

Mother, Jamie, and quite often the nanny began seeing the infant specialist twice a week. The specialist helped them work around Jamie's constitutional-maturational patterns and pull him into greater relatedness and shared attention. After five or six visits, they went to weekly sessions. The sessions focused on helping mother relax and experiment with variations in vocal pitch, emotional signaling, and tuning into the second or two when she could get Jamie's attention. She was able to become more animated and more varied in her voice and facial gestures, and over time she began eliciting faint smiles. A gentle and slow approach matched her style, but she found it "hard work" to counteract her natural depressive rhythm with more energy; she still tended to whisper and have lengthy pauses between her words.

The nanny adjusted more quickly once she realized that Jamie needed more, not less, interaction. She understood that looking at pictures in a book would not be as helpful for him as looking at her bright eyes and smiling face and hearing her changing vocal patterns. She began working with him for 20- to 30-minute intervals, three or four times a day. She encouraged him to look at her and show pleasure for 2 seconds, then 3 or 4, 5 or 6, and then 7 or 8 seconds. Mother did the same in the evenings when she got home from the office.

Within 2 months, the family, along with the nanny, returned to me for a follow-up visit, and mother announced that there had been "big improvements." She said, "I can sit down with him now without his crying, but I can't really calm him well yet." She described "magic moments," adding, "I now feel that I'm making it sometimes." Jamie was now a big 6-month-old showing a broad smile. He even made some vocalizations, moving his arms and legs in rhythm with his vocalizations and his smile. He was able to do this with mother, even though she was still a little slow in her rhythm, and her voice and facial gestures were not as varied as would be optimum (although much more so than in the first visit). With the nanny, Jamie smiled, vocalized, and moved very well. Meanwhile, father seemed to have learned something from mother and the nanny and was looking more at Jamie and making funny sounds and faces, although he seemed less able than the nanny to elicit smiles. Overall, the interactions were less tentative, with more affect, pleasure, and connectedness.

We got mother and baby down on the floor, nose to nose. She put her face 6 inches away from him and held out her finger, and he was able to reach for it while looking and smiling a little. At the end of the session, mother said, "When he cries, I will still have to give him to someone else, but I feel I'm making progress."

When I played with Jamie, he had nice motor tone and could smile, attend, and reach out for my fingers. However, given the amount of work I had to do to hold his attention for 4 or 5 seconds, along with his limited depth of pleasure and number of vocalizations, I concluded that a great deal of work was still needed.

The work continued with the infant specialist, and when the family came in a month and a half later, mother reported that Jamie no longer cried when he was with her. He was almost crawling, and mother felt that he showed more pleasure and was more attentive to her as well as to father and the nanny. In this session, while playing with mother, Jamie reached for her watch and her hair. He was very persistent in his intentionality, grabbing and looking at her and occasionally smiling when she made nice sounds. Mother's rhythm was still cautious (it had not improved as dramatically since the second visit as it had after the first), but she let him take her bracelet. He played with it and then gave it back to her. However, mother found it hard to get the idea of cause-and-effect, two-way interaction (which Jamie seemed capable of); she preferred just to smile and coo to get him to smile and attend.

Jamie's play with the nanny was more interactive. She took off her earrings and let him grab them. She hid them in her fist, and when he pointed in that direction, she opened it up and Jamie got a big smile on his face. Father, however, seemed very preoccupied and returned to his rough-and-tumble style of the first session, although with coaching he did some simple interactive games.

Jamie's progress was gradual but continual over the next 8 months. In a session when he was 15 months old, he walked in, gave me a nice (but quick) smile, and showed focused, organized behavior. He took toys out of the toy box and handed them to mother or me, then took them back from me, examined them, and handed them back to me. He responded to my gestures with his gestures and to mother's gestures with her gestures. Mother was still whispering in a low tone with long pauses, and Jamie himself had a calm, passive, slow-moving style. Yet he was clearly engaged, related, organized, focused, and capable of complex behavioral and emotional interactions.

What seemed to be missing was enthusiasm and robustness to his emotions and energy level. He treated mother rather like an acquaintance rather than someone he felt strongly about. He was able to warm up to me, but only slowly. He showed more intense pleasurable emotion with his nanny; he giggled and displayed complex behaviors and interactions. The main question now was how long the nanny would stay with them and what would happen if she moved on. There was the chance that she might leave in several months for a new job, although the parents hoped to keep her for another year.

Father was now more involved with Jamie, saying, "I think he likes me." He was proud that Jamie would run up to him as soon as he got home from work and might hand him a toy. Sometimes Jamie would take something that father brought home from the office and play with it. Father felt that there was some "acceptance now," and mother also took more pride in her child, feeling that they had a "real relationship."

It was clear, however, that although Jamie was now on schedule in terms of his major emotional milestones—he could attend and be warmly related and engaged and had mastered two-way communication and was moving into more complex forms of communication—he still lacked emotional range and depth, particularly with his parents. He was very calm and could recover from upsets or crying, but he still was disturbed by loud or high-pitched noises. He seemed to be bright in his approach to understanding the world, examining toys and searching behind things and under rugs for toys that I had hidden. His calm, methodical style helped him handle some of his auditory sensitivity to pitch and intensity, and he seemed to have good visuospatial skills, given his interest in figuring out how toys worked and his comfort in finding his way around my office and playroom. It seemed that Jamie had recovered from his early challenges and that his parents were getting more involved with him and feeling more confident in their parenting skills. However, many challenges remained in the family.

I continued to work with Jamie and his family regularly for another year. The work centered on facilitating and broadening his emotional range and depth as he mastered the next stages of his functional emotional developmental capacities. We worked on engaging him in a range of emotional interactions, from basic nurturing ones that supported comfort with dependency to assertive problem solving interactions where Jamie was challenged to "flex his muscles" and assertively master new terrains (e.g., treasure hunt games). As Jamie moved forward into using ideas, his parents were helped to continue broadening his emotional feelings and the depth of his feelings. In his pretend play, we now focused on following his lead but challenging him to "thicken the plot" as well. Themes of nurturing, conflict, and assertiveness as well as fear and anxiety were all increasingly elaborated in the pretend dramas Jamie and his parents orchestrated. Father's involvement was critical in helping Jamie get more comfortable with his assertive and aggressive feelings and being able to feel safe and secure in allowing them in pretend play.

Jamie continues to make progress with periodic follow-ups and is functioning in an age-expected manner emotionally, socially, and intellectually.

Jamie illustrates a type of interactive disorder, as described in our classification approach. His pattern is best captured by our category describing problems in age-expected emotional range and depth. This type of challenge occurs when the infant–caregiver relationship cannot negotiate the full range of expected emotional and social interactions in each stage of early development. This particular type of challenge, however, is well suited to an intervention approach that works on the caregiver–infant relationship patterns, with a focus on broadening and deepening the emotional range, flexibility, and stability at each of the functional emotional developmental levels. Taking into account the caregiver's personality patterns as well as the child's constitutional-maturational processing differences is vital to such an effort. In this case, mother's depression and father's relative lack of availability were critical factors.

References

Bowlby J: Forty-four juvenile thieves: their characters and home life. Int J Psychoanal 25:19–52; 107–127, 1944

Bowlby J, Robertson J: A two-year old goes to hospital. Proc R Soc Med 46:425–427, 1953

Carlson GA, Weintraub S: Childhood behavior problems and bipolar disorder: relationship or coincidence? J Affect Disord 28:143–153, 1993

Castillo M, Kwock L, Courvorise H, et al: Proton MR spectroscopy in children with bipolar affective disorder: Preliminary observations. Am J Neuroradiol 21:832–838, 2000

Coates S, Friedman R, Wolfe S: The etiology of boyhood gender identity disorder: a model for integrating temperament, development, and psychodynamics. Psychoanalytic Dialogues 1:481–523, 1991

Cytryn L, McKnew DH: Factors influencing the changing clinical expression of depressive process in children. Am J Psychiatry 131:879–881, 1974

Egland JA, Blumenthal RL, Nee J, et al: Reliability and relationship of various ages of onset criteria for major affective disorders. J Affect Disord 12:159–165, 1987

Geller B, Zimmerman B, Williams M, et al: Bipolar disorder at prospective follow-up of adults who had prepubertal major depressive disorder. Am J Psychiatry 158:125–127, 2001

Greenspan SI: Infancy and Early Childhood: The Practice of Clinical Assessment and Intervention With Emotional and Developmental Challenges. Madison, CT, International Universities Press, 1992

Greenspan SI, Glovinsky I: Children With Bipolar Patterns of Dysregulation: New Perspectives on Developmental Pathways and a Comprehensive Approach to Prevention and Treatment. Bethesda, MD, The Interdisciplinary Council on Developmental and Learning Disorders, 2002

Greenspan SI, Wieder S, Lieberman A, et al: Infants in Multirisk Families: Case Studies in Preventive Intervention. Clinical Infant Reports, No 3. New York, International Universities Press, 1987

Harrington R, Fudge H, Rutter M, et al: Adult outcomes of child and adolescent depression: II. Links with antisocial disorders. J Am Acad Child Adolesc Psychiatry 30:434–439, 1991

Lewis DO: From abuse to violence: psychophysiological consequences of maltreatment. J Am Acad Child Adolesc Psychiatry 31:383–391, 1992

Lish J, Dime-Meenan S, Whybrow P, et al: The National Depressive and Manic-Depressive Association (DMDA) survey of bipolar members. J Affect Disord 31:281–294, 1994

Radke-Yarrow M, Nottelmann E, Martinez P, et al: Young children of affectively ill parents: a longitudinal study of psychosocial development. J Am Acad Child Adolesc Psychiatry 31:68–76, 1992

Sigurdsson E, Fombonne E, Sayal K, et al: Neurodevelopmental antecedents of early onset bipolar affective disorder. Br J Psychiatry 174:121–127, 1999

Spitz RA: Hospitalism: An inquiry into the genesis of psychiatric conditions in early childhood. Psychoanal Study Child 1:53–74, 1945

Strober M, Morrell W, Burroughs J, et al: A family study of bipolar I disorder in adolescents: early onset of symptoms linked to increased familial loading and lithium resistance. J Affect Disord 15:255–268, 1988

Yeager CA, Lewis DO: Mental illness, neuropsychologic deficits, child abuse, and violence. Child Adolesc Psychiatr Clin N Am 9:793–813, 2000

8

Assessment and Treatment of Infants and Young Children With Regulatory-Sensory Processing Disorders

Regulatory-sensory processing disorders (RSPD) should be viewed on a continuum of regulatory-sensory processing variations. All children evidence unique regulatory-sensory processing profiles. They vary in the ways they respond to different sensations (such as touch and sound), comprehend these sensations, and plan actions. Some children, however, have processing differences that are extreme enough to interfere with daily functioning at home, in school, and in interactions with peers or adults, as well as with routine functions such as self-care, sleeping, and eating. As we describe regulatory-sensory processing in this chapter, note that although we focus on the disorders end of the continuum, the same patterns can characterize children without challenges and can be very helpful in understanding individual differences and the best ways to promote healthy emotional, social, and intellectual functioning. Although observations of variations in motor and sensory functioning in infants and young children have a long history (e.g., Ayres 1964), the concept of RSPD was first introduced in the 1980s and early 1990s when Greenspan introduced the concept of regulatory disorders (Greenspan 1992; Greenspan et al. 1987). Along parallel lines, the concept of sensory processing disorders has been developing since Ayres (1972). In 2004, a framework describing a new taxonomy for classifying classic patterns and subtypes of sensory processing problems was presented (Greenspan 1992; Miller et al. 2004).

Regulatory disorders as a diagnostic entity were subsequently incorporated into the diagnostic classification system of Zero to Three: National Center for Infants, Toddlers, and Families. More recently, the regulatory-sensory processing work group of the Interdisciplinary Council on Developmental and Learning Disorders (ICDL) has brought the two streams of thought together from the occupational therapy literature and the developmental, individual-differences, relationship-based (DIR) model of infant and early childhood mental health (Greenspan 1992) and reformulated and added to the description of RSPD.[1]

All children evidence their own unique regulatory-sensory processing patterns. These variations are always important to consider when constructing a developmental profile for a specific infant or child and his or her family. RSPD, however, should be considered when the child's motor and sensory differences are contributing to challenges that interfere with age-expected emotional, social, language, cognitive (including attention), motor, or sensory functioning. RSPD give rise to some of the same symptoms and behaviors as interactive disorders, including nightmares, withdrawal, aggressiveness, fearfulness and anxiety, sleeping and eating disturbances, and difficulty in peer relationships. However, RSPD involve clearly identifiable constitutional-maturational factors in the child.

Clinical Evidence and Prevalence of Regulatory-Sensory Processing Differences

There is now considerable evidence for the existence of regulatory-sensory processing differences in children with a range of mental health, developmental, and learning challenges and disorders. For an overview of this research, please see the *Interdisciplinary Council on Developmental and Learning Disorders Diagnostic Manual for Infancy and Early Childhood* (Interdisciplinary Council on Developmental and Learning Disorders 2005) section on RSPD. In understanding the contributions of regulatory-sensory processing differences to children's functioning, it's important to separate 1) research on the presence of these processes as important contributing factors and research that includes attention to these processes as part of a comprehensive, developmental, biopsychosocial intervention program (Greenspan and Wieder 2003) from 2) intervention studies that focus only on interventions for specific sensory processing dimensions.

---

[1]For a fuller description of this diagnostic category, please see Interdisciplinary Council on Developmental and Learning Disorders: *Interdisciplinary Council on Developmental and Learning Disorders Diagnostic Manual for Infancy and Early Childhood* (ICDL-DMIC). Bethesda, MD, Interdisciplinary Council on Developmental and Learning Disorders, 2005 (www.icdl.com).

Developmental Perspectives on Regulatory-Sensory Processing Disorders

To recognize problems as early as possible, it is important to emphasize that regulatory-sensory processing differences are evident very early in life. In a study of 8-month-olds (Doussard-Roosevelt et al. 1990; Porges and Greenspan 1990), we were able to show that a high percentage of the symptomatic infants had constitutional-maturational differences that contributed to their sleeping problems, eating difficulties, temper tantrums, and other symptoms (DeGangi and Greenspan 1988). The babies were either under- or overresponsive in some sensory modality or had sensory processing, muscle tone, or motor planning difficulties, in addition to difficulties with physiological regulation. These differences seemed to contribute to a skewing of parent–infant interaction patterns, which in turn affected the infants' personality development (DeGangi et al. 1991).

The infants' constitutional-maturational differences persisted and were evident at 18 months. The families also showed signs of distress (Portales et al. 1990). A small group of these infants who were followed to age 4 years displayed more behavioral and learning problems than a comparison group (DeGangi et al. 1993). Clearly, children with constitutional-maturational unevenness tend to be especially challenging. They have a harder time than other children in their relationships with caregivers, their families' functioning tends to be stressed, and they eventually may experience more behavioral and learning difficulties (Miller et al. 2004).

One can see how a child's constitutional-maturational characteristics influence interaction patterns, and hence the child's developing organization of experience, by considering a 15-month-old who has difficulty processing sounds she hears. At this age, children experiment with independence and negotiate separateness and connectedness by walking or crawling away from the parent while maintaining contact through glances and vocalizations. The child who cannot process sounds across a room, however, cannot obtain reassurance from the parent's voice. If her mother says, "Hey, that's terrific! Look how nicely you're walking!" the child, unable to decode the rhythm of mother's voice, is confused and may simply stare instead of smiling and brightening up. To feel secure, she has to come over and cling to her mother. If the mother is unaware of her daughter's difficulty in processing sound, she may feel angry or impatient at this clingy behavior and push the child away. When we talk on the telephone to a loved one far away, our ability to decode the affect in the voice allows us to feel warmth and connection. The child who lacks this ability has greater than average difficulty in developing independence.

Children with visuospatial processing impairments may have difficulty maintaining their internal representations, especially under the pressure of intense affects. If a child cannot maintain a mental image of her parents or other significant caregivers, she is likely to feel a sense of loss and may experience anxiety, fear, or depression. We hypothesize that the biological vulnerability for depression may be mediated in part through a visuospatial vulnerability that, in turn, creates vulnerability in the stability of mental representations. The loss of internal representations leads to dysphoric affects. The dysphoria experienced in depression is, in this model, in part secondary to the processing disturbance.

Regulatory-Sensory Processing Disorders

RSPD involve a distinct behavioral pattern *and* a sensory, sensory-motor, sensory discrimination, or attentional processing difficulty. When both a behavioral and a sensory pattern are not present, other diagnoses may be more appropriate. For example, an infant who is irritable and withdrawn after being abandoned may be evidencing an expectable type of relationship or attachment difficulty. An infant who is irritable and overly responsive to routine interpersonal experiences, in the absence of a clearly identified sensory, sensory-motor, or processing difficulty, may have an anxiety or mood disorder. Sleep and eating difficulties, in the absence of identifiable sensory responsivity or sensory processing differences, are classified as disorders in their own right. Further evaluation is then needed to determine whether the cause is an interactive disorder or some other underlying problem that does not fall within our three categories (interactive disorders, regulatory-sensory processing disorders, and neurodevelopmental disorders of relating and communicating).

Many attentional, affective, motor, sensory, behavioral control, and language problems that have traditionally been viewed as difficulties in their own right may in some children stem from a broader, more basic RSPD. General terms such as "overly sensitive," "difficult temperament," or "reactive" have commonly been used to describe infants and children with motor and sensory processing differences. But clinicians have tended to use such terms without specifying the sensory system or motor functions involved. There is growing evidence that constitutional and early maturational patterns contribute to the difficulties of such infants, but it is also clear that early caregiving patterns can exert considerable influence on how constitutional-maturational patterns develop and become part of the child's evolving personality. As interest in these children increases, it is important to systematize descriptions of the sensory, motor, and integrative patterns, as well as the caregiving patterns presumed to be involved.

For an RSPD to be present in an infant or young child, the clinician must observe one or more behavioral challenges *and* a sensory processing challenge including sensory modulation, sensory-motor, sensory discrimination, or attentional problems discussed below.

Types of Regulatory-Sensory Processing Disorders

Regulatory-sensory processing is an encompassing term referring to the way the nervous system manages incoming sensory information. It is the means by which sensory information is perceived and organized from external stimuli in the environment or from internal stimuli within the body to produce an adaptive response. In this context, *adaptive response* is defined as an effective behavioral response. Although traditionally considered from a behavioral perspective, adaptive responses may also be considered from a physiological perspective. From this perspective, adaptive responses include an efficient physiological response to a sensory challenge or demand.

Some individuals have difficulty processing sensory information and responding to it appropriately. When the sensory and motor difficulties are severe enough that an individual's daily routines and activities are disrupted and there are related emotional and/or behavioral challenges, the condition is considered an RSPD. Difficulties with motor, emotional, attentional, or daily living skills may be markers of how sensory stimuli are perceived and interpreted.

RSPD are divided into a number of specific disorders and also contain a category of "mixed" disorders based on the predominant characteristics of the child, including behavioral patterns and emotional inclinations, as well as motor and sensory patterns. Note that the descriptions of subtypes include a discussion of caregiving patterns (therapeutic strategies) that promote better regulation and organization in the child as well as caregiving patterns that intensify the child's difficulty. Because the daily routines of caregiving involve continual sensory, motor, and affective experiences for the infant and young child, irregular conditions in the environment, changes in routine, or handling that is not sensitive to individual differences can strongly affect infants and children with regulatory disorders as well as their caregivers.

There are a number of specific types of RSPD. Each is characterized by different types of regulatory-sensory processing and behavioral patterns. Although each type of disorder is identified separately, three broad patterns characterize each type:

1. Sensory modulation challenges, such as overresponsivity, underresponsivity, and sensory-seeking (Type I)
2. Sensory discrimination challenges (Type II)
3. Sensory-based motor challenges (dyspraxia and postural regulation difficulties) (Type III)

Sensory Modulation Challenges (Type I)

Sensory modulation challenges are characterized by an inability to grade the degree, intensity, and nature of responses to sensory input. Often the child's responses do not fit the demands of the situation. The child therefore demonstrates difficulty achieving and maintaining an optimal range of performance and adapting to challenges in daily life. Four subtypes of RSPD are related to sensory modulation challenges: 1) overresponsive, fearful anxious pattern; 2) overresponsive, negative, and stubborn pattern; 3) underresponsive, self-absorbed pattern; and 4) active, sensory-seeking pattern.

Overresponsive, Fearful, Anxious Pattern

Children who demonstrate overresponsivity to sensory stimuli have responses to sensations that are more intense, quicker in onset or longer lasting than those of children with typical sensory responsivity under the same conditions. Their responses are particularly pronounced when the stimulus is not anticipated. Children may demonstrate overresponsivity in only one particular sensory system; for example, "auditory defensiveness" or "tactile defensiveness," or they may demonstrate overresponsivity in multiple sensory systems. Overresponsivity to sensory stimuli in multiple modalities is often referred to as sensory defensiveness. Children are usually particularly overresponsive to specific types of stimuli within a sensory domain (e.g., in the tactile domain, they respond defensively to light touch but not to deep pressure), rather than to all stimuli within a domain.

Responses to sensory stimuli occur along a spectrum. Some children manage their tendency toward overresponsivity most of the time, whereas other children are overresponsive almost continuously. Responses may appear inconsistent because overresponsivity is highly dependent on context. Although children may generally attempt to avoid particular sensory experiences, sensitivities may vary throughout the day and from day to day. Because sensory input tends to have a cumulative effect, the child's efforts to control responses to sensory stimuli may build up and result in a sudden behavioral disruption in response to a seemingly trivial stimulus.

A child's behavioral characteristics when faced with uncomfortable stimuli can fall within a broad range. At one end of this spectrum, the child shows fearfulness and anxiety, often avoiding many sensory experiences. At the other end of the spectrum, the child shows negativity and stubbornness, or obstinacy exemplified by attempts to control the environment. (This latter tendency is described as a separate type in the following section, "Overresponsive, Negative, and Stubborn Pattern.") This range of responses is often termed the "fight, flight, fright, or freeze" response, and is attributed to sympathetic nervous system activation. Secondary behavioral characteristics include irritability, fussiness, poor adaptability, moodiness, inconsolability, and poor socialization. In general, children who are overresponsive to sensation have difficulty with transitions and unexpected changes.

Sensory overresponsivity is often seen with other sensory reaction patterns. For example, children may show overresponsiveness to tactile stimuli while seeking proprioceptive stimuli. Sensory overresponsivity also may be observed concomitantly with sensory discrimination problems and dyspraxia.

Behavioral patterns include excessive cautiousness, inhibition, and fearfulness. The child avoids sensation in an effort to limit unexpected incoming sensory stimuli. In early infancy, one sees a restricted range of exploration and assertiveness, dislike of changes in routine, and a tendency to be frightened and clinging in new situations. Young children's behavior is characterized by excessive fears or worries and by shyness in new experiences, such as forming peer relationships or engaging with new adults. Occasionally, the child behaves impulsively when overloaded or frightened. He tends to become upset easily (e.g., irritable, often crying); cannot soothe himself readily (e.g., finds it difficult to return to sleep); and cannot quickly recover from frustration or disappointment, especially in environments that include multiple or intense sensory stimuli. The fearful and cautious child may have a fragmented, rather than an integrated, internal representational world and may therefore be easily distracted by different stimuli.

Caregiver patterns that are characterized by soothing, regulating interactions; that respect the child's sensitivities; and that do not convey that the child has "bad behaviors" are helpful. Supportive parents anticipate noxious environments and minimize them or prepare the child for them. Enhancing flexibility and assertiveness in fearful and cautious children involves empathy, especially for the child's sensory and affective experience; very gradual and supportive encouragement to explore new experiences; and gentle, but firm, limits. Inconsistent caregiver patterns intensify these children's difficulties, as when caregivers are overindulgent or overprotective some of the time and punitive or intrusive at other times.

Overresponsive, Negative, and Stubborn Pattern

Children with the overresponsive, negative, and stubborn pattern tend to evidence the same physiological responses described above for children with the overresponsive, fearful and anxious type. However, rather than being overloaded and becoming fearful, anxious, and cautious, these children attempt to control their environments so that they can minimize fear and anxiety. Thus, these children may prefer repetition and the absence of change or, at most, change at a slow, predictable pace.

Behavior patterns may appear negativistic, stubborn, and controlling. The child can become aggressive and impulsive in response to sensory stimulation. He often does the opposite of what is requested or expected. Infants with this pattern tend to be fussy, difficult, and resistant to transitions and changes. Preschoolers tend to be negative, angry, and stubborn, as well as compulsive and perfectionistic. However, these children can display joyful, flexible behavior in certain situations.

In contrast to the fearful or cautious child, the negative and stubborn child does not become fragmented but organizes an integrated sense of self around negative patterns. In contrast to the impulsive, sensation-seeking child (described later in the section "Active, Sensory-Seeking Pattern"), the negative and stubborn child is more controlling, tends to avoid or be slow to engage in new experiences rather than to crave them, and is not generally aggressive unless provoked.

Caregiver patterns that enhance flexibility in the child's responses involve soothing and empathetic support of slow, gradual change and avoidance of power struggles. Caregivers can avoid power struggles by offering the child choices and opportunities for negotiation whenever possible. Caregivers can also help these children become more flexible by offering warmth; gentle, firm guidance and limits (even in the face of negative or impulsive responses that may feel like rejection); and encouragement of symbolic representation of affects, especially dependency, anger, and annoyance. In contrast, caregiver patterns that are intrusive, excessively demanding, overstimulating, or punitive tend to intensify negative patterns.

Underresponsive, Self-Absorbed Pattern

Children who are underresponsive to sensory stimuli are often quiet and passive, disregarding or not responding to stimuli of typical intensity available in their sensory environment. Alternatively, they may be so enthralled by a world of their own imagination that they have trouble engaging in the here and now. They may appear withdrawn, difficult to engage, and/or self-absorbed because they have not registered the sensory input in their environment. The term *poor registration* is often used to describe their behavior, as they do not appear to detect or register incoming sensory information. They may also appear apathetic and lethargic. They may seem to lack the inner drive that most children have for socialization and motor exploration when, actually, they do not notice the possibilities for action that are around them. Their underresponsivity to tactile and proprioceptive inputs may lead to poorly developed body scheme, clumsiness, or poorly modulated movement. These children may fail to respond to bumps, falls, cuts, or scrapes that can present a danger, and they may not notice pain, such as that from injuries to the skin and objects that are too hot or too cold.

Children who are underresponsive to sensation often do not seek greater intensity in sensory input even though they may require it for optimal environmental interaction. Children with this pattern may be overlooked or thought of as the good baby or easy child simply because they fail to make demands on people and things in the environment. These children often need high intensity and highly salient input in order to become actively involved in the environment, the task, or the interaction.

In some instances, children who are easily overloaded by sensory stimulation may appear to be underresponsive when in fact they are extremely overresponsive. The observable behavior is one that suggests withdrawal and shutdown, perhaps as a defense mechanism. Children with sensory underresponsivity also may have sensory discrimination challenges and dyspraxia.

Two patterns are observed. Some children tend to be self-absorbed, unaware, and disengaged, whereas others are self-absorbed, but very creative and overly focused on their own fantasy lives. Therefore, we describe two subtypes for the underresponsive self-absorbed pattern.

Self-absorbed and difficult-to-engage type.   **Behavior patterns** include seeming disinterest in exploring relationships or even challenging games or objects. Children may appear apathetic, easily exhausted, and withdrawn. High affective tone and saliency are required to attract their interest, attention, and emotional engagement. Infants may appear delayed or depressed and lacking in motor exploration and social overtures. In addition to continuing these patterns, preschoolers may evidence diminished verbal dialogue. Their behavior and play may present a limited range of ideas and fantasies. Sometimes children will seek out desired sensory input, often engaging in repetitive sensory activities, such as spinning on a Sit-n-Spin, swinging, or jumping up and down on the bed. The child needs the intensity or repetition of these activities in order to experience them fully.

Caregiver patterns that provide high-energy interactive input engage the child in activities and relationships and foster initiative. These patterns involve energized wooing and robust responses to the child's cues, however faint. In contrast, caregiver patterns that are low-key, laid-back, or depressive in tone and rhythm tend to intensify these children's patterns of withdrawal.

Self-absorbed and creative type. **Behavior patterns** of self-absorbed children, many of whom are also creative, include a tendency for the child to tune into his own sensations, thoughts, and emotions rather than to communications from other people. Infants may become interested in objects through solitary exploration rather than in the context of interaction. Children may appear inattentive, easily distracted, or preoccupied, especially when they are not pulled into a task or interaction. Preschoolers tend to escape into fantasy when faced with external challenges, such as a demanding preschool activity or competition from a peer. They may prefer to play by themselves if others do not actively join their fantasies. In their fantasy life, they may show enormous imagination and creativity.

Caregiver patterns that are helpful include a tendency to tune into the child's nonverbal and verbal communications and to help the child engage in two-way communication, that is, to open and close circles of communication. Caregivers should also encourage a good balance between fantasy and reality and help a child who is attempting to escape into fantasy stay grounded in external reality (e.g., by showing sensitivity to the child's interests and feelings; by promoting engagement and discussion of daily events, feelings, and other real-world topics; and by making fantasy play a collaborative endeavor between parent and child rather than a solitary activity). In contrast, a caregiver's self-absorption or preoccupation, as well as confusing family communications, tends to intensify the child's difficulties.

Active, Sensory-Seeking Pattern

Children with this pattern actively seek or crave sensory stimulation and seem to have an almost insatiable desire for sensory input. They energetically engage in activities or actions that are geared toward adding more intense feelings of sensation to satisfy a basic need or desire for sensory input. They tend to be constantly moving, crashing, bumping, and jumping; they may have a need to touch everything and have difficulty inhibiting this behavior; they may play music or the TV at loud volumes, may fixate on visually stimulating objects or events, or may seek unusual olfactory or gustatory experiences that are more intense and last longer than those of children with typical sensory responsivity.

Atypical responses occur along a spectrum; some sensory-seeking behavior is normal. Often these children prefer a higher level of arousal than adults feel is appropriate in a given environment. Sensory seeking may also be seen as a means to obtain enhanced input for individuals with reduced awareness of sensation. Sensory seeking may be done in an effort to influence (or increase) their level of arousal. For children who are sensory seekers, the need for constant stimulation is difficult to fulfill and may be particularly problematic in environments where children are expected to sit quietly, such as in school, in movies, and in libraries. Obtaining additional sensory stimulation, if unstructured, may increase the child's overall state of arousal and result in disorganized behavior. However, if directed, specific types of additional sensory input can have an organizing effect.

The behavioral characteristics of these children when their sensory needs are not met include demanding and insistent behavior. They may be impulsive, almost explosive, in their attempts to fill their quota for sensation. They have a tendency to "get in trouble," creating situations around themselves that others perceive as bad or dangerous. Secondary behavioral characteristics that describe these children include conduct that is overly active or aggressive, impulsive, intense, demanding, hard to calm, restless, overly affectionate, and craving attention. Extreme seeking or craving of sensory input can also disrupt children's ability to maintain attention for learning. Activities of daily living are frequently disrupted. Children may have trouble in school because they are distracted as they are driven to obtain extra sensory stimulation instead of focusing on tasks.

Behavior patterns involve high activity, with children seeking physical contact and stimulation, for example through deep pressure and intense movement. Frequently, the motorically disorganized child's tendency to seek contact with people or objects leads to disruptive behavior (e.g., breaking things, unprovoked hitting, intruding into other people's physical space). Behavior that begins as a result of craving sensations may be interpreted by others as aggression rather than excitability. Once others react aggressively to the child, his own behavior may become aggressive in intent.

Infants in this group are most satisfied when provided with strong sensation in the form of movement, sound, touch, or visual stimulation. They may be content only when held or rocked. Toddlers may be very active. Preschoolers often show aggressive, intrusive behavior and a daredevil, risk-taking style, as well as a preoccupation with aggressive themes in pretend play. When the young child is anxious or unsure of himself, he may use counterphobic behaviors, such as hitting another child first in anticipation of possibly being hit, or repeating unacceptable behavior after being asked to stop. When older and able to verbalize and observe his own patterns, the child may describe his need for activity and stimulation as a way to feel alive, vibrant, and powerful. Children who have extreme sensory needs that are not met may become demanding and insistent on getting their own way. They may be impulsive, almost explosive in their attempt to fill their quota for sensation. They have a tendency to get in trouble as they create situations around them that others perceive as bad or dangerous.

Caregiver patterns characterized by continuous warm relating, a great deal of nurturing, and empathy, together with clear structure and limits, enhance flexibility and adaptivity. Caregivers should understand the need for extra stimulation and give the child many opportunities to acquire more stimulation, preferably through interactive, modulated play. Encouraging the use of imagination and verbal dialogue to explore the external environment and elaborate feelings further enhances the child's flexibility. Advocacy in settings outside the home is required so that others understand the child's behavior, adapt these constructive caregiver patterns, and avoid labeling the child a behavior problem. In contrast, caregiver patterns that lack warm, continuous engagement (e.g., frequent changing of caregivers); that over- or underestimate the child; that are overly punitive; or that vacillate between overly punitive limit setting and insufficient limit setting may intensify the child's difficulties.

Sensory Discrimination Challenges (Type II) and Sensory-Based Motor Challenges (Type III)

As indicated earlier, in addition to challenges related to sensory modulation, there are RSPD related to sensory discrimination challenges and to sensory-based motor challenges (postural control problems and dyspraxia). For example, children with sensory discrimination challenges may find it difficult to determine what they are touching or how close to stand to someone else. Children with dyspraxia (i.e., motor planning and sequencing challenges) may find it difficult to carry out a multi-step task.

The two RSPD based on challenges in these processing areas involve inattentive, disorganized behavioral patterns and school performance and academic problems. Both these disorders may involve various combinations of difficulties in sensory discrimination, as well as sensory-based motor performance (including postural control problems and dyspraxia).

Inattentive, Disorganized Pattern

> With Sensory Discrimination Challenges
> With Postural Control Challenges
> With Dyspraxia
> With Combinations of All Three

Behavior patterns that are related to sensory discrimination, motor planning and/or postural control challenges include a tendency to be inattentive and disorganized. For example, the child may have difficulty following through on tasks or school assignments. In the middle of a homework assignment or household chore, the child may wander off to some other activity, seemingly unmindful of the original goal. In the extreme, the child's behavior may appear fragmented. As others put more pressure on the child, he may become more disorganized. When these challenges continue over a period of time, the child can easily become demoralized and feel depressed and/or angry. Impulsive or defiant behavior is not uncommon, nor are passivity, avoidance, and preference for activities such as video games, which are experienced as less demanding (in terms of sequencing and organizing complex plans of action).

When challenged to be involved in tasks that are difficult, one often sees increasing avoidance, fragmentation, and disorganization, as well as inattentiveness. It's not unusual for parents to describe a child as organized and attentive when getting ready to go to the video arcade or out for his favorite ice cream and yet fragmented, inattentive, and disorganized, when attempting a multistep math problem. Clinicians as well as caregivers often ask whether the behavior patterns described above are different from what are often described as attentional problems or attention deficit disorder. The descriptions of the different processing challenges that contribute to this type of behavior pattern help clinicians observe the relationship between specific regulatory-sensory processing patterns and attentional and organizational challenges.

Caregiver patterns that recognize the child's underlying challenges can help the child strengthen the processing areas contributing to his difficulties. In addition, while the child is working to strengthen underlying processing challenges, caregivers and educators who can help the child break down complex tasks into manageable steps and provide patient, multisensory support (visual, auditory, and motor cues) also tend to help the child make progress. On the other hand, caregiving patterns that characterize the child as unmotivated, bad, or lazy, and pressure and punish the child inevitably intensify the child's challenges, rather than help him set achievable goals that can be associated with a sense of mastery. The key to constructive caregiver patterns is to understand and strengthen the contributing processing differences that are described in this chapter.

Compromised School and/or Academic Performance Pattern

With Sensory Discrimination Challenges
With Postural Control Challenges
With Dyspraxia
With Combinations of All Three

Behavior patterns associated with motor planning and sequencing challenges (dyspraxia), postural control, and sensory discrimination difficulties may include circumscribed school performance or academic challenges. For example, difficulties with motor planning and postural control can make handwriting very difficult. Sensory discrimination difficulties may make distinguishing shapes or letters difficult. Visuospatial challenges may make lining up columns in math or in understanding concepts involving graphs or diagrams difficult. Motor planning and sequencing difficulties may also contribute to problems with sequencing ideas into sentences. If the processing contributions to these types of school performance and academic challenges are not addressed, the child may become avoidant, disinterested, and/or demoralized. A sense of failure, rather than a can-do, positive attitude may follow. School itself can become viewed as a place of failure and all activities in school, or school as a whole, may be avoided.

Caregiver patterns that recognize the processing contributions to the child's school performance and academic challenges and that provide supportive, stepwise help tend to improve the child's overall functioning. Caregivers who can break the challenge down into small enough steps for the child to experience a sense of mastery 70% to 80% of the time are likely to be especially helpful. Caregivers who are punitive, rejecting, or overly expectant often increase the difficulties. When a child has difficulty with a particular motor or sensory discrimination task, there is little intrinsic sense of mastery or pleasure in performing it. In comparison, when a child is naturally gifted at an activity, there is intrinsic pleasure in the activity itself. Therefore, support, guidance, incentives, and breaking down the challenge into easily mastered steps is essential to helping the child overcome his challenges and feel a sense of pride and accomplishment.

Mixed Regulatory-Sensory Processing Patterns

It is quite common for children to display mixed regulatory-sensory processing patterns. Combinations of patterns and/or subtypes in one child are common and differences among various sensory domains in the same child may be observed. For example, a child can experience sensory overresponsivity in the tactile system and sensory-seeking in the vestibular and proprioceptive systems. In addition, atypical response patterns to sensation can vary as a function of time or day, environmental context, stress, fatigue, level of arousal, and many other factors. Next, we outline a few of the common behavioral challenges that are often related to mixed regulatory-sensory processing patterns.

Common behavioral challenges related to mixed regulatory-sensory processing patterns. The mixed regulatory-sensory processing patterns described above can occur with and without behavioral or emotional challenges. A number of well-known symptom patterns are often related to mixed types of regulatory-sensory processing problems. A few of these are listed and briefly described below. However, it should be noted that these challenges may be related to interactive difficulties and/or unique motor and sensory processing challenges. Where the interactive elements (i.e., caregiver–child interaction patterns) are the predominant contributor, interactive disorders should be considered. Where the predominant contributor is a unique motor or sensory processing pattern, RSPD should be considered, and the clinician then should determine if the challenges are related to a specific pattern, such as sensory overresponsivity, or a mixed pattern, as described above. The challenges listed below are usually related to mixed regulatory-sensory processing patterns when this dimension is the main contributing factor. As with all mental health and developmental disorders in infancy and early childhood, there are always regulatory-sensory processing and interactive dimensions. The very common problems listed below are included in both the interactive and regulatory-sensory processing disorder categories because for different children, one or the other feature often predominates. It would, therefore, be an oversimplification to list these problems arbitrarily in only one or the other disorder category.

Attentional problems.   Children with problems in attending and sustaining their focus often evidence a number of regulatory-sensory processing challenges. Most children evidence difficulties with motor planning and sequencing. It is difficult for them to carry out a planned series of actions to solve a problem unless there is a great deal of structure guiding them. In addition, many children with attentional problems also evidence sensory discrimination difficulties, for example, in figuring out complex visuospatial patterns and solving visuospatial problems (searching systematically for a hidden object in all parts of a room). In addition, some children with attentional problems are sensory craving and, therefore, very active and sometimes aggressive. A small percentage of children with attentional problems are sensory overresponsive and, therefore, very distractible. They are distracted by different types of sounds or sights and easily become overloaded and more fragmented in a noisy or busy setting. Also, some children with attentional problems are sensory underresponsive and, therefore, ordinary sensations, such as the human voice, which would orient a child, don't draw their attention. Instead, they drift off into their own world. Some very bright children with this pattern wind up daydreaming a great deal. Clearly, many children with attentional problems evidence combinations of the above patterns, such as motor planning problems and sensory underresponsivity. Environmental and caregiving patterns may contribute as well.

Disruptive behavioral problems.   Toddlers and preschoolers with disruptive behavior often evidence sensory craving, which leads them to be very active and, at times, aggressive, even without necessarily intending to be so. Some of these children may also have areas of sensory underresponsivity where, for example, they may be relatively insensitive to pain, making this pattern even more intense. Some children also evidence sensory discrimination challenges, such as in auditory discrimination, making it harder to understand limits and guidelines. Each or any combination of these patterns can contribute to disruptive behaviors. Environmental, caregiver, and family patterns also contribute.

Sleep problems. Many children with difficulties falling asleep or sustaining sleep evidence some degree of sensory overresponsivity. Some also evidence sensory discrimination challenges. Others evidence a great deal of sensory craving and are, therefore, very active. Often, these sensory patterns are compounded by a variety of environmental factors and caregiving practices, which may contribute to the sleep challenges. From an early age, the child forms certain patterns with caregivers that reinforce sleep difficulties over time.

Eating problems. Many children with eating difficulties evidence sensory overresponsivity, especially in their oral cavity. Some also evidence low muscle tone, including low tone in their oral-motor area, as well as motor planning and sequencing challenges. Their oral-motor functioning challenges contribute to making eating a very difficult task. Other children are underresponsive to sensation in the oral cavity, also making eating difficult because expectable sensations from food are not occurring. Environmental and caregiving patterns may further contribute.

Elimination problems. Many children with elimination challenges evidence combinations of sensory underresponsivity, low muscle tone, and motor planning and sequencing difficulties. Some, however, are sensory craving and others are sensory overresponsive. Caregiver and environmental patterns contribute as well. For example, the child who is unable to sense when his or her bladder is full and who has a hard time regulating motor actions is more prone to having "accidents."

Elective mutism. Children with elective mutism are often sensory overresponsive and, therefore, highly anxious. Typically, a school environment is a challenging setting because of the noise and other sensations. Although overresponsivity is the largest contributor, children with elective mutism may also have dyspraxia. Attention to these differences, coupled with increasing the child's level of security and the gradualness with which the child enters a new setting, like school, can be very helpful.

Mood dysregulation, including bipolar patterns. Often infants and young children with fluctuating moods have an underlying challenge characterized by sensory overresponsivity coupled with sensory seeking. Therefore, when overloaded, instead of retreating and becoming cautious, they become more agitated and impulsive. As they become symbolic, this can take the form of shifting from fearful and depressive themes to angry and power-oriented themes. See Chapter 7 ("Assessment and Treatment of Infants and Young Children With Interactive Disorders") for a fuller description of infants and young children with mood fluctuations, including bipolar patterns.

Other emotional and behavioral problems related to mixed regulatory-sensory processing difficulties.   Children with mixed regulatory-sensory processing challenges may evidence emotional or behavioral problems or other symptoms not listed above. These may include anxiety, fearfulness, negativism, and so forth. Challenges or problems related to mixed regulatory-sensory processing challenges should be indicated in this category.

Mixed regulatory-sensory processing patterns where behavioral or emotional problems are not yet in evidence.   In the early years of life, many children present with mixed regulatory-sensory processing challenges but do not yet evidence clear emotional, social, and/or behavioral problems. Their regulatory-sensory processing challenges may be noted by their parent, early childhood educators, or their primary healthcare provider. For example, they may be overresponsive to light touch and have difficulty with sequencing motor responses. The recognition of these challenges provides an ideal opportunity for preventive work and family guidance that is geared to improving functioning in these and related areas and for preventing the emergence of emotional, social, and/or behavioral problems. Many parents and educators already implement such preventive strategies intuitively. However, identifying these patterns can help systematize these efforts and broaden the number of children who are helped.

Therapeutic Approaches

In contrast to the child whose developmental problems stem primarily from family interaction patterns, the infant or child with a regulatory disorder requires help in overcoming her own constitutional-maturational difficulties. However, the clinician must not attempt to address the child's regulatory capacities in isolation from child–caregiver interaction patterns. To succeed, treatment must address both.

The six-step developmental, individual-differences, relationship-based (DIR) intervention process described in Chapter 4 ("Therapeutic Principles") must be carried out with special attention to the child's sensory, sensory-motor, and organizational processing differences. Processing difficulties can interfere with a child's ability to negotiate the first two core developmental capacities: attending and engaging. In deciding on Floortime approaches that will best help the child focus, attend, and engage, it is helpful to incorporate the practical suggestions of occupational therapists trained in sensory integration work (Ayres 1964). The clinician needs to become familiar with the child's reactions to touch, sound, sight, smell, and movement. If a child is overly sensitive or reactive to tactile stimuli, the therapist may want to explore how he responds to firm pressure. Firm pressure, as part of rough-and-tumble play, helps some children normalize sensory input and fosters better focus and concentration. A child who is underreactive to sound may need to hear a stronger, more dramatic vocal pattern, whereas one who is overreactive will respond best to soft, soothing tones. Some children do better with low-pitched sounds, some with high-pitched ones. A child who has difficulty processing what he hears—that is, abstracting the sequence of sounds—may need simple rhythms with only one or two variations, whereas a child who processes sound easily may require the novelty of more complex vocal rhythms with four or five patterns. By observing whether a child has a knowing sense or a confused look about him, the clinician can gauge what type of vocal rhythm and sequence best fosters his attention and engagement. Similarly, the clinician will need to vary the brightness of lighting, the intensity of colors used in toys, and even the level of animation in his or her own face, depending on a particular child's sensitivity to different aspects of what he sees. As with sound, the complexity of visual input should vary according to the degree of visuospatial complexity the child can handle.

In the area of movement patterns, some children focus and attend best when involved in slow, rhythmic activities, such as swinging at a rate of four or five seconds per swing. Others do better when moved rapidly, at one second per swing. Still others do best when they have opportunities to experience both fast and slow rhythms. In addition to the rate and rhythm of movement, the position of the child can affect her ability to attend and maintain a calm, regulated state. An excessively finicky child may calm down most readily when resting on her stomach, over a parent's knees, with the parent's hands pressing firmly on her back while the parent uses his or her knees to move her in a slow, rhythmic way. Another child may do best in an upright position, resting against her parent's chest, with her head crooked into the parent's neck. This common upright position, however, is too activating for some children, who can better be calmed by a more horizontal position, particularly when they are feeling distressed.

Some children attend and focus best when they engage in large-muscle activities. For some, the optimal activity is one that combines large-muscle exercise with joint compression, thus giving the child sufficient receptor feedback. These children may find that jumping on a bed or trampoline helps them focus, attend, and engage.

Many children who are oversensitive to touch, sound, light, or their own movement patterns attend and engage best when they can be in charge of the interaction patterns. The more they can be in charge, the more they can regulate and monitor the sensory input and motor control they need. As infants grow into toddlers and develop better motor control, and thus better ability to take charge of their interactions, it is important to foster their initiative.

Many children who have regulatory difficulties also have difficulties with muscle tone and motor planning. They may have high or low tone or difficulty planning physical acts such as alternating hand movements when drumming on their own legs. As a baby, such a child may have trouble getting his hand to his mouth. As a toddler, he may knock things over: when he tries to grab one object, he knocks over another. Such a child needs practice in coordinating perception with motor acts. The clinician or parent should start with activities the child can master and work up to more challenging activities. Parents, teachers, and clinicians must understand that a child with low muscle tone will tire easily. He has to exert an enormous amount of energy and conscious effort to carry out routine activities that children with normal extensor tone do automatically, such as walking and climbing stairs. To develop extensor tone and help the child with coordination, strength, and stamina, one can use exercises such as having him lie on the floor on his stomach and pretend to be a boat, rocking back and forth and arching his back. In another exercise, "the bird game," the child scissors his feet around his parent's waist, arches his back, and flaps his arms as his parent spins around.

As always, one must help the child take one step at a time. First, build fundamental abilities by improving muscle tone and motor planning; then, expose the child to routine childhood activities that enable her to continue strengthening these abilities. Common play activities that build extensor tone and provide practice in motor planning include simple games of putting objects in certain places or taking them out; games that require the child to change direction rapidly, such as a game of tag in which the players do not run in a straight line; or activities, like the "bird game," in which the child puts her body into an extensor pattern. Such games and activities, together with the kinds of sensory-normalizing activities and interactions just described, will foster attention and engagement in both early and later stages of development.

As can be seen from the examples we have discussed, Floortime approaches that address a child's constitutional-maturational variations will directly foster his capacities for attention and engagement. As always, it is critical that the parents and clinician empathize with the child and follow his lead. A clinician who is naturally empathic and flexible will find it easy to engage a wide variety of infants and young children, whereas a clinician whose approach is more rigid will find it far easier to work with some children than with others. In general, the oversensitive, fearful, and cautious child requires a warm, available, yet cautious approach by the clinician. In working with an 8-month-old who is typically fearful and cautious when facing new experiences, for example, one should approach slowly, from afar, while vocalizing and giving the baby lots of flirtatious glances. The baby's probable expectation—that one is going to walk right over and try to pick her up—is thus not realized. As one moves across the room an inch at a time, making interesting gestures and facial expressions, the baby may relax and begin to flirt back for a second or two at a time, looking and then hiding his eyes in his mother's chest. One can sense when the child becomes apprehensive by the changed look in his eyes or by his averted gaze. At this point, one should stop advancing, hold one's position, and continue the flirtation. If the clinician now begins talking to the mother and only intermittently flirting with the baby, many 8-month-olds, even cautious and oversensitive ones, will begin seeking the clinician out with their eyes and sometimes with motor gestures. An important corner has now been turned. The relationship is moving ahead, and the clinician will soon have the opportunity to engage the child and foster his attention more fully. In many cases, what the clinician learns about the way to successfully approach a particular child proves very helpful to the parents, who may have felt frustrated, disappointed, or rejected because their previous attempts to woo their baby failed to elicit the bright smiles and warm interactions they expected.

For the child with a regulatory disorder, the second intervention step, problem solving, is oriented toward helping her anticipate, practice, and master the activities that are especially difficult for her. Problem solving can be employed at the early behavioral and gestural levels for the 6- to 18-month-old. For example, consider the child with tactile sensitivities who avoids touch and is cautious about any new toy, game, piece of clothing, or person. The parents should gradually introduce her to a new toy with new textures and allow her to play with it in whatever way she finds enjoyable. If her grandmother buys her a new shirt, she should not be expected to put it on immediately. Instead, a parent should let her play with the shirt, perhaps by engaging her in a game of pushing the shirt back and forth between them. If she enjoys the game, she will have the chance to see, touch, and smell the shirt and get used to its feel. Alternatively, her father might try putting the shirt over his head and allowing her to pull it off to see his eyes; caught up in this game, she may actually touch the shirt before realizing that it is something she might not have wanted to touch. Innumerable such opportunities exist to use behaviors and gestures to help the preverbal child anticipate and practice new experiences; the only limitation is the ingenuity of clinician and caregiver.

Children 2 years and older, and especially children from 3 to 4½ years old, can learn to use words and thoughts to anticipate difficult situations. A parent and child can, for example, discuss what is likely to happen at school the next day. The parent asks the child to imagine what feelings he might have and how he might behave in response to those feelings. Perhaps the parent engages him in reviewing similar situations from the recent past, in order to help him feel prepared for whatever uncomfortable sensations he may experience at school the next day and to reduce his likelihood of feeling surprised or shocked by them. In carrying out this exercise, many clinicians, parents, and teachers make the mistake of focusing only on situations and behaviors: "When you are in circle time, you will tend to sit in a corner by yourself." They fail to address the child's feelings: "When you are in circle time, you feel…how?" The child who can talk about feeling scared, "like I can't breathe," or "like my brain doesn't work" will have a great advantage over the child who discusses only situations and actions.

Examples of situations a child with a regulatory disorder might need to anticipate include putting on a new pair of shoes, circle time at preschool, times when everyone else is drawing and the teacher insists that she draw too, being pushed by another child, being surprised from behind by an adult or another child, hearing someone yell too loudly, being denied a toy by another child or an adult, and having a toy snatched away by a playmate. All of these experiences, so common in the life of any child, are especially challenging for the child with regulatory difficulties. By developing the ability to understand and verbalize how she is likely to feel and behave in each difficult situation, the child can approach such situations better prepared and begin to experiment with more adaptive coping strategies.

Trial runs in situations similar to those the child finds challenging are also enormously helpful. Suppose a preschooler who has difficulty in groups, because he is highly sensitive to noise and to being touched, is about to participate in circle time for the first time. In the weeks before this new experience, his parents can help him prepare by arranging play dates not with just one other child (assuming he already does well playing one on one) but with two or three playmates. In the familiar setting of his own home, with his mother or father present, he can experience situations in which he will bump shoulders with other kids, deal with competition and aggression, and hear loud noises. Having the children sit in a circle and listen to a story may be an effective culmination of the practice period. A child who has already had several such play dates may well feel more comfortable when he has to sit in a group at school. As long as the problem-solving discussions and practice sessions are tailored to be manageable for each child and are gradually made more challenging, they can effectively help children anticipate and prepare.

In the third intervention step, the child is helped to experience empathy for her own difficulties. For example, the clinician may express empathy for how a child feels when she has to sit in a group or hear loud noises. In many cases, the clinician must help the parents empathize as well. Accurately empathizing with children who have regulatory disorders can be difficult. It is hard to imagine how overwhelmed, disorganized, and fragmented a child who experiences sensory overload can feel if one does not have these sensitivities oneself. By interpreting such a child's behavior in light of one's own experience, one will likely misunderstand her. For example, a teacher may assume that a child who is behaving provocatively during circle time is self-centered and unwilling to share the limelight with other children. In fact, the child may feel overwhelmed and fragmented. The adult needs to listen carefully to the child to understand her actual experience, especially her experience of sensory overload.

Each child will develop his own fantasies that give meaning to sensory and affective experience. When a child who is oversensitive to sound hears voices that are too loud for his comfort, he may assume that the people around him wish to hurt him. Another child may imagine that people are trying to trick or manipulate him, and yet another may think that others hate him or want to deprive him of something. It is extremely important to help the verbal child sense that one understands not just the secondary fantasy but also the primary feeling of being overloaded and overwhelmed. This primary feeling is likely to stem from sensory and emotional overload of some kind.

When working with the preverbal infant or toddler, being empathic is especially difficult because the child cannot understand one's words even when one interprets her experience accurately. Nor can she use words to let others know what she is experiencing; the only clue may be a certain feeling tone in her body. It is one's emotional tone and attitude, rather than one's words, that communicate empathy to the preverbal child. A parent or clinician can convey empathy through facial expressions, gestures, and vocal tones that pick up the child's feeling states and convey understanding of them. When a child is feeling angry and belligerent, her empathetic expectations of the adult will be different than when she is frightened and overloaded, and these circumstances require different empathic responses. The angry child who starts to throw toys around may benefit from a firm, steady look that says, "You can't do that in here, and I'm here to make sure you can't." The frightened child may benefit from a gentle, tender manner and a concerned look that says, "I know it's scary."

In addition to demonstrating empathy, the adult should help the verbal child identify his core assumptions. Examples of core assumptions are "I shouldn't experience any pain" and "I'm entitled to escape whenever I feel uncomfortable." The parent or clinician needs to understand that the child's assumptions serve some important function for him. By learning to characterize his own assumptions, the child can begin to understand why he is doing the things he is doing.

Step four, breaking each challenge down into small steps, is critical for children with regulatory disorders. These children require more and smaller steps than many others; they can only put one toe in the water at a time. Whether a child's symptoms involve eating or sleeping problems, difficulty joining group activities, lack of assertiveness, temper tantrums, or inattentiveness, therapists and teachers need to develop a hierarchy of small steps, each of which is manageable for the child. If the child cannot manage the first step, it can be broken down into 10 smaller steps. The most important challenge for the child with a regulatory disorder is to transform her sense of standing still or sliding backward into a sense that she is making progress. It does not matter how small the steps are, as long as she can feel herself moving forward.

The fifth intervention step involves establishing a structure for the child that incorporates limits on disruptive behavior and incentives to work on the small steps that have been set up. Children with regulatory disorders may seem so overwhelmed, helpless, and unhappy that parents, clinicians, and teachers feel reluctant to set limits. However, limits on problematic behavior create a sense of security: the child knows that his aggressiveness cannot get out of control and that his environment cannot be completely manipulated by him. It is important to make limits sufficiently broad: one prohibits not only "biting" or "hitting" but instead "hurting other people." In addition, limits must be set in areas where one is fairly certain the child has the ability to stay within them. A child who has insufficient motor control to keep his food from falling on the floor will not benefit from limits related to eating more neatly. Another child with better motor planning abilities and coordination who ends up with food on the floor after each meal may indeed improve his eating habits with the help of such limits. Although it is generally important to set limits on children's capacity for or interest in hurting others and breaking objects, all other limits should be tailored to each child's capacities. Moreover, in most cases it is best to establish limits in only one or two areas at a time rather to than fight battles on four or five fronts at once.

Along with setting limits, one can provide incentives. These can take the form of stars, stickers, special privileges, or just expressions of warm admiration. Limits and external incentives can help a child progress toward a goal, particularly when she has not made that goal her own and therefore feels no motivation to achieve it for its own sake.

It is important to choose limits that do not compromise the first four intervention steps. A sanction that involves isolating the child and reducing his level of engagement with others will be unhelpful in the long run, as will a limit that is so concrete that it undermines the child's problem-solving abilities. Useful limits often arise out of problem-solving discussions during which the parent helps the child anticipate when he is likely to end up receiving limits and what the reasons for those limits will be. Once the child has done something that merits a limit, the parent can express empathy for his problem of having dug himself into a hole and having to be sanctioned.

As discussed in earlier chapters, every time limits or sanctions are introduced, Floortime should be increased. This important principle is especially hard to follow for parents and teachers of children with regulatory disorders, because the children tend to create a feeling of frenzied helplessness in the adults around them. The adults find themselves in continual power struggles with the children, forgetting that only a small percentage of time should be spent on limits. If a child is defeating the limits that have been set, it is necessary to find better and more effective limits rather than to spend more time futilely trying to enforce established ones. A good balance between setting limits and following the child's lead in Floortime is essential.

Sleep Problems

Sleep problems are extremely common in children; many bookstores devote a whole shelf to books advising parents on this topic. Most of these (Ferber 1985; Mindell 1997) offer a variation on the "cry-it-out" approach: let the child cry in bed for some period of time, say 5–10 minutes, then briefly look in to reassure her (and oneself) that she is okay, then leave her for a slightly longer period of time, and so on. Eventually, she will begin falling asleep without a parent present. This approach assumes that the child can indeed soothe herself to sleep but will not learn to self-regulate in this area as long as the parents remain continuously available.

At the other end of the spectrum (e.g., Sears 1999), parents are advised to take the child into their own bed and allow him to fall asleep beside them, offering whatever warm and supportive interventions prove helpful in soothing him to sleep. This approach assumes that the child will rely on the parents' presence and warmth as long as he needs to and will begin sleeping more independently when he is able.

A greater awareness of regulatory variations among children, however, points the way to an individualized approach in which parents attempt to figure out what is interfering with their child's sleep. The factors that interfere with sleeping are likely to interfere with other aspects of the child's development as well; identifying and altering these factors may be the easiest and most effective way to help the child not only sleep better but also mobilize her progressive developmental tendencies in general.

Many things can disrupt the sleep of a child who has a regulatory disorder. Common, day-to-day experiences will often upset his already fragile equilibrium. Exciting activities, especially late in the day, can make it hard for him to settle and sleep well. In children with dietary sensitivities, certain foods, especially if eaten late in the day, can disturb sleep. The texture or smell of sleepwear or bedding sometimes turns out to be the culprit. Other possible causes that must be considered include physical illness and side effects of medications. Some family interaction patterns, such as overstimulation, overprotectiveness, anxiety-ridden interactions, and marital conflicts, also can contribute to sleep disturbances.

When no simple cause can be identified, or when multiple causes are found but addressing them fails to help the child sleep through the night, the six-step DIR intervention approach may work. The parents begin using Floortime to help their child play out or discuss, in the light of day, whatever scary feelings she may be having at night. During Floortime, the child can get her dependency needs met in an atmosphere of warmth, intimacy, and collaboration with her parents, instead of demanding to have her needs met during nighttime power struggles. Through problem-solving time, the parents can help her develop initiative and mobilize her self-regulatory capacities. If a child has become accustomed to her parents taking care of her every need during the day, it is hardly surprising if she wakes up at night with the same expectation. As described in Chapter 4 ("Therapeutic Principles"), parents can use Floortime and problem-solving time to interact with their child in ways that foster her initiative. It is important that the parents facilitate, rather than block, the child's expression of feelings related to intimacy and aggression, especially anger about unmet dependency needs. A verbal child can be helped to describe how she feels upon waking alone in the middle of the night (if she can remember) and to anticipate how she is likely to feel the next night. Pretend play using animals and dolls to rehearse the nighttime situation will enable the empathic adult, by observing what scenarios the child creates, to discern the child's assumptions (for example, "Other people should help me when I feel uncomfortable").

The parent can then establish a goal: the child will learn to regulate himself during the day and the night. If the child is verbal, the specifics can be negotiated with or explained to him during problem-solving time. As always—and especially critical for the child with regulatory difficulties—the goal should be broken down into a series of small steps: if the child is waking up six times at night, the parents will start getting up and going to him only five of those times, then four, then three, then two, then one, then none. During the daytime, the parents can allow him to begin doing a few things for himself that he has been depending on them to do (e.g., picking up a toy that he drops, picking himself up after a minor fall). Once he is doing these things regularly, more tasks can be added to the list.

The goals, steps, and limits that are likely to succeed will vary depending on the regulatory profile of the child and the personalities of the parents. Parents who have a symbiotic orientation toward their children almost always need to take a very gradual approach to solving sleep problems. In such families, it often works best for a parent to stay in the child's room at first. The parent may progress from picking the child up when she wakes, to leaving her in bed and rubbing her back, to soothing her with kind words, to simply being present beside her bed. Alternatively, the parent can lie down on a cot in view of the child for the entire night. The parent must eventually extricate himself from the room entirely if the child is to learn to get back to sleep independently, but the weaning can be made so gradual that she may only whimper or cry for a few minutes when the parent does leave the room. Parents who feel more comfortable letting a child cry can break the goal of independent sleep into fewer steps. Such parents might start by leaving the room for 5–10 minutes before returning to check in, then increasing the interval to 15 or 20 minutes and so on.

Clinicians must be flexible in order to develop approaches that fit the needs of each child and family. The popular "tough-it-out" approach to sleep is seldom appropriate for children with severe regulatory disorders: they tend to cry for hours. Furthermore, parents cannot follow through on any plan that requires them to behave in ways that are very uncomfortable for them, nor should they be expected to. There are many ways to help a child learn better self-regulatory skills. For each child, an approach can be developed that will help him to feel warmly engaged and to practice assertiveness and self-regulatory skills during the day, while giving him experience in regulating his sleep at night, particularly in falling back asleep after waking up.

Eating Problems

Eating problems, like sleep problems, can be tackled in small steps using the six-step intervention approach. Again, parents or clinicians must recognize the regulatory component of the problem and carefully assess its nature and causes before attempting to intervene. Some children are extremely sensitive to certain textures and smells. For a child who has extreme tactile sensitivity around the mouth, or one who has difficulty chewing food because of low muscle tone or difficulties with motor planning, eating will be a far more difficult, unpleasant task than it is for the average person. Parents should experiment with different textures and odors and show their child that he can vary these; in this way, the child will learn that he can exercise some control over the eating situation and find ways to enjoy it. It is important that eating become pleasurable for these children. Involving an older child in menu planning and grocery shopping often helps. If a child's mouth is tactilely hypersensitive, the parent or clinician can use a thumb to apply deep pressure to his pallet before he eats: short bursts of pressure help to normalize sensation. As with any regulatory problem, parents should help the verbal child anticipate how he is likely to feel and behave during meals and in other situations involving food.

Attentional Problems

In a scenario that has become increasingly common, a young child is brought for evaluation by her parents because her teacher has advised them that she is "hyperactive" and "inattentive" in school and "needs medication" in order to focus. However, an attentional disorder is not a unitary entity: very different regulatory and interactional problems can give rise to similar "hyperactive" and "inattentive" behaviors. Medication may help one child but do nothing for another. A thorough assessment, with close attention to the child's self-regulatory strengths and vulnerabilities, is needed to determine the precise nature of and reasons for her inattentiveness.

As we saw in Chapter 5 ("Parent-Oriented Developmental Therapy"), the child who is inattentive, by definition, does not close many circles of communication. To be effective, intervention must give such a child a great deal of practice completing circles in the context of warm, supportive relationships with parents, teachers, and other significant adults. The goal is for the child to use purposeful activity and purposeful thought and to string together activities and thoughts as a way of sustaining attention. The strategies that are likely to prove successful in this area will differ from child to child, depending on the particular regulatory and interactional vulnerabilities that underlie the child's symptoms.

The following example illustrates how a clinician can employ a regulatory perspective in evaluating and treating children with attentional problems.

> Jacob, age 6 years, is referred by his teacher for an evaluation because he "spaces out" in school and gets "hyper" and "distracted" in groups. Although he can play calmly with a parent or with one friend at home, he has trouble in school, at birthday parties, and even when two or three peers come over to play.
>
> At the first evaluation session, Jacob comes in, says "hi," and looks warmly at the therapist. After an exchange of greetings, Jacob asks where the toys are. "Well, there are some toys in that closet," the therapist says. "Can I play with them?" "Oh, sure." Jacob goes to the closet and opens it. "What do you want to play with?" asks the therapist. Jacob takes out three or four trucks and starts rolling and crashing

them. The therapist comments, "Gee, it's fun to explore." Jacob then picks up a transformer truck and asks, "Do you know how this works?" He starts trying to figure out how the different parts of the truck relate to each other. "Can you help?" he asks the therapist. "Where do you need help?" "I don't know quite how to change this part." "Could you show me how you think it could be changed?" the therapist asks, and the two work on the truck together for a time. As the play session progresses, Jacob responds easily to questions about his family and peers. "My little sister makes me mad sometimes," he says. "What makes you mad?" "Well, she bugs me. She takes my toys and stuff." At school, he does not like it when other kids "poke fun at me" and "call me names." What he really likes, he says, is to go out with his father on Sundays. He spends some time describing the things he and his father do together.

Later in the session, Jacob draws. The therapist notes that his fine motor control lags behind his general intelligence. As the therapist and Jacob explore what happens at school, it becomes clear that Jacob has trouble comprehending complex questions and that, at times, he gives up trying to do so, opting instead to take a passive stance in the conversation, avoid the topic under discussion, or escape into fantasy.

At the end of the session, what else has the therapist learned? One on one, Jacob demonstrates many age-appropriate capacities. He is focused and attentive, engaged and related. He uses complex intentional gestures and represents wishes and feelings in an elaborate and organized manner. He gives hints of having difficulty with competition and aggression (e.g., "other kids poke fun at me"), but further evaluation is needed to determine how he handles these and other emotional themes. In getting Jacob's history from his parents, the therapist learns that Jacob has always had some trouble with auditory processing and fine motor skills. He is also hypersensitive to touch and therefore easily gets overloaded by tactile input; when he feels overwhelmed, he tends to withdraw and look distracted. Clearly, there are regulatory components to Jacob's attentional difficulties. His parents are warm and supportive. They are able to address complex feelings with Jacob in the symbolic mode, as evidenced in part by his ability to describe feeling "angry" or "needy."

Based on the information gleaned from the clinical evaluation sessions, history, and observation of the family, the clinician decides to intervene on several fronts at once. He organizes a program to remediate Jacob's constitutional-maturational difficulties: a speech pathologist will work with Jacob on auditory processing, and an occupational therapist will work on motor planning, fine motor control, and sensory reactivity. The clinician will help the school to adjust to Jacob and to teach him in ways that best fit his information-processing tendencies. When Jacob's parents and teacher ask about medication for him, the clinician suggests that this issue be put on hold while they see what can be accomplished through a psychotherapeutic and educational program.

The clinician will coach Jacob's parents in floor-time and problem-solving approaches that can help Jacob learn to attend and focus even when he is feeling anxious. The clinician will also help the parents to become aware of their own feelings and of any counterproductive patterns in their interactions with Jacob (e.g., over-stimulating him, withdrawing from him, being too concrete with him) that may interfere with his ability to complete circles of communication.

Working directly with Jacob, the clinician will help him stay organized at both the gestural and the representational levels by helping him learn to open and close increasingly long chains of communication circles. He will also help Jacob identify and label feelings that decrease his desire to stay focused and lead him to "tune out." Whenever a child has both constitutional-maturational problems and maladaptive responses to anxiety, these challenges will interact, and both need to be dealt with.

The therapist notices that when he and Jacob discuss a subject that makes Jacob uncomfortable, Jacob stops completing circles. The manner in which a child's processing difficulties and ways of coping with anxiety combine to produce "inattentive" behavior can be seen in the following exchange. As Jacob and the therapist talk about a situation at school, Jacob abruptly reaches for the transformer truck and begins examining it. The therapist says, "Gee, since you were telling me about school, I'd like to hear more about what happens there." Jacob says, "Oh, look at this transformer!" "It's an interesting transformer, but we were talking about school and your friends." "Oh! Can I play with that game over there?" No doubt Jacob's auditory processing vulnerability plays some role in his continuing to ignore what the therapist says. In addition, however, he is deliberately avoiding the topic of what happened at school. In a sense, Jacob intensifies his processing weakness whenever he feels anxious.

At this point, the therapist can try engaging Jacob in self-observation about the communication process, rather than the content: "Gee, let's see if I've got this right: I want to talk about your friends and school, but you would prefer to ignore that I'm even asking you the question and just play the game." Jacob might confirm or deny the statement, thus successfully closing a circle, but he might ignore the statement and continue talking about the game. The therapist could then focus on a new theme: how Jacob has such a hard time completing a circle, and how a complex statement containing three or four sentences seems to make him feel lost. The therapist might ask, "When I ask you a question, what happens to your thoughts?" Jacob might answer, "My mind is just empty. I feel lost." As the therapist shifts gears again and helps Jacob describe how he feels lost, the two can progress to looking at different situations and feelings that make him feel lost and then to considering how he behaves when he feels this way.

The therapist will also coach the parents in keeping the logic of conversations going with Jacob by closing circles with him. When Jacob goes off on a tangent, the parents, like the therapist, must address with Jacob the process he is using to cope with information and interaction. The parent can acknowledge to Jacob that he seems to prefer talking about something else, or that he seems lost, and then try to bring Jacob back to the original topic. If Jacob says, "I don't want to talk about that!" he has closed the circle. He is getting practice in logical thinking and communication; he has identified and voiced an intention; and he has, for the moment, stopped "spacing out."

In working with parents, the therapist should help them determine which emotional themes trigger their child's avoidant behavior. Is she more likely to cut off communication when discussing rivalry with peers, the teacher's disapproval of her, or her feeling of being overwhelmed by all the noise in her classroom? Therapist and parents can explore with the child how she typically feels and behaves in whatever situations she finds overwhelming. If the problem is all the noise at school, how does she feel when people are making noise? One child described her reaction this way: "It feels like there are a thousand bees in my head. I can't hear anything else, and I don't know what I'm doing. It's awful." A therapist could respond, "Well, tell me more about what that awful feeling is like" and proceed to help the child describe the feeling using as many metaphors as she can. The better and more extended a description she gives, the more she learns to understand and anticipate the painful feeling. Equally important, she is getting practice in staying with the feeling instead of escaping it by withdrawing and "spacing out." She can then be helped to consider what maneuvers she typically uses to flee from such feelings. It is important for parents (and therapists) to understand that a child's ability to identify and describe her tendencies does not mean that they are deliberate or that there is no constitutional-maturational component to her difficulties. It only means that she can use her capacities for self-observation and symbolization to become more flexible in her coping style.

Like "spacey" behavior, the forgetfulness displayed by many children with attentional problems can reflect both processing difficulties and the child's maladaptive ways of coping with anxiety. A focused, well-organized child tends to ask himself questions throughout the day, especially at transitions such as the end of the school day: "What homework do I have to do tonight? Which books do I need to take home? Do I have my sweater with me?" The forgetful, inattentive child fails to cue himself in this way; he simply walks out of school thinking about the green leaves on the trees outside or the friend he wants to talk to on the school bus. The books he needs for his homework do not enter his thoughts until an angry parent is standing over him, yelling. In our clinical work with inattentive children, we have noticed that as the children learn to ask themselves these rhetorical questions, their apparent inattentiveness abates. It is equally important, however, to help the child become aware of his own desire to be forgetful, avoidant, or passive in response to painful feelings. One child put it beautifully: "When the work gets too hard and too much, I just chuck it over my back by forgetting everything."

The role of self-cuing in the ability to attend suggests that attention and concentration are not a natural ability but rather an active process that depends on logical, purposeful thinking. Because many "inattentive" children can think quite logically and purposefully, particularly when they are highly motivated, they may be more capable than is commonly thought of applying the same active thinking process to transitions throughout the day.

Mood Dysregulation: A Unique Type of Interactive and Mixed Regulatory-Sensory Processing Disorder Characterized by Bipolar Patterns

In recent years, there has been growing interest in early identification and treatment of bipolar-type mood dysregulation in children (Carlson and Weintraub

1993; Cytryn and McKnew 1974; Egland et al. 1987; Geller et al. 2001; Lish et al. 1994; Radke-Yarrow et al. 1992). In children, manic or hypomanic states often cause aggressive behavior or agitation rather than the frantic, grandiose thinking commonly seen in adults. Diagnosing bipolar patterns in children is therefore difficult (Harrington et al. 1991; Strober et al. 1988). We do not have a clear understanding of the antecedent variables leading to bipolar disorder in children, although a host of neuropsychological vulnerabilities or deficits has been suggested, including problems in the areas of language, motor development, perception, executive functioning, and social functioning (Castillo et al. 2000; Sigurdsson et al. 1999). Furthermore, a comprehensive intervention program that addresses family interactions and educational issues as well as biochemical treatments has not been formulated.

We propose a novel hypothesis: bipolar patterns in children can be understood as arising from a unique configuration of antecedents involving sensory processing and motor functioning, early child–caregiver interaction patterns, and early states of personality organization. Specifically, we suggest that children at risk for developing bipolar-type mood dysregulation share the following characteristics:

1. An unusual processing pattern in which oversensitivity to sound, touch, or both coexists with a craving of sensory stimulation, particularly movement. This sensory craving is usually associated with high activity and aggressive, agitated, or impulsive behavior (in contrast, most oversensitive children are more fearful and cautious). Therefore, when overloaded with stimuli, oversensitive children with this unusual combination of processing differences cannot self-regulate by withdrawing, as a cautious child might. Instead, they become agitated, aggressive, and impulsive, thereby overloading themselves even more.
2. An early pattern of interaction, continuing into childhood, characterized by a lack of fully coregulated reciprocal affective exchanges. In particular, caregivers are unable to interact with the infant or child in ways that help her "upregulate" and "downregulate" her moods to modulate states of despondency and agitation.
3. A personality organization in which the fifth and sixth functional emotional levels of development have not been mastered. Emotions either are not addressed at the symbolic level, instead remaining at the level of behavior or somatic experience, or are represented as global, polarized affect states rather than in integrated form.

The DIR assessment of a child and family will determine whether the child has this combination of characteristics. A comprehensive, developmentally based intervention program must address all three issues. A program can be designed to head off the interactive experiences that intensify the child's sensory processing difficulties, and the child can be helped to understand her particular processing challenges and to prepare herself for situations in which these challenges will likely pose a problem. A child with constrictions at the early, presymbolic level of two-way affective interaction can be helped to master the capacity for long sequences of coregulated affective exchanges necessary for a more stable mood. For example, when she begins to show more agitation in her voice and movement, the therapist might deliberately shift to a more soothing, comforting tone to "downregulate" the intensity of affect. When she becomes more apathetic and self-absorbed, the therapist might employ a more energetic rhythm of preverbal and verbal exchange, speaking faster and using more animated hand gestures to "upregulate" the child's mood. The therapist might also explore, with a verbal child, how she feels during these shifts of affective rhythm and intensity. During such discussions, the child can be helped to symbolize and reflect on the feelings she is experiencing.

A child who can use words to describe actions but who cannot symbolize emotions can be helped to advance through the stages of language development described in Chapter 2 ("The Functional Emotional Stages of Development"): first, to begin using words to describe feelings as concrete entities, which are close to action and which demand action ("I'm mad," "I'm hungry"); second, to use affects as a signal of internal experience ("I feel mad," "I feel hungry"), thus making possible reflection and problem solving.

A developmentally based treatment program for a child with patterns suggesting a bipolar disorder might involve several components, including individual psychotherapy for the child, perhaps twice a week; weekly sessions with her parents to help them create a family environment that will facilitate her development; and work with the school to help staff understand and adapt to her. It might also include specialized educational programs to strengthen processing weaknesses and facilitate social and emotional growth in the school setting.

By ensuring that the parents fully understand their child's developmental profile and therapeutic goals, the therapist can increase the likelihood that they will support the long-term, comprehensive approach that is necessary to help a child with bipolar patterns. Having very specific goals that are easily understood but that nonetheless embrace complex psychological processes (e.g., the child will begin naming, and later reflecting on, intense feelings) will help the parents to participate effectively and to monitor their child's progress. The therapist will also need to help the parents work through whatever conflicts may previously have precluded a commitment to long-term therapy.

Family Interaction Patterns and Regulatory Disorders

Clinicians treating regulatory disorders in children are likely to see certain kinds of parental feelings and fantasies, caregiver–child interaction patterns, and family dynamics. Parents and other caregivers of an infant with regulatory problems commonly feel frustrated because their efforts to calm their baby and elicit his attention are unsuccessful, making it hard for them to enjoy the new relationship. The parents' frustration may escalate as their toddler, from about 15 months onward, begins to exhibit irritability, temper tantrums, and aggression. When parents cannot help a child control and regulate his own body, they often feel a profound sense of failure and conclude that they must be "bad parents." If the child wakes frequently at night, the parents are likely to feel chronically tired. When physical exhaustion is coupled with feelings of frustration and failure, the situation can become explosive, putting the child at risk of abuse. Some parents have their own histories of regulatory dysfunction; if they tend toward aggressive behavior themselves, the clinician must be alert to the possibility of physical abuse. If parents exhibit patterns of withdrawal, avoidance, and depression, the clinician must watch for various forms of neglect as well.

In families that do not experience such extremes, the clinician is likely to see one of several patterns of response by parents and caregivers to a child's regulatory difficulties. Some parents become overly controlling and punitive, insisting that the child self-regulate by adhering to certain standards that the parents have defined. They may try instituting a structure of punishments and sanctions. When the child fails to respond to their best attempts to establish control and order, they respond with increasingly punitive measures until they decide that they can go no further; it is at this point that some families seek professional help. By this time, the child's regulatory problems may have gotten so severe that the situation appears out of control.

Other parents vacillate between overly controlling, punitive responses and states of withdrawal. One day, they feel energized, determined to make their child pay attention, eat, sleep, and behave; the next day, they give up, shrug, and say, "He'll have to do this on his own, when he wants to." Some parents become very fragmented in their thinking, particularly if they have regulatory problems of their own; their behavior begins to mirror the fragmented behavior of their child. Needless to say, a fragmented set of responses by the parents, vacillating between punitive control and lack of availability, provides an extremely unstable, confusing environment for an infant or young child.

Some parents begin to feel hostility and a desire to reject their child. Such parents may be very aware of their fantasies of escape. They may voice these aloud or otherwise convey them to the child. Other parents defend against the wish to escape, because experiencing it consciously would stir guilt or other unpleasant feelings; these parents may become rigidly and somewhat mechanically nurturing toward their child. They are likely to feel highly anxious and to overprotect the child, denying her the opportunity to develop self-sufficiency. Even parents who lack the underlying wish to flee sometimes transform their frustration into anxiety and overprotective behavior.

Any of the parental responses we have described can intensify the child's difficulties with self-regulation. When parents respond in erratic, labile, fragmented ways, an infant or child becomes more erratic and labile than he might otherwise be. When parents are overly punitive and controlling, the child may escalate his negative, avoidant, or defiant behavior. Parents who are anxiously overprotective and controlling may elicit passive, compliant, or avoidant patterns.

In families coping with regulatory dysfunction, family dynamics may take on characteristic patterns that extend beyond the parent–child relationship. In many such families (particularly those in which the mother assumes most of the responsibility for childrearing), the mother feels chronically exhausted and the father feels neglected and spends as much time as possible at his workplace to avoid the battle zone of the family. Mother then feels neglected and unsupported by father. Each feels that the other is not caring or nurturing enough, there is no sexual intimacy or warmth between them, and they become highly critical of one another. The anger they both feel toward the child may get displaced onto each other; their anger at each other may get played out toward the child. Older siblings can be drawn into this pattern, too: they feel ignored on one hand and frazzled and caught up in the chaos on the other. They may begin to behave in challenging ways themselves.

Bear in mind that although we have identified family patterns that commonly accompany regulatory dysfunction, this is by no means an exhaustive list of possibilities. Each child and each family is unique, and there are an infinite number of variations in parental fantasies, parent–child interactions, and family dynamics. Whatever the patterns identified, it is critical to work with each of them at the same time as one addresses the child's constitutional-maturational challenges. Using the approaches we have described in this book, one works with the parents and child to strengthen the child's constitutional-maturational capacities and to foster more flexible, age-appropriate patterns of relating. As the infant or child is helped to negotiate each of the six core developmental capacities, to incorporate the full range of emotional themes in her relationships, and to strengthen her constitutional-maturational capacities for attention, engagement, and information processing, the pressures on the family will decrease. At the same time, in separate meetings with the parents, the clinician helps them explore and understand their own feelings, especially their feelings toward their child, as well as their interactions with each other and the family dynamics as a whole. By working on both fronts at once, one can help the parents begin to feel hope and to experience gradual improvement in family functioning.

For infants and young children who evidence significant constitutional-maturational variation as part of their regulatory disorders, it is very helpful to arrange at least a consultation with an occupational therapist trained in sensory integration work. The occupational therapist can evaluate the contributions of sensory over- or underreactivity, sensory processing, muscle tone, and motor planning difficulties to the child's regulatory disorder. In addition to providing a better understanding of the child's symptoms, and thus a more complete picture of the kinds of intervention needed, the occupational therapy consultation can help self-blaming parents begin to understand that their child has certain characteristics of which they may have been unaware and that these have made their job as parents especially challenging. Parents who have been mystified by their child's seemingly inexplicable responses and behaviors can begin to feel hope as they learn that there are specific reasons for their child's troubles and specific interventions that can help.

The amount of occupational therapy involvement that should be arranged, beyond the initial consultation, will depend on the clinician's own skill in working with sensory and motor patterns, the severity of the child's constitutional-maturational challenges, and the degree to which the parents are gifted and diligent in carrying out initial suggestions. Where a child has a significant developmental delay involving muscle tone or motor planning, however, it is almost always useful to arrange follow-up occupational therapy sessions. If sensory reactivity problems are extremely severe, it is useful to have the occupational therapist play a very active role and participate in follow-up meetings with the parents and the clinician.

Where the child evidences receptive or expressive language impairments, speech pathologists should also be consulted during the assessment phase. Depending on the severity of the impairments, the family's competencies, and the clinician's experience in working with language development, the speech pathologist may need to play a role in the treatment phase as well.

Case Illustrations

Justin

When 4½-month-old Justin was brought to me (S.W.), mother explained that they were worried because he cried excessively (despite a pacifier) and needed to be held "all the time." When upset, he was hard to comfort even when held; he flailed his arms and disliked being on his back. He woke up four times a night and had a hard time getting back to sleep. Father added that Justin seemed to prefer looking around at his environment to interacting with his parents.

Justin was a reserved child; it was hard for anyone to get him to smile. He looked at us but did not reach out with a smile or any other expression. When offered a pen or a shiny object, such as a spoon, he would increase his attention on the object and the person holding it and smile faintly, but he never reached out. He did watch his parents' movements, such as when his father left the room and when his mother switched chairs.

Mother reported that Justin cried if she put him down, and if she then left the room, he'd cry even harder. She felt that he was not relating to her much and that it would get worse when she went back to work in 3 weeks. Their live-in helper, who was not present at this meeting, had similar patterns with Justin, mother thought.

The pregnancy and delivery had been unremarkable. Justin's birth weight was 8.5 lb and his Apgar scores were 9/9. They left the hospital after a few days, and

Justin had been physically healthy since. Mother reported that he had good muscle tone after he was born; he could hold his head up and put his hands in his mouth. He ate well and was gaining weight.

As I observed mother interacting with Justin, I saw that she used an intermittent fast tone followed by complete silence, then another fast tone and silence. She tried putting a rattle in his hand; he eventually took it and looked at it. He got upset when mother moved him up and down, and when she stroked his arms to relax him, he was clearly uncomfortable, evidencing some tactile sensitivity. When father took Justin, he did not try to interact with him much, he just held him on the shoulder and comforted him.

Upon examination, I found that Justin had slightly low muscle tone and showed a slight delay in motor development in terms of his ability to hold his head up securely, but he coordinated his arm movements with things he was interested in. He was quite sensitive to touch on his back and a little less so on his arms and legs. He could respond to a range of vocalizations at both high and low pitches but needed a lot of vocal input before he looked and smiled a bit; he seemed to be somewhat underreactive to vocalizations (although he did not become distant when vocal cadences got complicated). He responded best to steady, persistent vocalizations of a medium pitch and volume. With facial animation, he was also under- rather than overreactive; he did better with a lot of animation, which made him look and smile more. He responded reasonably well to a range of lighting situations, without any difficulty with bright lights.

My impression was of a baby at some risk: slightly low motor tone and slow in motor development, reserved and somewhat underreactive to auditory and visual input and overreactive to touch. Mother was worried and clumsy in her interaction patterns, unconfident in her wooing ability, and was planning to go back to work. In this session, I did not learn much about mother's own background and why she was uncomfortable with the baby. Father seemed uncomfortable as well, but more easily satisfied by whatever small comfort Justin achieved.

We discussed Justin's reactivity pattern and his need for a lot of persistent, calm, and slow auditory and visual input, and that he needed to be held firmly and not rubbed lightly on the back or the arms (he tolerated light touch better on the abdomen, however). We discovered that he responded slightly better when I bounced him in my lap and then hugged him. His attention also improved with gross motor activity and joint compression along with firm pressure. I demonstrated how to get him to smile more deeply with persistent overtures—I used vocalizations and interesting facial expressions as well as firm pressure on the back or arms, and bouncing in the lap followed by joint compression.

Toward the end of the session, mother talked about wanting Justin to be less clingy; she wanted him to love her, but she also wanted to get back to work full-time as soon as possible. She explained that her income was essential for the household, to "put food on the table," but admitted that she could begin at half-time and gradually work up to five-eighths time so that she could be home a large part of the afternoon. I agreed that this was a good idea, given that she and Justin were still working out their relationship patterns. Both of them would feel more comfortable with more time together. I also suggested that mother and baby work on interaction patterns with a colleague of mine a few times a week, so that mother could learn to help Justin calm down and be more attentive and engaged, using the procedures we had discussed.

After working on their patterns, mother returned with Justin 6 weeks later. She said that he still cried a lot when he was alone and was easily frustrated, but she was pleased that he was trying to crawl and was relating to her more, looking and smiling and even interacting a bit. However, he still woke up four or five times a night; mother and father were becoming exhausted. Also, despite his increased interaction, Justin often would not look at mother: "Particularly when I come home from work, he will ignore me for the first hour or so. He takes a long time to warm up." I empathized, pointing out that Justin was a reserved baby and was probably still very sensitive to separation. Rather than showing his sensitivity through anger, he showed it through withdrawal.

As they played together, I observed that Justin was much more engaging and smiling than when he came in the first time. When his mother talked to him for a minute or two, he responded well with a nice organized look and a big smile. He had a pattern of smiling and looking for a few seconds, then looking away for a second or two, then coming back. He seemed to need a break from intense looking and smiling more often than other babies his age; although he needed a lot of wooing and input, he got overloaded more quickly than other babies. Many underreactive babies can sustain their attentiveness and pleasure once they are engaged, whereas overly sensitive babies will tune out after just a few seconds of engagement. Justin had some elements of both; he had a narrow zone that took him a long time to get to, then he could focus and enjoy. Yet when he got overloaded, he needed time out to regroup.

Justin looked at and followed his mother as she moved around the office. He followed toys to the floor and handed his rattle to mother. She took it, looked at it, and handed it back to him. He also reached for a little, brightly colored toy globe that could spin around, and he and mother smiled as they exchanged it with each other. However, mother was still quite uncomfortable interacting with him; she alternated between nice moments and passive silence. She would look confused and overload Justin with too quick a cadence of words or hand him too many things in a row. She could slow down and maintain a nice reciprocal rhythm for isolated moments, then she acted awkwardly. When she went too fast or withdrew, Justin tuned out quickly and looked blankly around the room, unfocused and disinterested. Nonetheless, they had made impressive gains.

Father did not come to this session. Mother thought that he felt too uncomfortable to participate and reported that he had been doing a lot of holding and cuddling but was reluctant to try more interaction.

I spoke with mother about her history. She said that she had been an only child of aloof, formal parents. She suspected that her mother had been depressed during her childhood and that there was a family history of depression, but she was not sure because the family was so "secretive and closed." She felt that she and her husband had a friendship—"We don't fight very much"—but not a deep or passionate relationship. Her background made her feel ill-prepared for a baby who was "changing his mind all the time." I empathized with how hard it must be, with no preparation in terms of younger brothers and sisters to take care of, to be the mother of a challenging baby. We talked about how she and Justin could learn about relationships together, and she seemed reassured by this idea.

When I saw Justin as an 8-month-old, mother was still worried about his lack of sustained attention. "He doesn't attend to me as long as I would like," she said. "He looks at me, may smile at me and may even interact, but then he looks away."

The live-in housekeeper was also at this session; mother was worried that Justin attended longer and seemed to respond more deeply to this helper, who spent the greater part of the day with him because mother was working.

Mother reported that Justin was crying less and played a little more independently. He was also sleeping better, and mother was more comfortable letting him cry on his own at night if he woke up, because he could now cry himself back to sleep after 5 minutes or so. She would look in on him to see if he could settle himself down and only had to go in to him two or three times a night rather than four or five. Justin continued to be a good eater.

Watching mother play with him, I saw that she still had the pattern of intruding—using quick vocalizations, trying to force him to hold something, or handing him too many objects in a row—and then becoming passive. She had the same anxious quality as before, and an uneven rhythm, although she vocalized her discomfort. When she overwhelmed him, Justin would turn from her and look around the room, then try to look back to her and smile and engage. Nevertheless, they had some moments of warm engagement when exchanging objects, smiles, or sounds.

I then watched the housekeeper interact with Justin. She was very laid back but could persistently woo and engage him. They had wonderful, warm, mutually attentive engagements, with peek-a-boo games and exchanges of objects and smiles. He disengaged less from her than from mother, and only after 30 or 40 seconds of engagement. When he looked away, she would calmly re-engage him. She seemed ideally suited to him.

Playing with me, Justin was very happy and vocal and motorically interactive. He smiled deeply and was highly contingent. His motor tone was improving and he tolerated a little more touch on his arms and back. I could hold his attention for a full minute, and he gave me several deep smiles, particularly if I sat him on my lap, bouncing and holding him firmly on his arms, with my fingers on his back. He responded to a wide range of vocalizations and facial expressions and engaged me in peek-a-boo. We handed various objects back and forth, and he was generally flirtatious, with subtle smiles.

I got down on the floor with him and noticed that he was not quite yet able to crawl. He reached objects by slithering forward. When I went head-to-head with him, he assertively moved toward me; he seemed to enjoy being on his stomach and interacting from that position. I had mother and the housekeeper interact with him that way, too. Mother felt uncomfortable but was willing to practice; the housekeeper felt more at ease with it. We talked about giving Justin more practice now that his motor tone was better and he was almost ready to crawl.

Mother surprised me by saying that she was thinking of stopping work entirely, or reducing her time, in order to form the relationship she wanted with her baby. She thought that she and her husband could afford it after all, because they had some savings. Without pressuring her, I empathized with the pleasure I thought she would be having being close to the baby during this special time in his life and supported her in considering all the options. I also helped her elaborate on her worries about not being a good mother. She said, "If I do stay home and still can't get into a good relationship with him, then I really will feel terrible." When I asked her in what way she would feel terrible, she talked about times in her childhood when she felt clumsy and couldn't get other children to like her; she felt she hadn't had the natural abilities that other children had. She now blamed this on her parents for being so formal and uncomfortable with their emotions. Mother then had some very warm interactions with Justin. I drew her attention to them, and she smiled and became hopeful that they could learn to be close together.

Mother returned when Justin was 10 months old. She reported that he was continuing to make progress: he was now sleeping through the night (although there had been a few difficult evenings, when she had let him cry for 15–20 minutes, before he adjusted). She felt more confident in helping him to take this final step, because he was more adept at self-calming and more independent. (In general, it is more helpful to work on mastering separation challenges "in the light of day" before attempting to address the same issue in the evening.)

In this visit, mother talked again about leaving work entirely. She had already reduced her work schedule back to half-time from two-thirds. She was also contemplating getting pregnant again, so that by the time Justin was 2 years old he might have a brother or sister. She seemed comfortable with these plans and hoped that she and Justin would become even closer once she was home with him full-time. She reflected on her jealousy toward the caregiver, but in a constructive way, admitting, "I can't expect him to prefer me if I'm not home with him as much as she is."

While they played, mother picked up a doll that Justin was investigating. She rocked it close to her, and he crawled over and grabbed at it. They had a very interesting interaction: mother was talking to the doll and vocalizing for it, but soon after Justin came over to play with it, she got distracted and tuned him out; she looked for another toy rather than staying with the first one. I pointed out, "You just had a beautiful moment, but then for some reason you decided to disengage. This time, you did it before Justin did it to you." Mother said that she had not been aware of it, but on reflection, she wondered whether she was doing to Justin exactly what he did to her. She thought that perhaps she did this at home, too, that she had become so sensitive to his rejection that she rejected him first. She realized that she did this only in the microcosm of play, because she was dutifully attentive to him generally. She remembered how sensitive she was as a teenager to boys not liking her or rejecting her. "I would often try not to like them first," she said.

Shortly afterward, Justin crawled over to mother and started touching a Snoopy doll just as she touched it. Mother spontaneously made Snoopy talk to him, making silly sounds and asking, "Do you want to give me a hug?" Much to the surprise of me and mother, Justin looked, smiled, and started imitating the sounds mother was making for Snoopy—"ga-ga, boo-boo," and "da-da" and "ma-ma"—although he could not repeat the exact words mother used. This was by far their best interaction ever, and a momentous occasion. Mother smiled deeply and warmly and for the first time felt "fully like a mommy," as she told me later. It was not so much that Justin had imitated her words, but that the level of warmth and connectedness between them was deeper than ever before. Mother's relaxation and creativity in the way she made Snoopy talk had drawn Justin in for this wonderful moment, in which they had not only cause-and-effect interaction but also emotion, vocalization, motor manipulation, and the beginning of a psychological drama.

After this interaction, Justin was his usual self. He disengaged and relaxed for a while, looking at different things. When he rejoined mother with nice reciprocal behavior, vocalizations, and emotional gestures, she was able to stay with him. They exchanged sounds together directly—"ba-ba," "da-da," and "ma-ma"—and then played a little game of hiding and saying "bye-bye." Justin tried to find mother when she hid behind a chair, playing out separation themes in the safety of the office.

As they played, the same subtle disengagement issue emerged. Sometimes in the middle of peek-a-boo, or chasing his mother behind the chair, Justin would disengage and get distracted by something else. Mother would look pained for a second, then turn away from him and start talking to me, or fumble in her purse for something. When Justin turned and looked eagerly at her, ready to reengage, she was still preoccupied. Mother was missing the fact that Justin needed to take time out when he got overexcited; his disengagement was a way to take a break, but she took it as rejection. When I pointed this out to her, she was able to see it much more readily, and related a few instances at home when she felt she might have done the same thing. She was much more self-observant now and could regroup more quickly.

We discussed how she could remain engaged so that Justin could take his time out and then reengage. They were already successfully sustaining periods of engagement, as well as adding on periods of shared attention. They had nice, complex two-way communication patterns in which Justin opened and closed at least four or five circles in a row and used motor actions, vocalizations, and a range of emotion; he was looking more and more age appropriate.

Mother continued her progress, and about 6 weeks later she stopped working entirely. She felt more relaxed and self-assured as a mother and more comfortable with spontaneous emotion. Although father did not rejoin our sessions, mother reported that their relationship was better and warmer, and she was more comfortable taking the lead and drawing father in.

They returned when Justin was 14 months old; he was walking now and went immediately for some toys. He became fascinated with a toy whale. Mother jokingly started a game, saying that she was hiding the whale and putting it behind my chair. Justin made some wonderful facial gestures, looking puzzled and curious, and then started searching. He found the whale and brought it to mother. When I asked if he would bring it to me too, he grinned and giggled and brought it to me. I said, "The whale wants to give you a kiss," and he put his cheek up and let the whale touch him. He then took the whale and wanted to touch it to my face.

He was beginning to use a few words, like "mom" and "that." Mother reported that she had counted 20 different words already, and that his language acquisition had grown dramatically since she had stopped working. He looked more deeply content than I had seen him before, and mother felt that he had gotten "happier and happier" with her home full-time. He only occasionally woke up at night. If he cried for a while, she was comfortable in letting him cry it out, although she would go in and comfort him if she thought he was having teething pain. "He still demands my attention too much some of the time," she said, "and won't let me go out of the room. He pulls my newspaper or magazine if I am trying to read, or pulls on my leg if I am talking on the phone. He cries if I don't give him the attention he wants."

We discussed that it was time for mother to help Justin use the "distal communication modes" to learn how to be close to her even when she was not holding him. Eventually he would become more secure in his ability to comfort himself. We talked about communicating with Justin through vocalizations and facial and motor gestures when he was across the room. If mother was reading a magazine, for instance, she could look up every few minutes and make some distal communication with him while he played. She had been getting into a pattern, common to many parents, of letting him pursue her until she felt that she had to flee for a few moments of peace. Justin sensed her desire to get away, which made him more ardent in pursuing her. We came up with the idea of giving him 20 or 30 minutes of full, intense Floortime, focusing on distal communication interactions. Then mother would take an organized time out for herself, on the phone or with the newspaper, but every few minutes she would look up and interact with him using gestures and words.

In the play part of this session, mother and Justin had nice reciprocal interactions. He took a little doll and put it in the truck she was playing with and pushed it around. Then he took her hand and showed her how to put a man in the car. With a look of great satisfaction, he indicated that he wanted her to put a man in another car so that they could make a kind of train. They exchanged many affective, vocal, and motor gestures together, closing at least five or six circles in a row. Mother was pleased by the initiative and leadership Justin was showing.

Near the end of the session, mother needed further reassurance that she could set limits on Justin when, after a half-hour of Floortime and lots of distal communication, he continued to interfere with things she wanted to do. It was now appropriate for her to say "no" or "wait," and Justin could understand what these words meant. The idea of learning to wait would be an important element of their distal communication.

This case illustrates preventive intervention with a child who had risks from two sides—his low muscle tone and slightly delayed motor development and his underreactive auditory and visuospatial sensory processing patterns—which made it hard for him to engage and stay engaged. Also, his tactile sensitivity made it hard for his mother to comfort him. He was unusual in having a very narrow comfort zone for receiving information. It took a lot of visual and auditory input to woo him; he would engage for a few seconds and then become overloaded and need to disengage and look around.

His unique constitutional-maturational pattern aggravated the family's psychological patterns. Mother, due to her upbringing with very formal parents, was uncomfortable with closeness and emotion. She was very sensitive to rejection, often rejecting first before she could be rejected. Father tended toward massive avoidance when confronted with psychological challenges and was also uncomfortable with emotions. The housekeeper was much more consistent and persistent but tended toward passive comforting and did not have a lot of wooing power. Thus, Justin's own pattern made it hard for him to engage the world and led him to disengage quickly after being engaged, and mother's sensitivity to rejection and difficulty with emotions made it hard for her to woo her son.

Working with both sides of the equation enabled this family to make gradual progress. By the middle to the end of the first year, Justin was becoming increasingly richly engaged, attentive, and more interactive. He was still rather passive and reserved, finicky and fussy, and having sleep problems, and mother was still feeling uncomfortable with her mothering abilities. However, toward the beginning of the second year, Justin was taking over the interactions more and showing greater initiative. Mother became comfortable enough with her mothering role to give up work in order to prepare for a new child and to fully consolidate her relationship with Justin so that he would not be more involved with the housekeeper than with her.

This case shows how slow such progress can be, but it also shows that slow, gradual progress can be the best because mother and Justin fully worked through their differences and challenges. By the early part of the second year, they both experienced a great deal of competency. Justin was able to catch up to healthy, age-appropriate toddler patterns that included behavior and emotional complexity and interaction, built on a foundation of solid attachment and capacity for shared attention.

Justin's case illustrates the DIR approach and the use of the new classification of regulatory sensory-processing disorders. We worked to foster Justin's progression to higher levels of functional emotional development (D) by working with his individual processing differences (I) and tailoring learning relationships (R) to his individual differences and developmental level. In terms of our new classification of regulatory sensory-processing disorders, it can be seen that Justin illustrated challenges in a number of categories. He had patterns of underreactivity (sounds, Type 2); overreactivity (touch, Type 1); and muscle tone and motor planning and visual and spatial processing problems (inattentive, disorganized with both difficulties in motor planning and in sensory discrimination, Type 4). Most infants and children will show a mixture of contributions from the different subtypes of regulatory sensory processing disorders.

In this case, we observe unique opportunities presented when we can work with an infant and his or her family in the first year of life and begin addressing the regulatory sensory-processing challenges early. It enables us to help the infant and family negotiate their early functional emotional developmental capacities—that is, the foundation for healthy relationships and social and intellectual skills before problems become chronic. It also enables us to help set in motion healthy family patterns by addressing both the parents' ways of interacting with their baby and the perceptions and expectations they are beginning to form that can influence their interaction for years to come. Being present in these early formative months, therefore, provides a very valuable opportunity for preventive work. Justin continued to do well once his healthy foundations were established.

Ryan

Ryan was 22 months old when his parents first brought him to me (S.W.). Mother, a busy journalist, complained, "He refuses to eat, he's hyperactive, and he won't sleep for more than an hour or two at a time." She added that she was "depressed" and father was "frustrated and fed up." She was also worried that Ryan was very small for his age and not adequately gaining weight.

Mother reported that Ryan had had many difficulties as a baby. The pregnancy had been planned, full-term, and unremarkable. Early feeding problems, however, led to a number of evaluations and diagnostic procedures.

Ryan slept for only an hour at a time and refused to feed. One of the consultations determined that Ryan was allergic to milk and soy. He was put on Nutramagin but only took 20 ounces a day, with a little cereal added. He never slept through the night; by the time he was 4 or 5 months old, he slept for 2–3 hours, was up for a half-hour, and then went back to sleep. He remained highly distractible and irritable.

When Ryan was 15 months old he weighed only 18 pounds. He did not enjoy eating and would scream and try to get out of his chair. He also had difficulties with his attention span and activity level. Various additional consultations and elimination diets were only partially helpful and no specific cause for his ongoing challenges was found.

When I saw Ryan at 22 months, his mother's main concerns were Ryan's sleeping and eating patterns along with his activity level and irritability. "He won't sit down," she said. "But when he does, he will take three or four bites of something and then get up, and two minutes later may sit down again." She felt that she spent all her time trying to feed him. She spent much of the day running back and forth between her high-pressure job and her son. She was involved with the different helpers she had for him but wondered if she should quit her job or switch to working part-time.

Mother was understandably overwhelmed and close to tears, but she was dedicated and could "stay in there" under dire circumstances. Father was calmer and organized but more impersonal. He seemed concerned but was less involved with Ryan and separated from the day-to-day experiences of his family.

Ryan was a small 22-month-old. He seemed organized and connected to mother and to me but was bland and unenthusiastic in his relatedness, without any sense of emotional intensity or warmth. He could be purposeful in his play with toys, and intentional in his gestures and simple use of words, but about half the time he would tune out, going in and out of attention and relatedness.

Mother reported that a live-in helper had been with the family for about 9 months. She was organized, somewhat passive and sedate, and patient; she could spend an hour and a half giving Ryan his lunch, distracting him to help him eat. Distracting him was key to successfully getting him to eat; without that, mother said, "Forget it." She said he took 1.5–2 hours to fall asleep, and she would often have to stay with him for the first 45 minutes. After he woke up at 6:30 A.M., he could be hyper the rest of the day and sometimes did not even take a nap.

As she talked, mother would occasionally say things like, "I don't care about my job," "It's a no-win situation," "I can't control him," and "I don't know what to do." At times, she would throw her hands up in defeat. As I observed her playing with Ryan, I noticed that she was quite laid back but would occasionally push her face right up to his. She vacillated between being overly passive and overly intrusive. Her depression and long silences between vocalizations did not give Ryan a rhythm he could easily connect to: two or three words, long silence, then two or three more words. Her gestures had the same pattern.

Their verbal interaction seemed somewhat fragmented: "What's this?" mother asked. "Crayon," Ryan answered. "Why don't you write on this?" she directed him. Ryan picked up a doll instead, saying "Anna baby," giving it a name. Then he handed a Transformer to mother and said, "Go car." He turned to color something with the crayon, and mother said, "Make a picture for me." He was very slow, passive, and unexpressive but methodical and attending. He responded to mother with gestures and looks and had an overall sense of relatedness. For example, when mother said, "Put the lady doll in there," Ryan put the doll in a carriage. After he had picked up several dolls, mother asked him, "How many do you have?" and he counted, "One, two, three, four."

I was impressed with Ryan's gestural organization and two-way communication, but he showed little affect or enthusiasm. When mother asked him, out of the blue, "What did you tell Santa you wanted?" (it was near Christmas time), he answered, "Bike, car." Then she asked, "Where does Santa come from in the house?" and he said, "Fireplace." He was cognitively quite sophisticated and able to answer her questions. Shortly after this, he took out the whale puppet. Mother took it from him, saying, "He will bite you." Ryan took it back and then pretended that it was biting mother. Mother reacted with "Ouch!" This was their best sequence of pretend play and showed what the dyad was capable of in terms of fantasy and elaboration. In general, however, they did not match this level of representational interaction. There was a subdued quality between them, with each rather uninvolved with the other. They had some vocal and gestural interaction, but without much enthusiasm, emotional depth, or vocal intensity. Ryan generally would not close mother's circles when she verbalized; he would continue what he was doing, such as taking out toys and manipulating them or putting them in the house or into cars and carriages. Their capacity for opening and closing symbolic circles was for the most part latent, as evidenced by the sequence with the whale; this sequence also showed, perhaps, why they were a little scared of and avoided each other.

I suggested that mother engage Ryan more energetically, if it would not be too draining for her, given the effort it took to get him to eat. Mother quickly responded, "He rejected me as a baby by tuning me out and turning away, so I became passive." I found this statement very revealing. Mother was not stating it as an insight about her feelings but as a statement of fact.

Mother and son then started playing again. Ryan put a baby doll in a truck, and mother asked him if the baby wanted to go into the house. As he put the baby in the house, she said, "Very good." He then identified another toy as a "camera," and mother said, "Give it to me. I'll take a picture of the baby." He complied, and she took a picture. I observed that perhaps they were ready to develop some pride in each other.

As Ryan and father played together, they engaged well and were organized in terms of behavior and gestures. Ryan used sentences and phrases, but sometimes without clarity. For example, he said to father, "Get toy for me." Father would identify different objects, such as a car, and Ryan would nod yes or no. He was very direct in his instructions to father. Father was gentle and warm, very patient, and contingent. When Ryan was already looking at the house, he said, "Let's look at this house," and they would examine it together. As Ryan took toys out of the chest, father helped him identify them, how they worked, and whether or not they fit in the house. Father was more even and laid back than mother, and somewhat responsive, although he did not show a wide range of emotion or much enthusiasm. I asked father if he were enjoying the play, and he admitted that sometimes he found it repetitive and boring and did not usually play with Ryan. We talked about the value of his playing with Ryan at home as well.

The parents and I discussed using Floortime to work on the intensity of Ryan's engagement and affect. I mentioned that although they seemed quite related, with good two-way gestural communication with him, mother and father were not very enthusiastic when helping Ryan use emotional ideas in his play. I explained that he was available for more elaborate drama, and by joining energetically in the drama with him, they could create interactive opportunities. Ryan might then play out some of the issues on his mind, as he seemed able to play out his feelings. Mother dutifully agreed to try, and father reluctantly said he would spend more time on the floor with Ryan. He recognized that he had left a lot of the childrearing to mother, who was overwhelmed.

We also decided to try an elimination diet to see if other foods were contributing to Ryan's sleeping and eating difficulties and his irritability (which I did not observe). The different groups to withhold for 10 days, and then reintroduce as challenges, were sugars, additives, preservatives, and dyes; salicylate-containing fruit; peanuts and nuts; dairy products; eggs; soy; wheat and yeast. I suggested that they be alert to other groups to which he might be sensitive.

We decided to postpone direct treatment for Ryan's sleep disturbance. However, I recommended an occupational therapy evaluation to look for sensory reactivity difficulties, particularly in the oral area, and any other subtle issues around motor tone and motor planning.

Within a few weeks, the parents discovered that the removal of milk, eggs, and soy from Ryan's diet reduced his diarrhea and gas, his hyperactivity, and his wakefulness at night. They had not yet eliminated sugar, wheat, and fruit.

The occupational therapy evaluation and ongoing follow-up work revealed that Ryan had severe hypersensitivity to touch around his mouth and postural insecurity and insecurity with movements in space, particularly swinging, orbital and circular spinning, and movement into an inverted position. Ryan preferred self-generated movement to movement on playground equipment or by a person. The occupational therapist recommended eliminating peripheral distractions at feeding time (only a few toys would be allowed on the food tray), expanding the number of meals to three complete meals and two snacks, cutting back on Ryan's evening bottle to reduce risk if he vomited at night, and placing Ryan in his high chair and providing social interaction during feeding time.

Talking with the parents further about their own family backgrounds revealed a history of depression on mother's side but no history of mental illness on father's side. Mother delved into the subject of her depression, expressing "feelings of giving up." "I don't care," she said. "I can't make decisions." Later she added, "I'm overwhelmed emotionally." Father felt that family life was too hectic and that work was an escape. His wife was always worried and complaining, and his son's constant neediness for feeding and attention interfered with any time alone for the couple. Mother and father had had a nice, but not very intense, emotional relationship with each other before Ryan was born; they felt ill-equipped to deal with such a challenging child. They were committed to each other and their marriage but felt they were simply living "day-to-day," with no sense of pleasure or relaxation in their lives. Father wanted mother to be firmer with Ryan and enforce limits, whereas mother felt that she was "the cause of his difficulties" and did not want to make them worse. She realized that he was "a very sensitive baby."

By this follow-up session, the elimination diet had been completed; in addition to milk, eggs, and soy, salicylate-containing fruits, chemicals, and sugar were problems for Ryan. They intensified his irritability and wakefulness. Now that they were removed, he was sleeping a bit better and was less active and more focused. Mother wondered about going all the way to organic foods for him to eliminate chemicals.

Mother also reported that the occupational therapy sessions were helpful. She had learned exercises to reduce Ryan's oral tactile hypersensitivity and normalize oral sensation, such as rubbing the soft and hard palate. In addition, she had learned to vary food textures so Ryan would experiment with them. By putting different types of pressure on the hard and soft palate and on the lips, some textures would be normalizing. She felt that this was somewhat successful in terms of Ryan taking over more of his feeding. However, father thought she was going to too many therapists.

Talking about Ryan's developmental history, mother said that he had been very socially alert from the age of 4 months or so but that he had also been very clingy. He wanted to go with her into the bathroom and insisted on being held day and night either by mother or the woman who was helping to care for him. Mother had breastfed him for 6 weeks and then weaned him onto the bottle. Yet even though he was so clingy during his first year, Ryan had been willing to vocalize when mother vocalized. He would reach out in a controlling, rather than interactive, way, but he was "quite intentional." In his second year, Ryan had asthma, eczema, and diarrhea—as a result of his diet, mother thought. He was up about every 2 hours, a pattern that continued until the present time.

As I watched Ryan play with his parents over the next few sessions, a pattern became clear. Mother would alternate between silence—while Ryan moved cars in and out of houses or identified toys on his own—and being intrusive, anxiously opening and closing her own circles. For example, she would ask, "What's this?" and if Ryan did not answer immediately (which was often the case) she would say, "That's the boy doll. What does he want to do with the little girl?" Before he could respond, she would be telling him something else. She often touched him as she spoke. When he occasionally put his fingers in his mouth, she would quickly pull them away, saying that he would get "some germs."

Ryan would sometimes respond to her gesturally, but in a negative way, such as by turning his body away avoidantly. For example, at one point mother put a puppet on her hand and asked Ryan, "What are you going to say to the puppet?" When he did not reply, she said, "Say hi to the puppet. Say hi." Ryan turned away and said, "No," then put a block onto another block and toppled them over. Occasionally he would acquiesce and respond as mother wanted, but in general during their play he showed very little assertiveness, enthusiasm, or depth of emotion, either pleasurable or angry. Even though he could speak in short phrases, his representational or symbolic play was minimal. Although he was very gesturally sophisticated and intentional, he rarely closed gestural or verbal circles, except by sometimes turning away from or acquiescing to mother. More often, however, he shifted themes by turning his body away and changing the subject, usually in reaction to mother's intrusiveness.

Father's pattern with Ryan was somewhat similar. Although he was less intrusive, anxious, and fragmented, he tended to control the rhythm of the interaction and to do things for Ryan. There was also less relatedness than Ryan had with mother, despite Ryan's negative affect with her.

Playing with me, Ryan tended to be shy. He handed me things, made gestures, and occasionally said a word or two to me, but it was clear that it would take him a long time to warm up to me. Mother said that Ryan was also cautious and avoidant with other children, with whom he would parallel play.

At the end of this preliminary evaluation, it appeared that Ryan—a bright, cognitively age-appropriate child—was functioning slightly below age levels in terms of his emotional organization. He was functioning at the early representational level, between 18 and 20 months, rather than 22–24 months. Because he was enormously constricted in the range and depth of affect in his representational elaborations, his relatedness was globally constricted. In addition, he was locked into a passive, avoidant, negative pattern of interaction with mother, who alternated between intrusiveness and depression; the pattern was similar with his somewhat uninvolved, partially related father.

Ryan was engaged and capable of two-way communication and early representational capacity but had massive constriction of each developmental level he had achieved. As a result, he had little ability to negotiate emotions, even though he had had access to age-appropriate developmental levels for such negotiation. Because he lacked an ability to elaborate either pleasure or assertion/aggression, he was left to negative, avoidant postures, such as reacting to being fed and negatively self-regulating with sleep. It would not have been surprising if other disturbances in somatic regulation emerged, given his lack of representational or prerepresentational depth and range.

In addition to the family dynamics that contributed to Ryan's pattern were his individual constitutional-maturational differences. His constitutional vulnerability was not, however, as overwhelming as I had suspected when learning about his symptoms and history; I expected to find much more tactile sensitivity and problems with motor tone and motor planning. He did, however, have hypersensitivity to touch in the oral area (which accounted for his mouth being a target organ for his negativism and avoidance), while postural insecurity contributed to his being unsure of his body in space. This insecurity also contributed to his comfort with passivity and not taking risks in terms of motor assertiveness. These constitutional variables intensified his interactional limitations. Furthermore, Ryan's early history of medical procedures had undoubtedly contributed to his developmental difficulties and accentuated his constitutional and interactional patterns.

Ryan's treatment plan included various elements, beginning with the ongoing occupational therapy sessions, which focused particularly on feeding and better postural control. As noted earlier, mother was learning new ways of feeding Ryan to help normalize sensation in his mouth. I also suggested motor exercises (which mother could practice during Ryan's weekly occupational sessions) that would gradually help him with posture and to feel more comfortable in space.

The treatment also involved working on parent–child interaction patterns. Mother and father would each do Floortime with Ryan for at least a half-hour every day and in regular consulting sessions. They would use these experiences to better understand their relationships with Ryan and how they were undermining or supporting his development. In these sessions, mother's alternating depression and intrusiveness (and her son's concomitant negative and avoidant patterns) and father's lack of involvement were explored, along with the parents' own emotional reactions to these patterns.

Over time, mother learned to establish a consistent rhythm, giving Ryan more space and time to respond and lead rather than just react against her. We focused on his opening and closing of gestural circles and then symbolic circles. Mother would have to figure out what Ryan was trying to do before she could move in and give him several new options or answer the questions that she herself had raised. After working on this, mother smiled and recalled how, as a child, she had been "the boss and the queen bee" among the other children, directing the drama. Her own mother had been "aloof, yet controlling"—she "gave me nothing in terms of warmth but made me very tough [and] controlling…. I would never let her control or exploit me," mother explained.

Mother began to relax, smile, and even giggle during her play with Ryan. Ryan started taking the lead; for example, in one session he put the whale puppet on his hand and held his mouth open. Instead of trying to act out a feeding scene, mother asked, "What does the whale want?" Ryan answered that the whale was hungry. Mother asked him what food he would like, and Ryan determined which of the pretend food items he wanted to eat. Although simple, this interaction showed a major improvement in mother's ability to wait for Ryan to direct the drama. In a subsequent session, when Ryan had the whale eating food, mother wondered aloud how the whale felt when it was spitting the food out. Ryan, now almost 30 months old, said, "Well, mad." Mother asked what the whale wanted to do, and Ryan then made the whale bite everything in the room, knock down toys, and even throw toys. Mother and I empathized with how mad the whale could get, and Ryan's affect broadened and brightened; it was the first time he had dealt with his anger representationally. He was also much more gesturally animated, using his complex gestural system to deal with anger. After this, he was more relaxed about assertiveness, and mother's rhythm had fewer silences and less intrusion; she showed more respect for her son's initiative. Mother's relationship with me and with her husband was also easier.

Father, on the other hand, had less trouble being unintrusive, and although he knew intellectually how to relate to Ryan, it was very hard for him to get deeply involved. Initially, he was reluctant to do Floortime and was against mother receiving occupational therapy support or her own counseling. "She should be able to handle it on her own," he said. He had almost no awareness of the depth of his wife's depression. On one occasion, when father was not in the room, mother confided that "the marriage was just like two roommates, with little love or intimacy or warmth." She felt that she only stayed in it because of her depression and general sense of hopelessness.

The work with father included addressing the whole issue of what pleasures he felt with his family, particularly as he was reluctant to do the Floortime with Ryan and to be more involved with his wife. We explored his early family upbringing, including the fact that he had a self-centered, anxious, and needy mother and that his father had passed away when he was 9 years old. He felt fortunate that his older sister had been there to help take care of his mother. He admitted that he had buried himself in books and avoided intimacy, which had depth of feeling. He had always had some friends and had dated in high school and college, but he avoided intense relationships, he felt, partly because they reminded him of his mother's helplessness. He was confused about the fact that he had married a fairly depressed and fragmented woman; he had thought that she could be competent because she was a journalist. He had not focused on his wife's similarities to his mother (although his wife was in some ways very strong despite her depression).

As father looked at these patterns in his life, he relaxed a bit and started enjoying his Floortime with his son. Ryan began experimenting with motor assertiveness—roughhousing typical of children this age—and father even went to one occupational therapy session, where he learned how to help Ryan do this roughhousing as a way of improving postural control. Slowly, Ryan increased his intimacy in play with his father. Initially, he just gave more looks and smiles and showed greater intensity of affect, then his overall quality of relatedness grew more animated and his symbolic play evolved. For example, in one session with father, Ryan was being somewhat cautious and whiny. He noticed a flashlight and asked what it was. Father, in his own quiet but now warmer style, responded, "Let's see if we can figure it out" and began pressing the different switches. He showed it to

Ryan, who started pressing buttons himself and suddenly pressed the button that made the light go on. He enjoyed shining it at father, and every time he did, father made a funny face and Ryan started giggling. Then he gave father the flashlight, and when father shined it at him, Ryan made funny faces. He started ordering father around, saying, "Do it more," and "Put it over there." Then he imitated a television character and had father hide behind the chair and shine the light at him so he could pretend he was on stage. He had gotten some of the puppets and was starting a puppet show when the session ended. Ryan's taking charge was impressive, and I admired how, with father warmly supporting and shining light on him, Ryan had given the light over to father in order to perform.

In a session with mother, Ryan (who was now more than 2½ years old) came in eager, alert, warm, and verbal. He got out the toys and told me to put the doll in the chair. Talking in complex sentences, he took charge of the drama, involving me and mother. He identified one of the toys as a boat and another as a truck and announced that one part of the room would be where the boat was going (water) and that the truck was going near the water. The dolls on the chair were to go on the water first and then into the truck. He decided that I would manipulate the car while mother manipulated the boat; he handed each of us toys and dolls from the "shoreline" (the chair) to take into our different vehicles. Again, what was impressive here was his control of the drama; he was animated, smiling with pleasure and mastery. Meanwhile, mother was able to follow and take pride in his initiative.

At that point, Ryan was eating much better and gaining weight more readily, sleeping through some nights and only waking up once during other nights. He was still somewhat cautious and shy with other children; a goal was to have other children whom he enjoyed visit several times a week to give him more practice in one-on-one situations where he could learn to relax in interactive play, just as he now could with mother and father.

Ryan was still not comfortable with assertiveness in all situations. He was, however, gradually becoming more comfortable, showing pleasure and joy, a sense of mastery, and assertiveness in situations where he felt comfortable and trusting, such as sessions in my office. I discussed with the parents having Ryan's teacher draw him more into peer-to-peer activities in his class, where he tended to avoid the assertiveness and unpredictability of the group.

Ryan showed gradual, steady progress over a period of 10–12 months. With his parents' help, he was able to overcome many of his original symptoms and—both gesturally and representationally—expand the range and depth of both plea sure and assertiveness, and he began experimenting with aggression. He was confidently approaching age-appropriate patterns in terms of his developmental level and the range and depth of experience he could organize and communicate.

Ryan's case illustrates a number of important principles imbedded in the DIR approach. It shows how important it is to work with the family and interactive patterns, especially when there are clear regulatory sensory-processing challenges, so that the young child can master his basic emotional, social, and intellectual capacities— that is, his functional emotional developmental capacities. Importantly, as children master these critical functional capacities, they are better able to find ways of coping with their constitutional and maturational variations. A comprehensive approach— involving, in this case, interactive work, family work, and occupational therapy to work directly on the regulatory sensory-processing challenges—all came together to help this young child make significant progress on a number of significant challenges.

In terms of our classification model, Ryan demonstrated patterns consistent with sensory hyperreactivity (Type 1) and postural insecurity and insecurity in moving in space (Type 4).

Eating problems can be among the most difficult for both parents and professionals. There is a tendency to focus narrowly only on the symptoms without a full understanding of the regulatory sensory-processing, emotional, social, and family contributions. A comprehensive approach most often provides the best opportunity for both mastering the symptoms and promoting overall adaptive development. Ryan continued to do well with periodic follow-up and moved ahead nicely into the next stages of development.

References

Ayres AJ: Tactile functions: their relation to hyperactive and perceptual motor behavior. Am J Occup Ther 18:6–11, 1964

Ayres AJ: Sensory Integration and Learning Disabilities. Los Angeles, Western Psychological Services, 1972

Carlson GA, Weintraub S: Childhood behavior problems and bipolar disorder: relationship or coincidence? J Affect Disord 28:143–153, 1993

Castillo M, Kwock L, Courvorise H, et al: Proton MR spectroscopy in children with bipolar affective disorder: preliminary observations. Am J Neuroradiol 21:832–838, 2000

Cytryn L, McKnew DH: Factors influencing the changing clinical expression of depressive process in children. Am J Psychiatry 131:879–881, 1974

DeGangi GA, Greenspan SI: The development of sensory functioning in infants. Phys Occup Ther Pediatr 8:21–33, 1988

DeGangi GA, DiPietro JA, Greenspan SI, et al: Psychophysiological characteristics of the regulatory disordered infant. Infant Behav Dev 14:37–50, 1991

DeGangi GA, Porges SW, Sickel RZ, et al: Four-year follow-up of a sample of regulatory disordered infants. Infant Ment Health J 14:330–343, 1993

Doussard-Roosevelt JA, Walker PS, Portales A, et al: Vagal tone and the fussy infant: atypical vagal reactivity in the difficult infant (abstract). Infant Behav Dev 13:352, 1990

Egland JA, Blumenthal RL, Nee J, et al: Reliability and relationship of various ages of onset criteria for major affective disorders. J Affect Disord 12:159–165, 1987

Escalona S: The Roots of Individuality. Chicago, IL, Aldine, 1968

Ferber R: Solve Your Child's Sleep Problems. New York, Simon and Schuster, 1985

Geller B, Zimmerman B, Williams M, et al: Bipolar disorder at prospective follow-up of adults who had prepubertal major depressive disorder. Am J Psychiatry 158:125–127, 2001

Greenspan SI: Infancy and Early Childhood: The Practice of Clinical Assessment and Intervention With Emotional and Developmental Challenges. Madison, CT, International Universities Press, 1992

Greenspan SI, Wieder S: Infant and early childhood mental health: a comprehensive developmental approach to assessment and intervention. ZERO TO THREE 24:6–13, 2003

Greenspan SI, Wieder S, Lieberman A, et al: Infants in Multirisk Families: Case Studies in Preventive Intervention. Clinical Infant Reports, No 3. New York, International Universities Press, 1987

Harrington R, Fudge H, Rutter M, et al: Adult outcomes of child and adolescent depression, II: links with antisocial disorders. J Am Acad Child Adolesc Psychiatry 30:434–439, 1991

Interdisciplinary Council on Developmental and Learning Disorders Diagnostic Manual for Infancy and Early Childhood Workgroups: Interdisciplinary Council on Developmental and Learning Disorders Diagnostic Manual for Infancy and Early Childhood Mental Health Disorders, Developmental Disorders, Regulatory-Sensory Processing Disorders, Language Disorders, and Learning Challenges. Bethesda, MD, Interdisciplinary Council on Developmental and Learning Disorders, 2005

Lish J, Dime-Meenan S, Whybrow P, et al: The National Depressive and Manic-Depressive Association (DMDA) survey of bipolar members. J Affect Disord 31:281–294, 1994

Miller LJ, Robinson J, Moulton D: Sensory modulation dysfunction: identification in early childhood, in Handbook of Infant, Toddler and Preschool Mental Health Assessment. Edited by DelCarmen-Wiggins R, Wiggins A. New York, Oxford University Press, 2004, pp 247–270

Mindell JA: Sleeping Through the Night. New York, Harper Collins, 1997

Murphy LB: The Individual Child (Publication No. OCD 74–1032). Washington, DC, U.S. Department of Health, Education, and Welfare, 1974

Porges SW, Greenspan SI. Regulatory disordered infants: A common theme. Paper presented at the National Institute on Drug Abuse Research Analysis and Utilization System (RAUS) Review Meeting on Methodological Issues in Controlled Studies on Effects of Prenatal Exposure to Drugs of Abuse, Richmond, VA, June 8–9, 1990

Portales AW, Porges SW, Greenspan SI: Parenthood and the difficult child (abstract). Infant Behav Dev 13:573, 1990

Radke-Yarrow M, Nottelmann E, Martinez P, et al: Young children of affectively ill parents: a longitudinal study of psychosocial development. J Am Acad Child Adolesc Psychiatry 31:68–76, 1992

Sears W: Nighttime Parenting: How to Get Your Baby and Child to Sleep. New York, Plume, 1999

Sigurdsson E, Fombonne E, Sayal K, et al: Neurodevelopmental antecedents of early onset bipolar affective disorder. Br J Psychiatry 174:121–127, 1999

Strober M, Morrell W, Burroughs J, et al: A family study of bipolar I disorder in adolescents: early onset of symptoms linked to increased familial loading and lithium resistance. J Affect Disord 15:255–268, 1988

9

Assessment and Treatment of Infants and Young Children With Neurodevelopmental Disorders of Relating and Communicating

Neurodevelopmental disorders of relating and communicating (NDRC) involve problems in multiple aspects of a child's development, including social relationships, language, cognitive functioning, and sensory and motor processing. This category includes earlier conceptualizations of multisystem developmental disorders as characterized in *Infancy and Early Childhood* (Greenspan 1992) and *Diagnostic Classification: 0–3* (DC:0-3; Diagnostic Classification Task Force 1994). Additionally, NDRC include the DSM-IV-TR (American Psychiatric Association 2000) category of pervasive developmental disorders, also referred to as autism spectrum disorders. The main distinction between NDRC and the earlier conceptualizations is that the NDRC framework enables a clinician to more accurately subtype disorders of relating and communicating in terms of the overall level of social, intellectual, and emotional functioning and the associated regulatory and sensory-motor processing profile. This framework helps differentiate the profiles of children commonly considered on the autism spectrum and with other special needs conditions and helps define the variations seen among the children with the same diagnosis. This differentiation is important for both intervention planning and research purposes.

Since the description of multisystem developmental disorders in 1992 and later in DC:0-3 and of pervasive developmental disorders in DSM-IV-TR, we have developed a broader framework to allow consideration of the full range of problems in relating, communicating, and thinking.[1] Thus, the large degree of individual variation in infants and young children who ultimately evidence common features of difficulties in forming relationships, communicating at preverbal and verbal levels, and engaging in creative and abstract reflective thinking can be captured. These children typically evidence a type of static encephalopathy (i.e., nonprogressive central nervous system dysfunction) that interferes with the expected progression of these core capacities. Children within this broad category, however, evidence wide variation in the degree to which they relate to others and master early communicative and thinking skills, as well as in their most basic ways of processing sensation (e.g., some are sensory overresponsive and others are sensory underresponsive; some have relatively strong visual memory whereas others have relatively weak visual memory). Therefore, we believe it is important to have the broadest possible conceptual framework within which to capture the full range of individual variation.

As we look at this full range of variation (i.e., at all possible subtypes), we discover that numerous biological and overall developmental pathways are associated with these types of challenges. For example, difficulty in connecting affect to perception and motor action, and subsequent difficulty in relating, communicating, and thinking may be the result of several neurodevelopmental pathways, each with its own genetic or constitutional-maturational variations (Greenspan and Shanker 2004). Therefore, we suggest a broad category of NDRC to facilitate advances in research, evaluation strategies, and clinical intervention programs.

As indicated, NDRC may be viewed as part of the broad neurological category of nonprogressive disorders of the central nervous system. The technical term in the international diagnostic system, ICD-10 (World Health Organization 1992) is *static* (nonprogressive) *encephalopathy* (disorder of the central nervous system).

In diagnosing NDRC, it is important to understand how regulatory-sensory processing disorders differ from NDRC. Although regulatory-sensory processing disorders involve deficits in processing capacities, unlike NDRC, they do not derail a child's overall relating and communicating. NDRC combine regulatory-sensory processing problems with significant developmental delays and dysfunctions. The child's biologically based processing difficulties contribute to his relationship and communication difficulties. A complete evaluation of the child's regulatory-sensory processing capacities is necessary to understand their contributions to NDRC.

---

[1]For a fuller description of NDRC, please see Interdisciplinary Council on Developmental and Learning Disorders: *Interdisciplinary Council on Developmental and Learning Disorders Diagnostic Manual for Infancy and Early Childhood* (ICDL-DMIC). Bethesda, MD, Interdisciplinary Council on Developmental and Learning Disorders, 2005 (www.icdl.com).

It is also important to recognize that developmental impairments may result from severe environmental stress and trauma. For example, in what has been described as failure-to-thrive syndrome and in severe deprivation patterns, an infant's motor, cognitive, language, affective, and physical growth may slow down or cease altogether. Persistent abuse or neglect can produce a similar global disruption in development and functioning.

The developmental, individual-differences, relationship-based (DIR) approach helps us understand the relationship between adaptive capacities and pathological symptoms in each infant or child. For example, an infant's impairments in auditory-verbal, visuospatial, or perceptual-motor processing can make ordinary relating and communicating extremely difficult. Even reasonably stable, supportive, and empathic parents may be unable to find some special way to capture their child's attention, engage him, and interact with him. The resulting lack of appropriate human interaction will likely prevent vital social learning during key periods of development. Between 12 and 24 months of age, for example, most children develop several critical skills at an especially rapid rate—reciprocal affective and motor gesturing, comprehending the "rules" that govern complex social interactions, pattern recognition, a sense of self, and early forms of thinking. A deficit in these skills can easily look like a primary deficit rather than a consequence of underlying biologically based processing impairments.

The DIR model is especially helpful in understanding how genetic and/or other biological patterns interact with environmental patterns in the formation of a disorder. For example, an infant with low muscle tone and sensory underreactivity becomes increasingly self-absorbed if his primary caregiver is depressed and unavailable.

Interestingly, many families of children diagnosed with autism or related disorders report—and have videotapes to confirm—that in the first year of life, their children were engaged and beginning to participate in reciprocal interactions. Although these early patterns may have shown some vulnerabilities, only in the second year did the child clearly begin disengaging. We hypothesize that a combination of two events may derail the child's forward momentum between 16 and 24 months.

The first is the child's own emerging capacities for higher-level presymbolic, symbolic, and cognitive functioning. Because these new capacities are emerging on a vulnerable foundation (such as a weak capacity for intentional two-way affective communication), they contribute to the child's becoming overloaded with new information about the world. Around this time, for example, the toddler is developing a sense of his physical relationship to surrounding space, and this leads to a greater awareness of his potential vulnerability. Such cognitive advances may, paradoxically, overwhelm a child with severe vulnerabilities in earlier developmental capacities, causing him to regress in his behavioral organization, self-regulation, interpersonal patterns, motor control, and language abilities.

New capacities alone seem to be enough to derail some children. In some cases, however, a second event might occur. Careful history taking reveals that during the same period of development, the child experienced one or more stresses, such as the loss of a caregiver, a parent's return to work, a parent's preoccupation with the birth of a sibling, a challenging physical environment, and so forth. For children who already have a tenuous hold on their interpersonal relationships and developmental competencies, the combination of emerging capacities and environmental stresses may be overwhelming.

As the child becomes increasingly challenging, the parents may find him so confusing, frustrating, and anxiety-provoking that there are further compromises in attempts at shared attention, engagement, and preverbal and verbal communication. Many parents report growing feelings of alienation, anger, and loss. The child, as he loses whatever level of engagement and purposeful relating he had previously enjoyed with his caregivers, seems to spin more and more idiosyncratically out of control. Prerepresentational children may exhibit increasing motor and behavioral randomness, whereas children who have achieved some degree of representational capacity begin using words and ideas in more fragmented and personalized ways or they may lose the capacity for speech and representation altogether. In either case, the lack of an intentional, organizing human relationship may further contribute to the child's biologically based primary vulnerabilities.

We have recently formulated a new hypothesis to understand the core biological and subsequent experiential relationships in the developmental pathway leading to autism spectrum disorders. In this hypothesis, which we call the affect-diathesis hypothesis (Greenspan and Shanker 2004; Greenspan and Wieder 1999; Interdisciplinary Council on Developmental and Learning Disorders 2000), we suggest that the core biological deficit expresses itself as a difficulty for the infant in connecting emerging affects to sensation (or perception) and to emerging sensory motor patterns (forming a sensory-affect-motor pattern). Later on, this same difficulty compromises the toddler's capacity to connect affect to complex problem-solving motor patterns and emerging symbols in language.

Typically, infants evidence a sensory-affect-motor connection as they begin to attend to the world. For example, turning to look toward mother's smiling face and pleasurable vocalizations requires perception (taking in pleasurable sensations), pleasurable affect (the sound of her voice, the sight of her face), and motor action (turning toward the pleasurable face and voice). This sensory-affect-motor connection becomes especially important as the infant engages more and more in reciprocal social and emotional interchanges in the second half of the first year of life. In these interchanges, affect clearly guides purposeful motor actions, such as exchanging vocalizations, trading funny little grins, reaching for the piece of banana in mommy's mouth, and so forth.

By the early part of the second year, the child's ability to connect sensation, affect, and motor action becomes even more vital as the toddler engages in shared social problem solving—for example, taking a caregiver by the hand, gesturing to the toy area, pointing to a particular toy that is out of reach, and making numerous back-and-forth gestures to get the parent to pick him up to reach the desired toy. In such interactions, as in earlier developmental stages, the child's purposeful or intentional behavior is clearly fueled by his affect (i.e., the desire for that toy). Yet now the child's affect is involved in many back-and-forth interactions in a row, and in this way affect guides the relationship between perception (i.e., seeing the toy) and a complex, multistep social and motor action to get the toy. The vast majority of children with autism spectrum disorders, even when these disorders are diagnosed at later ages, are reported by their parents to have had difficulty in mastering this early capacity for shared social problem solving (i.e., a continuous flow of back-and-forth affective signals) (Greenspan and Wieder 1997).

Therefore, we hypothesize that a biologically based difficulty with forming an early sensory-affect-motor connection (and subsequent difficulties with connecting affect to complex motor patterns to facilitate motor planning and sequencing and shared social problem solving) is an important contribution to the pattern of challenges and symptoms we observe in autism spectrum disorders. As the capacity to repeat words emerges, this same difficulty compromises the child's learning to connect affect to words to give them meaning (e.g., the child repeats words without clear affective intent).

Children vary, however, in the degree to which this fundamental capacity is disrupted and also differ in basic motor, sensory modulation, visuospatial, auditory processing, and language capacities. However, without the capacity to connect affect or intent to these fundamental capacities, especially the initial motor capacities, these related capacities are not developed in an appropriate manner. For example, children with relatively strong auditory processing and verbal capacities may repeat whole books because of their strong auditory memory, but at the same time, they may be unable to use language meaningfully. Similarly, children with relatively strong motor capacities may line up their toys but are often unable to engage in motor-based interactive problem solving. Children with relative weaknesses in these related developmental capacities may evidence little or no verbal behavior at all and perform only simple repetitive or aimless motor behavior.

We have found that children with relative strengths in their related developmental capacities tend to make progress more rapidly once we are able to engage them in a comprehensive intervention program that works with their core difficulty in connecting affect to sensations and motor actions. We have also observed that the relative deficit in connecting affect to sensations and motor actions often improves with an intervention program that focuses on affective learning relationships that consider the child's unique developmental profile. Children appear to have the flexibility to develop side roads even when the main highway evidences relative impairment (Greenspan and Wieder 1997, 1998, 1999).

As this discussion suggests, NDRC can be more fully understood from the perspective of a developmental biopsychosocial model. Applying the DIR model has enabled the development of a classification system that attempts to capture individual subtypes based on a more complete understanding of the developmental pathways that lead to significant challenges in relating, communicating, and thinking. These pathways, characterized by individual processing differences, include the following:

- *Sensory modulation*—the ability to modulate or regulate sensation as it is coming in
- *Motor planning and sequencing*—how we act on our ideas or on what we hear and see
- *Auditory processing and language*—the way in which we receive information and comprehend and express it
- *Visuospatial processing*—the ability to make sense of and understand what we are seeing

We propose four types of NDRC that cluster the major profiles that we have observed in children with significant challenges in relating, communicating, and thinking. It is important to remember that these types and their associated features are on a continuum. As children make progress, receive intervention, and move forward, we see movement within each type, as well as from one type to another. Each type is described below, along with a brief clinical illustration. These illustrations highlight the main features and quality of the relationships and functioning and are not complete.

Types of Neurodevelopmental Disorders of Relating and Communicating

Type I: Early Symbolic, With Constrictions

Children with Type I disorders exhibit constrictions in their capacities for shared attention, engagement, initiation of two-way affective communication, and shared social problem solving. They have difficulty maintaining a continuous flow of affective interactions before intervention and can open and close only four to ten circles of communication in a row. A circle of communication is a back-and-forth interaction where the infant or child responds to the caregiver's gestures or overtures, and vice versa. Often, children with Type I disorders also evidence perseveration and some degree of self-absorption. At initial evaluation, one sees islands of memory-based symbol use, such as labeling pictures or repeating memorized scripts, but the child does not display a range of affect expected for his age and has difficulty integrating symbol use with other core developmental capacities and engaging in all processes simultaneously.

With an intervention program that addresses the child's individual processing differences and promotes shared attention and reciprocal affective communication, children with Type I difficulties tend to make rapid progress. Often, one sees a child move from constricted patterns of interaction, perseveration, self-stimulation, and self-absorption toward warm, pleasurable engagement and a continuous flow of affective interactions. The child begins initiating such interactions by spontaneous use of language and maintaining the flow of interactions at the levels of two-way problem-solving communication, creating ideas, and building bridges between ideas. Even when language is delayed, the child is able to sequence complex gestures (signs) and use toys to convey symbolic ideas until language is strengthened. Thus, the child moves toward abstract and reflective levels of symbolic thinking. His more robust capacities enable him to develop healthy peer relationships and participate in typical activities.

Eventually, with appropriate intervention, children with Type I difficulties can usually participate fully in a regular academic program. Often an aide may be required for a period of time to help with regulatory-sensory processing and related attentional challenges. In addition, because academic skills and abstract thinking depend on processing abilities, educational interventions to address specific learning difficulties may be required.

Clinical Illustration

David, age 2½ years, was self-absorbed, perseverative, and given to self-stimulation. He did not make eye contact with his parents or exhibit much pleasure in relating to them, nor did he play with other children. During his evaluation, David spent most of his time reciting numbers or the alphabet in a rote sequence, spinning and jumping around randomly, and lining up toys and cars while making self-stimulatory sounds. When he was extremely motivated, he could blurt out what he wanted. He occasionally showed affection by hugging his parents and tolerated their hugs, although he never looked at them. He could imitate actions, sounds, and words and recognize pictures and shapes.

David presented both challenges and strengths in his regulatory and sensory processing profile. He was a highly active child who was interested in learning about the world, even though he could do so in only a fragmented and fleeting way, as he flitted around the room flapping his arms searching for something familiar. His intense movement also served to increase his muscle tone and energy. When something captured his attention, he explored the object briefly, sometimes blurted out its label, but had no communicative intent. He could recite memorized letters and numbers that never changed, but he could not process (comprehend) when others spoke to him. By his third year, he became increasingly self-absorbed and would resort to exciting himself with his recitations. He was unable to engage in any two-way communication or even respond to his name. David also demonstrated some visuospatial strength in that he could randomly discriminate objects in his environment and later locate them again. He sought out mirrors to reflect what he was doing and used them for visual feedback, because he could not process incoming auditory feedback from others. He also manipulated toys, indicating he understood what they represented and could use them in simple sequences (e.g., to eat the pretend food or push the car), suggesting he had the rudiments of con-

necting purposeful intent to motor planning. This ability was also seen in his spontaneous imitations of new actions with toys and ritualized movements to songs. It
was also evident that David had strong affect and showed great pleasure when
happy—even in his self-absorbing pursuits—and intense anger or avoidance when
thwarted. His ability to initiate and connect affect to intent was his strongest asset.
Although auditory and visual processing capacities were significantly challenged,
he still showed relative strengths and weaknesses.

With a comprehensive intervention program, David quickly became more engaged, entered into a continuous flow of affective interactions, began initiating
long pretend-oriented sequences, and gradually began using language purposefully
and creatively. His early perseverative interest in cars transformed into their use for
elaborate symbolic dramas and remained a special interest for several years during
which he became the resident "expert" on brands and models. This gave way as he
expanded his emotional range and emotional interests, as well as motor planning
abilities. He used Floortime sessions to spontaneously explore and rehearse new
emotional themes, and he became an abstract thinker. He could also reflect on his
feelings and was highly empathic with others.

In the pattern of progress described above, his developing capacities enabled
him to begin relating more to both parents and peers. At present, as a teenager,
David attends a regular school, where he excels in English as well as math. He continues to have some difficulty with fine motor sequencing (e.g., with penmanship).
Although he did not become an athlete, he enjoys shooting baskets or playing tennis with friends and writes the sports feature in his school paper. He is still active
and quite enterprising, now looking for opportunities to do "business." Although
he tends to become somewhat argumentative in competitive situations, he enjoys
close friendships, has a great sense of humor, and shows insights into other people's
feelings.

Type II: Purposeful Problem Solving, With Constrictions

Children with Type II disorders, when seen initially (often between ages 2 and 4
years), have significant constrictions in the third and fourth core developmental
capacities: purposeful, two-way presymbolic communication and social problem-
solving communication. They engage in only intermittent interactions at these
levels, completing at most two to five circles of communication in a row. Other
than repeating a few memorized scripts from favorite shows, they exhibit few islands of true symbolic activity. Many of these children show some capacity for engagement, but their engagement has a global, need-oriented emotional quality and
is on their terms. They often evidence a profile of moderate processing dysfunctions in multiple areas.

Children in this group face greater challenges than those in Type I and make
slower, but consistent, progress. Overcoming each hurdle requires a great deal of
time and work. Over time, they can learn to engage with real warmth and pleasure.
They gradually but steadily improve their capacities for purposeful interaction and
shared social problem solving, learning to initiate and sustain a continuous flow of
affective interactions. The slow development of this continuous flow prevents a

more robust development of symbolic capacities; these capacities also improve, although these children tend to rely on imitation of books and videos as a basis for language and imaginative play. As the children gradually progress through each new capacity, they begin creating ideas and may even reach toward building bridges between ideas in circumscribed areas of interest. However, they do not display an age-appropriate depth and range of affect, and their abstract thinking is very limited and focused on real-life needs.

Although many children in this group make continuous progress, most cannot participate in all the activities of a regular classroom with a large number of children. They can, however, benefit from appropriately staffed inclusion or integrated programs or from special-needs classrooms in which language development is emphasized and the other children are interactive and verbal.

Clinical Illustration

Three-year-old Joey was extremely avoidant, always moving away from his caregivers and making only fleeting eye contact with them. He displayed considerable perseverative and self-stimulatory behavior, such as rapidly turning the pages of preferred books or pushing his toy train around and around the track. He also chose books and figures from his favorite shows, such as Barney or Winnie the Pooh, and had them board his trains. No one dared to touch his figures because he would throw a tantrum instantly when he thought the figures would be taken away. He could purposefully reach for his juice, put out his arms to get dressed, or give and take an object from his parents, but he could neither negotiate complex preverbal interactions nor imitate sounds or words, although he vocalized some. The only pleasure he showed with his parents was during roughhousing or tickle games and when his mother sang to him as he fell asleep.

Joey relied on visual information to deal with his environment and had a remarkable memory for things and places. He was underresponsive to words spoken to him but overresponsive to sudden high pitched or vibrating sounds, which continuously distracted or alarmed him and kept him vigilant. He relied on ritualized patterns in daily life and protested changes he could not understand. Although he seemed to somehow find his favorite books or figures, he did not search for things in any planned way, leading to frustration and tantrums. He also found obstacle courses hard to do, and, rather than follow the other children in the gym, he would collapse on the floor and watch them. These patterns reflected the multiple sensory and motor processing challenges (auditory, visuospatial, and motor planning), compounded by over- and underresponsiveness and low muscle tone. Life became increasingly challenging for him and his family as he grew and pulled away from relationships and their increasing expectations.

Joey's intervention program addressed each of the processing areas in individual therapies and a home program. The emphasis was on expanding pleasurable interactions and establishing a continuous flow of interactions through affect cuing and problem solving. As he became more engaged and began to expand his play, it became evident that Joey had islands of receptive symbolic understanding suggested by his early interest in Barney riding his train. He began to use figures from various books and shows, first scripting and then recreating real-life experiences such as birthday parties. Visual strategies and oral motor treatment helped reduce his frustration.

Now, at age 6½, after nearly 4 years of intensive intervention, Joey can relate with real pleasure and joy and use complex gestures and words to negotiate with his parents. He can describe what he wants in sentences ("Give me juice now—I'm thirsty!"); respond to simple questions ("What do you want to do?" "Go to Disney World on my trains!"); and have conversations involving four or five exchanges of short phrases giving his opinion or making a plan for the day. He enjoys listening to and reading story books and is beginning to read sight words. He also engages in early imaginative play with great joy and delight, throwing grand birthday parties, dressing up, and making his action figures fly around the room. Joey insists on being the superhero but does not always have a motive even when he has a destination (to get the "bad guy").

Although he cannot yet consistently answer abstract "why" questions, Joey can do basic real-life reasoning about safety. He is able to play with peers and run with the crowd in the context of action or structured games and with some adult involvement. He is now in an inclusion kindergarten program and participates in preacademic activities, with relative strengths in visual thinking and math. He also enjoys play dates with his classmates. Joey continues to make progress at a slow but consistent pace. Interestingly, Joey's perseverative, self-stimulatory patterns have largely abated and appear only occasionally.

Type III: Intermittently Engaged and Purposeful

Children in the Type III group are very self-absorbed. Their engagement with others is extremely intermittent, having an in-and-out quality. They display very limited purposeful two-way communication, usually in pursuit of concrete needs or basic sensory-motor experiences (e.g., jumping, tickling). They may be able to imitate or even initiate some rote problem-solving actions, but they usually evidence little or no capacity for shared social problem solving or for a continuous flow of affective exchange.

With affect-based intervention, children with Type III difficulties can become more robustly engaged in pleasurable activities, but their capacity for a continuous flow of affective interactions improves very slowly. They can learn to convey simple feelings such as happy, sad, and mad, but the in-and-out quality of their relatedness constricts the range and depth of affect they can negotiate. Over time, they can learn islands of presymbolic purposeful and problem-solving behavior. These islands may, at times, also involve the use of words, pictures, signs, or two- to three-step actions or gestures to communicate basic needs. Receptive understanding of often-used phrases in routines or when coupled with visual cues or gestures can become a relative strength.

Some children in this group will use toys as though they are real (e.g., they will try to eat pretend foods, feed a life-size baby doll, or put their feet into a pretend swimming pool as though they could go swimming). They do not usually reach the level of truly representing themselves using toys or dolls.

Multiple severe processing dysfunctions, including severe auditory processing and visuospatial processing difficulties and moderate-to-severe motor planning problems impede the continuous flow of purposeful communication and problem-solving interactions. Some children in this group have severe oral-motor dyspraxia and do not speak more than a few ritualized words, if they speak at all. They may, however, learn to use a few signs or to communicate using pictures or a favorite toy.

Children in this group require very individualized educational approaches and may eventually learn to read words through motor pathways and to understand visuospatial concepts. It is important that they be included in hybrid programs to encourage social activities, ritualized learning, and the development of friendships.

Clinical Illustration

Sarah, age 3 years, ran into the playroom looking for Winnie the Pooh, climbed up on the stool in front of the shelves, but could not move the little figures around in the basket to search for her beloved character. The next moment, the basket was pulled off the shelf and all the figures fell out. Without bothering to look on the floor, Sarah began searching in the next basket. Her mom ran over before the second basket was dropped and offered to help. Sarah echoed, "help!" and grabbed her mother's hands and put them in the basket. Her mother had to point to the Pooh figure before Sarah actually saw it. She grabbed it and ran off to lie on the couch. Mom then brought Tigger over to say hello; Sarah grabbed Tigger and ran to the other side of the room. She held her figures tightly and turned away when her mother came over again. Mom then took the Eeyore figure and started to sing ring-around-the-rosy while moving Eeyore up and down. This time, Sarah looked and filled in "down" to "all fall down." She then moved rapidly away and went over to the mirror. This pattern of flight and avoidance after getting what she wanted, followed by not knowing what to do next, was typical of Sarah.

With a comprehensive intervention program, Sarah slowly learned the labels for things she wanted. She learned how to protest rather than scream. She recognized and could say familiar phrases like "come and eat," "go out," and "bath time." She became quite engaged when involved in sensory-motor play and loved to be swung and tickled. She even began to play with toys, first dipping her toes into the water of the play pool and then letting Winnie jump in. She began to imitate more words and actions. She tried to initiate problem-solving interactions to get her figures, but only when she was very motivated or very mad and usually only after energetic sensory-motor play had pulled her in. Her expressive language expanded to include more and more phrases indicating what she wanted, but her weak receptive processing made it difficult for her to answer any questions, and she relied on visual and affect cues to understand what was said to her. This transferred to puppet play and even simple role playing, in which she took the part of a cook or doctor. Problem solving progressed very slowly because of Sarah's very poor motor planning, but she became more easily engaged and more responsive to semi-structured and structured approaches to learning. Between ages 4 and 5, she learned to count and to identify colors, and she loved to paint and cut with scissors. At age 6½, Sarah demonstrates some preacademic abilities, including reading some sight words. She attends a special education class that integrates activities with typical peers. She enjoys being with other children and joins the crowd in running around, hiding, and chasing, but she does not yet play interactively. She has, however, learned various social rituals of greeting, sharing, protesting, and so on. Sarah can also spontaneously communicate with a big smile, "Feel happy!" or with a frown, "Feel mad!"

Type IV: Aimless and Unpurposeful

Children in the Type IV group are passive and self-absorbed or active and stimulus seeking; some exhibit both patterns. They have severe difficulties with shared attention and engagement unless they are involved in sensory-motor play. They tend to make very slow progress, and developing expressive language is very challenging for them.

With intervention, children with Type IV difficulties can become warmly engaged and intermittently interactive through use of gestures and action games. Through their ability to relate and interact, they can learn to problem solve. The goal is to challenge them to open and close many circles of communication in a row so that they can progress as much as possible in their problem-solving ability.

Some children learn to complete organized sequences of the sort needed to play semistructured games or carry out self-help tasks, such as dressing and brushing teeth. Many of these children can share with others the pleasure they experience when they can use their bodies purposefully, to skate, swim, ride bikes, play ball, and so on. These meaningful activities can be used to encourage shared attention, engagement, and purposeful problem solving.

Children in this group have the most severe challenges in all processing areas. Many have special challenges in motor planning, including oral-motor dyspraxia. As a consequence, their progress is very uneven. They have the most difficulty with complex problem-solving interactions, expressive language, and motor planning. They may have periods of progression and regression. Regressions can occur for unknown reasons. Sometimes regressions appear to occur because the environment is not sufficiently tailored to the child's processing profile.

Educational approaches need to be very meaningful to the child in order to pull these children in. Both visual and motor pathways must be found to help the child focus and learn.

Clinical Illustration

Harold, at age 3½ years, progressed only very slowly to imitating sounds and words, even with an intensive program to facilitate imitation. He could say one or two words spontaneously when he felt mad or insistent on getting something, but otherwise he had to be prompted and pushed to speak. Every utterance was extremely difficult for him, and he would sometimes stare at a caregiver's mouth to try and form the same movements. His severe dyspraxia also interfered with his engaging in pretend play, although from his various facial expressions and the gleam in his eye when he engaged in playful interactions with his parents, it appeared he was playing little "tricks." He sometimes held onto toy objects, like a soft sword or a magic wand, and used them in ritualized ways—but he could not use toys to sequence new ideas. He could become engaged and even initiated sensory-motor interactions involving the expression of pleasure and affection. Although games with his brother had to be orchestrated, he did enjoy running around the schoolyard and the pool with other children.

In the second year of intervention, at age 5 years, he was able to interact and communicate with three or four back-and-forth exchanges about what he wanted (e.g., pulling his dad over to the refrigerator and finding the hot dogs). He could even retrieve a few words at such moments: "hot dog"; "what else?"; "french fries." Harold became more consistently engaged over time, developed islands of presymbolic ability, and tuned in to more of what was going on around him. He no longer wandered aimlessly and could be observed picking up trucks to push, putting together simple puzzles, or engaging in other cause-and-effect play. He let others join him but invariably turned the interaction into sensory-motor play, which brought him great pleasure.

As indicated, each type, in addition to being characterized by its functional emotional developmental capacity, should also be characterized in terms of its regulatory-sensory processing profile. Chapter 8 ("Assessment and Treatment of Infants and Young Children With Regulatory-Sensory Processing Disorders") highlights the different regulatory-sensory processing domains that should be considered. A full clinical understanding of the child requires this profile, in addition to the type designation described above.

For research purposes, the regulatory-sensory processing profile can be simplified. For example, most children with NDRC (including autism spectrum disorders) evidence challenges in language and visuospatial thinking, but differ enormously in their auditory memory and visuospatial memory capacities, as well as in their motor planning and sensory modulation capacities. Therefore, those features that capture important clinical and, most likely, etiological pathway differences, must be highlighted. Table 9–1 summarizes both the NDRC types and their regulatory-sensory processing profile in terms of these dimensions, and Table 9–2 summarizes the motor and regulatory-sensory processing patterns that are helpful in profiling the child. These summaries are provided to facilitate the use of this framework in a variety of clinical and research settings.

Other Neurodevelopmental Disorders (Including Genetic and Metabolic Syndromes)

The four types of NDRC described above can be used to describe children with any category of nonprogressive developmental disorder, including many of the well-known genetic syndromes. These syndromes involve problems with communicating and language, thinking (i.e., cognitive challenges), sensory and motor

---

TABLE 9–1.   Overview of clinical subtypes of NDRC and related motor
                 and regulatory-sensory processing profiles

Type I—Intermittent capacities for attending and relating; reciprocal interaction; and,
   with support, shared social problem solving and the beginning use of meaningful ideas
   (i.e., with help, the child can relate and interact and even use a few words, but not in a
   continuous and stable age-expected manner).
Children with this pattern tend to show rapid progress in a comprehensive program that
   tailors meaningful emotional interactions to their unique motor and regulatory-sensory
   processing profile.

Type II—Intermittent capacities for attention, relating, and a few back-and-forth
   reciprocal interactions, with only fleeting capacities for shared social problem solving and
   repeating some words.
Children with this pattern tend to make steady, methodical progress.

Type III—Only fleeting capacities for attention and engagement. With lots of support,
   occasionally a few back-and-forth reciprocal interactions. Often no capacity for repeating
   words or using ideas, although the child may be able to repeat a few words in a memory-
   based (rather than meaningful) manner.
Children with this pattern often make slow but steady progress, especially in the basics of
   relating with warmth and learning to engage in longer sequences of reciprocal
   interaction. Over long periods of time, these children often gradually master some words
   and phrases.

Type IV—Similar to Type III above, but with a pattern of multiple regressions (loss of
   capacities). May also evidence a greater number of associated neurological challenges,
   such as seizures, marked hypotonia, and so forth.
Children with this pattern often make extremely slow progress. The progress can be
   enhanced if the sources of the regressive tendencies can be identified.

Note.   NDRC = neurodevelopmental disorders of relating and communicating

---

processing, and sometimes relating. Children born with these syndromes, including Down, Rett, Angelman's, Prader-Willi, Turner's, fragile X, and others, may
have relative strengths in relating but often have compromises to different degrees
in various developmental capacities. As with the other NDRC, it is important to
evaluate auditory processing and language capacities; visuospatial processing; sensory modulation; and motor planning and sequencing, including oral-motor.
Only such a comprehensive evaluation permits the construction of an optimal intervention program. When a child evidences a well-identified genetic or metabolic
syndrome, the syndrome should be identified as well as the type of NDRC that
best describes the child's functioning. In this way, the child can be described both
from the perspective of the etiology of his disorder and the developmental profile
that characterizes it.

   It should be emphasized, however, that as with all infant and early childhood
disorders, attempts at categorization should not substitute for constructing a de-

---

TABLE 9–2. Overview of motor and regulatory-sensory processing profile

---

Children with NDRC (which include children with autism spectrum disorders) tend to evidence very different biologically based patterns of sensory reactivity, processing, and motor planning. These differences may have diagnostic and prognostic value, and therefore it may be helpful to describe them. The child's tendencies can be briefly summarized in the framework outlined below. *Note:* Almost all children with an NDRC diagnosis evidence language and visuospatial thinking challenges.

The patterns listed below are the ones that tend to differ among children. Please check all boxes that apply and, if sufficient clinical information is available, also use the box to indicate the degree to which that characteristic applies on a 1 to 3 scale (with 1 indicating minimum and 3 indicating the maximum degree).

Sensory Modulation

☐ Tends to be overresponsive to sensations, such as sound or touch (e.g., covers ears or gets dysregulated with lots of light touch)

☐ Tends to crave sensory experience (e.g., actively seeks touch, sound, and different movement patterns)

☐ Tends to be underresponsive to sensations (e.g., requires highly energized vocal or tactile support to be alert and attend)

Motor Planning and Sequencing

☐ Relative strength in motor planning and sequencing (e.g., carries out many-step action patterns, such as negotiating obstacle courses or building complex block designs)

☐ Relative weakness in motor planning and sequencing (e.g., can barely carry out simple movements and may tend to simply bang blocks or do other one- to two-step action patterns)

Auditory Memory

☐ Relative strength in auditory memory (remembers or repeats long statements or materials from books, TV, records, etc.)

☐ Relative weakness in auditory memory (difficulty remembering even simple sounds or words)

Visual Memory

☐ Relative strength in visual memory (tends to remember what is seen, such as book covers, pictures, eventually words, etc.)

☐ Relative weakness in visual memory (difficulty remembering even simple pictures or objects)

Note. NDRC = neurodevelopmental disorders of relating and communicating

---

velopmental profile of the child that includes the perspective reflected in each of the axes of the recommended multiaxial framework. This emphasis is especially important for many of the syndromes described in this category because, as indicated above, some children with a number of developmental challenges are very warm and engaged and have a real strength in their capacity for intimacy and, at the same time, evidence marked difficulties in motor functioning, language, and/or areas of cognitive functioning.

In addition, although many of the developmental disorders referred to above are best described in terms of the category of NDRC (in addition to their etiologically based diagnoses), some children may be best described in terms of their regulatory-sensory processing patterns and more closely approximate the criteria for this category. For example, a child may be very warmly related and comfortable with intimacy, using emotions or affect to signal, and may easily participate in back-and-forth reciprocal social interactions. However, he may also show marked motor and cognitive challenges, as well as language delays (using whatever language is at his disposal creatively and meaningfully). This child may be described best in terms of his etiologic syndrome and the regulatory-sensory processing categories that capture his unique individual differences.

Therefore, it is helpful to consider all nonprogressive developmental disorders within the multiaxial framework presented in this manual. The goal is to describe each child's unique characteristics as a basis for constructing a comprehensive, developmentally based intervention program.

Therapeutic Principles

The most important therapeutic principle is to facilitate the child's moving toward an adaptive, developmental progression with a focus on the fundamentals of forming relationships, communicating with social and emotional gestures, and learning to use ideas meaningfully. Before elaborating on this principle, let us first look at some of the obstacles to effective intervention.

The biggest obstacle to the successful treatment of NDRC is delay in detecting deficits in the building blocks of relating, thinking, and communicating and initiating a program to reestablish an adaptive developmental process. When problems are detected early, caregivers and children can, to varying degrees, learn to work around regulatory dysfunctions and their associated relationship and communication problems. They can, again to varying degrees, form warm, empathetic, and satisfying relationships. (For descriptions of the degrees and rates of progress that are possible, see the classification system outlined later in this chapter.) In many cases, however, parents suspect that something is wrong when their child is 13 or 14 months old, but they wait to investigate. Perhaps someone advises them that the child "will grow out of it." At about 20 months, many parents arrange a developmental assessment but lose another 4–5 months waiting for speech therapy and occupational therapy workups and for neurological and genetic consultations. All of these assessments may be helpful, but they should take place within a week so that treatment can begin promptly. At this age, every month that passes is worth years later on. If the child finally gets a therapist's attention at 2 years of age, she has lost important time. (Our clinical experience with 2- to 3-year-olds, however, shows that with the help of an intensive intervention program, many can still learn gestural communication, adaptive emotional expression, and eventually symbolic communication. The earlier such a program is started, however, the quicker we see progress.)

Treatment should have one simple goal: to get the child back into, or to establish, a continuous flow of natural, warm communication. To accomplish this goal, treatment must help the child learn to attend, engage, interact purposefully, experience a range of feelings, and ultimately think and relate in an organized, logical manner. In short, treatment must help the child master the six core developmental capacities outlined in the DIR model. Caregivers must be helped to provide the kinds of interactive experiences necessary for the child to master these capacities. Finally, an educational setting must be selected or tailored to meet the child's need for both special teaching expertise and peer interaction that provides the kind of feedback the child needs to develop his capacity for intentional relating.

Before describing effective treatment more fully, let us consider some common approaches that are often ineffective.

Fragmented, Rigid Approaches

Perhaps one of the most common unhelpful approaches is to teach discrete skills in an isolated or fragmented way. This haphazard approach invariably leads to educational, therapeutic, or parental interactions that are stereotyped, controlling, or avoidant. For example, suppose a therapist is trying to get a child to put a square block in a square hole, but the child is looking out the window, staring at the ceiling, or banging the block on the floor. Frustrated by his inattentiveness, the therapist may finally hold his face and insist that he look at her. Next, she tries to get him to listen by speaking slowly and firmly, perhaps in a repetitive monotone: "Look at me. Look at me. Look at me." She may reason that this way of speaking provides the child with a simple, clear stimulus and will thus help him plan and carry out the desired behavior. If the therapist has been influenced by behavioral schools of thought, she may add a reward, such as a piece of candy or verbal praise (also delivered in a computer-like monotone), every time the child looks at her. Because parents often copy the therapist's way of speaking and relating to the child, the child is likely to experience the same kind of mechanical interactions at home.

Any objective observer, seeing an adult sit next to a child and talk in a computer-like voice, would hardly be surprised at the child's lack of interest. Who wants to talk to a machine? The adult has given the child no real incentive or reason to pay attention. Clearly, children who tend to be aimless and self-absorbed and adults who tend to be rigid and stereotyped cannot assist one another in genuine relating.

It may be that most adults who work with such children begin inadvertently to copy the child's perseverative and stereotyped speech and behavior. The adult tends to be perseverative and stereotyped in a rigid, focused way, whereas the child vacillates between rigid, focused perseverative activities and more aimless, distractible, self-absorbed behavior. Nonetheless, one observes a remarkable similarity in the behaviors of adult and child.

Perhaps such identification with the child should not be surprising. The child is not providing the kind of feedback most adults expect. Even therapists working with very anxious, conflicted children get lots of affective and behavioral responses from them. Parents are probably biologically programmed in some way to respond to the feedback they get from their children, and this feedback keeps them engaged and interacting. The smiling baby, the eagerly pointing toddler, or the chattering preschooler elicits certain feelings in her parents that in turn lead the parents to behave in ways that promote developmental capacities in their child. A smiling baby promotes a smiling parent. When the adult receives only aimless, perseverative, or self-absorbed feedback, he or she is unprepared and will likely feel confused. The natural response to this confusion may be to either become overly rigid and controlling or to withdraw. One sometimes sees a similar pattern when a child who is developing in a healthy fashion interacts one on one with an aimless and perseverative child: the healthier child may, like many therapists, begin intruding and pressuring the other child to give some response.

Some clinicians and programs rationalize such intrusive, stereotyped behavior as "therapeutic." It is important to understand, however, that although this behavior may be a natural, biologically driven tendency in anyone faced with a child who is not providing the expected feedback, it is not therapeutic.

Another overly rigid, stereotyped approach is the use of a strict behavior-modification program. Systematic reinforcers are employed to promote certain positive behaviors, whereas time-outs and certain abstinence procedures are employed to discourage or extinguish negative behaviors. The very systematization of such approaches, and the mechanical quality of the resulting interactions between child and adult, may promote rigid, stereotyped interactions rather than genuine relatedness.

The widespread use of such approaches may help explain why children with pervasive developmental disorders and autism often look increasingly unusual as they grow older. They commonly become more stereotyped and more perseverative. Even children who develop certain "splinter skills" and intellectual capacities, such as reading or arithmetic, may nonetheless exhibit increasingly rigid and stereotyped social responses. (The movie *Rain Man*, starring Dustin Hoffman as a high-functioning man with autistic-type patterns, provides a good example.) We need to consider the possibility that the types of interventions that have been organized on behalf of these infants and children tend to promote rather than to remedy their more mechanical qualities.

If every time we wish to help a child copy a particular motor sequence or perform a particular academic task, we can simultaneously work on his core developmental competencies in a spontaneous way that promotes his initiative, we may see a progression toward greater flexibility, warmth, intimacy, and spontaneity.

Working Above the Child's Developmental Level

Parallel Commentary

A tendency exists even among the most relationship-oriented therapists to ignore the delayed child's core needs and employ therapeutic tactics taken from intervention with developmentally more advanced children. One such error, also mentioned briefly in Chapter 4 ("Therapeutic Principles"), involves parallel play and commentary. Suppose a particular child is not only nonverbal and nonrepresentational but also is not yet capable of complex interactive gestures. He can react to someone else's overture by taking a block that is offered to him, but he cannot initiate giving the block back and will not look at or vocalize to the giver. A therapist trained to work with neurotic 2-, 3-, and 4-year-olds may assume that she can form a relationship simply by sitting next to the child and commenting on what he is doing. "Oh, Johnny is putting one block on top of the other. Oh, he's knocking it down now. Now he's building it up again." The child, meanwhile, shows no emotion and may not even take in what the therapist says. No interaction is taking place, and the child's developmental capacities are not being furthered. A therapist and child may go on this way for weeks, months, or even years with little or no movement or gain.

Searching for Underlying Conflicts

A therapist watching the child just described might also make the mistake of reasoning, "Ah ha, this child is building up and breaking down with his blocks. This looks to me like a conflict involving aggression and castration anxiety. Or a conflict involving loss. Or a conflict involving growth and destruction." The therapist may begin to comment to the child that he is destroying his blocks, or destroying his family with the blocks, or building up the blocks and then destroying them. She may comment further on fears of destruction or of growth. Yet as she pursues alleged underlying conflicts, the therapist misses the fact that this child is not even functioning at a level that enables him to understand symbolic verbal communications. She erroneously assumes that even though the child has not spoken a word or interacted gesturally, he has a preconscious or unconscious capacity to understand everything she is saying. Even if the therapist tried to ask, simply and directly, "Why do you like to knock down the blocks?" she would still be working well above the capacities of someone who is barely gesturally, and not at all verbally, interactive.

Focusing on Splinter Skills

"Splinter skills" are isolated cognitive abilities often acquired through rote learning methods. Parents, understandably, want their cognitively and linguistically delayed children to appear more normal. Therapists may long for some sign of intellectual brilliance from a delayed youngster. Together, they may try to help the child master specific skills, such as reciting the days of the week, recognizing letters or words, or memorizing the contents of a book. Some of the rigid, stereotyped methods described earlier, such as holding a child's face or using candy as a reward, can enable the child to perform specific tasks under certain circumstances and with certain cues. However, a change of location, context, or even the verbal sequence used to cue the behavior will take away the child's ability to recognize the letters or read the book in any but the most concrete and perseverative way. Splinter skills may boost the morale of the parent, educator, or clinician, but rarely do they help the child much.

Certain mechanical skills, however, may help a child mobilize her core developmental competencies. As long as the *method* of teaching is not overly mechanical, learning sounds or words that she can use to signal needs or desires—as a less delayed child might do with complicated hand gestures or facial expressions—can only be helpful. Later on, the same words may become part of a more complex symbolic capacity. Similarly, concepts such as "more" and "less," "up" and "down," as well as social behavior such as sitting and concentrating, can be helpful if they are taught in ways that promote the child's spontaneity and initiative. However, if the teaching of such skills is overly stereotyped and not integrated with efforts to promote the child's core developmental competencies, those competencies may actually be undermined.

Working Below the Child's Developmental Level

At the other extreme, some clinicians make the mistake of focusing only on developmental competencies that the child has already mastered. Using the example of the child playing with blocks, suppose this child loves to cuddle with his parents and hug them. He is happy to lean against his dad while he perseveratively stacks up and knocks down his blocks. A therapist who focused her efforts only on warmth, security, and cuddling would be working below this child's developmental level. Fostering emotional closeness might not do any harm, but it accomplishes nothing more than helping the child practice something he is already comfortable with. As implied in the previous sections, a treatment plan appropriate for this child's level of development would focus first on fostering intentional two-way communication—that is, the therapist would actively attempt to help the child open and close increasing numbers of communication circles in a row.

Principles of Effective Intervention

Perhaps the primary goal in working with children who have NDRC is to enable them to form a sense of their own personhood—that is, a sense of themselves as intentional, interactive individuals. As we have discussed, infants and young children with these disorders tend to operate in an aimless, fragmented, idiosyncratic, and impersonal manner. If one tries to imagine what their internal experience is like on the basis of their behavior, it seems that they organize fragments of experience around basic needs and stereotyped interactions with their physical world.

In normal development, we hypothesize, a young child's sense of self evolves from her ability to abstract from repeated experiences of human interaction. From infancy, a child has a seemingly infinite number of interactions with her caregivers. The sense of personhood that she abstracts from this accretion of experiences does not initially exist at a symbolic, or representational, level. In its earliest form, it likely organizes itself around physical sensations, a sense of being connected to others, and the affects associated with this sense of connection or engagement. Later, as a result of increasingly complex experiences of two-way purposeful communication, the child's sense of personhood widens to encompass a sense of intentionality. At higher levels, as the child uses symbols and organizes and differentiates these, she develops an increasingly complex, nuanced symbolic sense of self. In a child's development of a sense of personhood, as in her development of all other capacities, earlier levels serve as a foundation for higher levels.

In designing interventions for children who have delays and dysfunctions in their capacities for relating and communicating, it is critical to remember that their sense of self derives not simply from language functioning, motor functioning, or cognition. Addressing any or all of these in isolation may only reinforce a child's sense of fragmentation. Instead, one must consider how any proposed intervention affects the child's ability to abstract from human interaction, to organize an emotional, sensation-based experience of his own being. Because children with NDRC often lack the most basic foundations of interpersonal experience (e.g., many are not interactive in the purposeful way that ordinary 8-month-olds are), much of the experience they would otherwise use to abstract a sense of self is unavailable to them.

A Comprehensive Program

A comprehensive program is based on our DIR model. This model includes a focus on three vital dimensions—functional, emotional, and developmental capacities.

A DIR-based comprehensive program involves a number of components, including an *intensive* home program with parents and other caregivers, an educational program, appropriate therapies, and if indicated, biomedical interventions.

All elements of the program need to focus on helping the child build the core foundations for relating, communicating, and thinking as well as for overcoming symptoms. The home program is especially important because of the amount of time children spend with caregivers and their emotional importance.

All the elements in the DIR model (Table 9–3) have a long tradition, including speech and language therapy, occupational therapy, special and early childhood education, and Floortime–type interactions with parents (which is consistent with the developmentally appropriate practice guidelines of the National Association for the Education of Young Children [Bredekamp and Copple 1997] and pragmatic speech therapy practices, both of which attempt to foster preverbal and symbolic communication and thinking). The DIR model, however, contributes to these traditional practices by further defining the child's developmental level, individual processing differences, and the need for certain types of interactions in terms of a comprehensive program where all the elements can work together toward common goals.

In this model, children and their parents are engaged in emotional interactions that use their emerging, but not fully developing, capacities for communication (often initially with gestures rather than words). The longer such children remain uncommunicative, and the more parents lose their sense of their children's relatedness, the more deeply the children tend to withdraw and become perseverative and self-stimulatory.

Such an "intensive" approach is not intended to overwork or stress children. Their state of mind is considered and the interactive activities recommended are part of playful interactions in which their interests and initiative are followed and opportunities are created for joyful, soothing, and pleasurable interactions. When the children are tired, the playful interactions might involve them showing or verbalizing to their parents where it is best to rub their back or feet. Passive television watching (except for one half-hour a day) and rote memory exercises such as memorizing letters or numbers are not recommended.

The DIR intervention is fundamentally different from behavioral, skill building, or play therapy or psychotherapy. The primary goal of this intervention (sometimes referred to as *Floortime*) is to enable children to form a sense of themselves as intentional, interactive individuals; to develop cognitive language and social capacities from this basic sense of intentionality; and to progress through the six functional emotional developmental capacities.

Cornerstones of the Home and School Program

Next, we discuss some of the elements in a comprehensive program in the context of the DIR model. We begin with the types of interactions that should characterize a home and school program to master the functional emotional capacities and build a sense of self, as well as the abilities for relating, communicating, and thinking.

TABLE 9–3.   Elements of a comprehensive program

I.   **Home-based, developmentally appropriate interactions and practices (Floortime)**

   A.   Spontaneous, follow-the-child's-lead Floortime (20- to 30-minute sessions, 8–10 times a day)

   B.   Semistructured problem solving (15+ minutes, five to eight times a day)

   C.   Spatial, motor, and sensory activities (15+ minutes, four times a day), including

   1.   Running and changing direction, jumping, spinning, swinging, deep tactile pressure

   2.   Perceptual motor challenges, including looking and doing games

   3.   Visuospatial processing and motor planning games, including treasure hunts and obstacle courses

   4.   The above activities can become integrated with the pretend play

II.   **Speech therapy** (typically three or more times a week)

III.   **Sensory integration-based occupational therapy and/or physical therapy** (typically two or more times a week)

IV.   **Educational program** (daily)

   A.   For children who can interact and imitate gestures and/or words and engage in preverbal problem-solving, either an integrated program or a regular preschool program with an aide

   B.   For children not yet able to engage in preverbal problem-solving or imitation, a special education program in which the major focus is on the following: engagement; preverbal purposeful gestural interaction; preverbal problem solving (a continuous flow of back-and-forth communication); and learning to imitate actions, sounds, and words

V.   **Biomedical interventions**, including consideration of medication, to enhance motor planning and sequencing, self-regulation, concentration, and/or auditory processing and language

VI.   **A consideration of**

   A.   Nutrition and diet

   B.   Technologies geared to improve processing abilities, including auditory processing, visuospatial processing, sensory modulation, and motor planning

---

Functional Emotional Developmental ("D") Capacities: Mastering the Foundations of Relating, Communicating, and Thinking

Levels 1–4: Attention, Engagement, Two-Way Intentional Communication, and Problem-Solving Interactions

For children with NDRC, the earliest therapeutic goals must target the earliest developmental capacities: focus and concentration, engagement with other humans, and two-way intentional communication. Addressing these capacities is easier said than done: a child who is tuning out, wandering apparently aimlessly around the room, banging on the windows, touching the floor, and repeatedly opening and closing doors hardly appears interested in focusing, engaging, and interacting. The same tactics that help foster attention and engagement in children with regulatory disorders will be helpful here. How does this child process experiences of sound, touch, and other sensory stimuli? Can she focus better on loud voices or soft ones, in a brightly lit room or a dimly lit one? What kinds of motion or physical activity seem to help her focus best? As mentioned in Chapter 8 ("Assessment and Treatment of Infants and Young Children With Regulatory-Sensory Processing Disorders"), an occupational therapy consultation may help answer such questions: many occupational therapists are especially gifted at finding ways to help infants and children focus and engage.

Whatever specific tactics are required, it is always best to employ these in the context of spontaneous interaction with the child. Forced, mechanical intimacy of the kind described earlier—for example, holding a child's head or rewarding the child with candy for looking at the adult—is not true intimacy and probably does not yield the kind of visceral pleasure that occurs in routine development. It is critical to create opportunities for the visceral feeling of pleasure and intimacy that leads a child to *want* to relate to the human world.

To foster this feeling parents, therapists, and teachers need to take advantage of each child's natural interests and inclinations. Consider the example of a father who had tried unsuccessfully for weeks to attract his son's attention. The toddler had a habit of turning a toy wheel around and around for long periods of time. One day, the father discovered that by reaching over and turning the wheel in the opposite direction, he could finally arouse his son's interest and curiosity. Whose hand was this turning the wheel, and whose face was connected to the hand? For the first time in his life, the child looked up at his father with a warm, alert expression. He was experiencing interaction and a feeling of connection through a mechanical motor activity, one that was actually perseverative in nature, because his father had joined in the perseveration. In cases where such an opening does not seem to present itself, and the child is actively avoiding human interaction by engaging in some solitary perseverative activity, the adult must physically get in the child's way. For example, one boy wanted only to scratch the floor with his fingernails. His mother wisely did not intrude in an overly vigorous way, but she made her presence felt by placing her hand in each spot her son wanted to scratch. Each time, he looked annoyed and pulled her hand away. Annoyance is a type of engagement, and by pulling his mother's hand away, the child was interacting with her. As the mother playfully varied her intrusions—for example by pulling her hand away at the last second—she actually got a grunt of pleasure from the toddler.

This response took many weeks to elicit. However, the days, weeks, and even months needed to foster a spontaneous sense of pleasure and engagement are time well spent, because these capacities are the foundation of all subsequent learning. The child cannot abstract a sense of self from human experiences that he has never had. Skipping the earliest therapeutic steps and starting with more "advanced" goals will set the child up for failure.

The third step in the early therapeutic sequence involves fostering simple, and then more complex, gestural communication. When a child already has some linguistic skills, such as reciting letters and numbers, it can be tempting to base interactions on these. As discussed earlier, the therapist who does so is working above the child's level. Instead of starting at the verbal or symbolic level, one must get simple gestural exchanges going with the child first. One then builds on these to stimulate more complex gestural communication. One uses symbols only as they relate to gestures already operative. A clinical example illustrates this principle well:

Bobby, a 28-month-old boy diagnosed with pervasive developmental disorder, was playing with a car on the floor during an assessment session. He moved it back and forth, examined how it worked, and began rolling it again. His father tried to engage him by commenting, "That's a nice car. Look how Bobby is moving it. Now it's going fast. Now it's going slow." Although the father was talking warmly to his son, nothing was happening between them. The therapist suggested that he try to be more interactive. He then did what many parents and therapists would do: he continued to talk to his son about the car, asking, "Can you move it here?" He cupped his hands, pretending they were a house, and said, "Look, move the car into my house." Bobby continued to ignore him. The father, beginning to look discouraged, kept experimenting with different tactics. He made a tunnel with his hands and suggested that Bobby put his car in the tunnel. Exasperated, he began saying in a commanding tone, "Bring the car here. Give it to me!" Finally, in disgust, he took the car from his son and tried to hide it. Bobby got angry, threw a mild tantrum, and then refused to touch the car further, causing his father to feel even more discouraged. The father's attempts included two of the ineffective, but common, approaches discussed earlier: parallel verbal commentary and trying to interact with verbal or symbolic signals pitched at a higher level than the child can handle (e.g., using one's hands as a make-believe house). As often happens, the father's frustration led to abrupt, intrusive action.

Bobby's therapist then helped the father start with simple gestural exchanges of which Bobby was already capable. He advised the father to follow Bobby's lead. Because Bobby had resumed moving and examining the car, the therapist told his father, "Speak, and use any words you want, but make the interaction a very simple, gesture-to-gesture interaction. Use your words only as icing on the cake, an elaboration of the gestures. Use your motor system in interaction with Bobby's motor system." The father looked perplexed. The therapist explained, "You can take out other cars and aim them in his direction, or you can play with this car with him. The idea is to get some simple interaction going between you, no more complicated than rolling a ball back and forth." The father again tried cupping his hands and getting Bobby to send the car his way. The therapist commented, in a supportive manner, that this gesture had not worked before, either because Bobby did not want to respond or because he did not understand the complex gestural communication or the implied symbolic communication involved. The father then tried something much simpler: he gently put his hand on the car as Bobby was examining it and pointed to a particular part, as if to say, "What's that?" In pointing, the father actually moved the car, so that Bobby felt the car moving in his hands and noticed without upset his father's involvement, because it was gentle, slow, and unobtrusive. Bobby took the car back but looked at the spot his father had touched with his finger. The father's more physical, nonsymbolic gesture had succeeded in getting Bobby to close a circle of communication.

After getting this minimal interaction going, and when Bobby had started rolling his car again, the father got a second car and started moving it back and forth next to Bobby's. He moved his car toward Bobby's but did not crash into it. Bobby first pulled his car away, then moved it fast toward his dad's. Now three or four circles had been closed, and a real interaction was under way. Within a few minutes, father and son were involved in a game where they moved their cars toward each other, sometimes slowly, sometimes fast, and sometimes even crashing them. Then Bobby's father tried using his hands again, but he did not try to create a house or tunnel; he simply made a barrier, and Bobby closed another circle by trying to get his car around it.

Toward Level 5: From Gestures to Symbols

As they played with their cars, Bobby was exhibiting some focus and concentration, he was experiencing a degree of pleasure and engagement, and he and his father were exchanging simple and complex gestures. It was now appropriate to try exploring Bobby's symbolic capacities, but only in relation to the action he was involved in. The therapist said to the father, who had continued some commentary during the play, "If you like, you could now add words in a more interactive and intentional way. Just experiment with different words to see what he can understand." The father started to say "fast" while moving his car fast, and "slow" while moving it slowly. After he had done so four or five times, Bobby boomed his car into his father's and said "fast," without pronouncing it quite clearly. The father beamed, amazed that his son could learn a new word and use it appropriately so quickly. The therapist commented that words and symbols *can* be learned quickly as long as they are related to the child's experiences and built on his gestures. Words in isolation carry no meaning for him.

Bobby had very good fine motor skills, despite gross motor clumsiness and delays in all other areas. Later in the assessment session, Bobby's father wanted to show off how well Bobby could identify and draw different shapes. When he tried to get Bobby to say "square" or "circle" or told him to draw a shape, however, Bobby did nothing. The therapist again suggested that they get complex gestures going first. The father took a pencil and started scribbling circles. Bobby, who had already begun scribbling on the paper, responded by drawing a circle, a remarkably nice one. His father smiled as if to say, "See, I told you so!" Bobby had apparently done the same thing many times at home. As his father continued to scribble circles, Bobby responded to each circle by drawing one of his own, right next to his father's. Once this game was under way, the therapist suggested that Bobby's father might now try to introduce words, because the deed was firmly in place. The father started to say "circle" each time he drew one; much to our surprise, after three or four repetitions of this, Bobby himself started to say "circle" as he drew each circle. Each time he uttered the word, Bobby grinned with satisfaction toward his father.

Later on, Bobby drew a circle on his own while I was talking with his parents. He looked up at them to call their attention to it. He was now initiating gestural and early symbolic communication.

The experience of Bobby and his father illustrates the principle that as one succeeds in helping a child open and close circles of communication at the gestural level, one should begin moving into the more complex gestural and early symbolic realms. It is extremely important that these capacities be joined.

Levels 5 and 6: Fostering the Use of Representations (Ideas) and Logical Thinking

As children with severe difficulties in relating and communicating gradually learn to represent their experience, they typically start off representing it in a highly fragmented and at times emotionally intense or labile way. Some previously withdrawn, aimless children become so connected to their caregivers that they cling, demand, and talk all the time, even though a year earlier they were not speaking a word. It is as though having discovered that the human world is a wonderful place, they want to make sure they do not lose it. The child's new, intense relatedness and verbosity tend to operate in short bursts of ideas or fragments of higher-level concepts. A child may talk to herself about cars crashing, then suddenly say, "Look at the leaves out the window," and then, "Give me my juice!" Immediately after uttering these words, she may start playing out a scene of dolls having a tea party. Each burst of symbolic activity may last only 30 seconds, and there may be no logical bridges between one burst and another. However, this driven quality should be understood as an important progression beyond the child's previous withdrawn, aimless state. The use of fragmented ideation suggests that the child's capacity for symbolization is developing. The task now is to foster more differentiated, abstract, and logical use of ideas while continuing to promote the child's spontaneity and initiative. The parent, clinician, or teacher must walk a fine line between empathizing and following the child's lead and actively helping her to become more logical.

Self-Absorbed Thinking

As we discussed in Chapter 8 ("Assessment and Treatment of Infants and Young Children With Regulatory-Sensory Processing Disorders"), a child with receptive language impairments has a much easier time attending to his own thoughts than to the words and ideas of other people. Most children with NDRC have difficulty with auditory-verbal processing, and some also have difficulty processing visuospatial information. Children with these patterns have to work much harder than most people to take in verbal and sometimes visual information from caregivers, therapists, and others. As intervention helps them begin developing the capacity for symbolic thought, they experience an excitement and ease in tuning into their own emerging thoughts, especially because these have been so long in coming. They will often use intense ideation as a way of keeping themselves interested and excited and practicing a new skill, but they will also use it as a substitute for taking in the ideas of others. At this stage, a child remains engaged at the behavioral level but is disengaged at the symbolic level. For example, he may physically cling to his parents but speak and play according to his own game plan, without taking in and responding to his parents' symbolic-level feedback. He can sit in his mother's lap and tell her a story about a tea party, but if she asks, "Who's coming to the party?" or "What's going to happen next?" he ignores her inquiries and continues as though no one else had spoken. If this pattern continues too long, the result may be a child who, although very related and engaged, is idiosyncratic in his thinking and speech. He never begins differentiating between fantasy and reality, between his own thoughts and the outside world.

It is the taking in of symbolic-level feedback that enables the child to categorize her symbolic-level experiences. The parent or caregiver becomes the representative of what is outside the child and thus the foundation for reality. In other words, if there is a symbolic "me" and a symbolic "you" interacting, this forms the basis for more differentiated, cause-and-effect symbolic interactions. If the child experiences only the "me" in interactions, she cannot progress toward differentiating self from other at the representational level, even though she differentiates these at the earlier level of somatic and behavioral experience.

As we discussed earlier, it can be difficult to enter the behavioral world of a child with multiple severe developmental delays. It may be even harder to enter his symbolic world. In Floortime and during problem-solving discussions, the parent must persist in trying to bring the child back to the parent's comment or question until the child closes the symbolic-level circle. The parent can try spending about half the time gently playing dumb, like the television character Columbo. Suppose the child has just pretended that his puppet bit a cat, and the parent plays the role of the cat, saying, "Ouch! You hurt me." If the child then looks out the window, the parent can ask, "But what about the cat? What about his ouch?" If the child responds, "I'll give another ouch," and has the puppet bite the cat again, he has closed the circle. If he goes back to gazing at the trees outside and the parent says, "Don't you want to talk more about the cat?" and the child replies, "No let's look at the tree," he has closed another circle and created a logical bridge between one set of ideas and another.

Floortime and pretend play, talking about food or friends, negotiating bedtime, or just watching a cartoon on television can all provide opportunities for helping a child to open and close circles at the symbolic level and to differentiate and connect ideas. Because the child with auditory processing delays finds it so much easier to march to her own drummer, parents and clinicians can easily find themselves slipping into conversational patterns that do not help the child maintain an increasingly long flow of interactions at the symbolic level. For example, the adult may ask the child an endless series of discrete questions that do not support a long chain of communication circles: "What color is the car?" How fast is the car going?" Where is the car driving to?" Such conversation, even when successful in getting the child to respond, tends to take on a mechanical, singsong quality. It does not help the child build logical bridges.

As the adult succeeds in helping the child to become more verbal, the adult must balance focus on the content of the child's verbalizations with interest in the child's feelings and emotional intentions. In the following exchange, the adult succeeds in avoiding a mechanical exchange focused only on content and instead addresses the child's real affective drama:

> Child: Look at my car!
> Adult: I see it.
> Child: It goes fast—zoom!
> Adult: I can see that. It looks exciting that it's going so fast.
> Child (with a big smile): Watch, I can make it go like a rocket ship!
> Adult: Wow, that's a powerful rocket.
> Child (beaming with pride): Here it comes!

By attending to and empathizing with the child's affect, the adult supports the child in connecting a series of ideas that develop the theme of power. To accomplish this, an adult needs to be relaxed, curious, and spontaneous and to choose simple words that do not overwhelm the child's vulnerable receptive language capacities. Some adults make the mistake of talking very slowly and clearly, which can cause their speech to take on a mechanical, contrived quality. Slow, mechanical sentences are actually harder for the child to understand because they lack the rhythmic variations that support the meaning of the words. (A string of numbers recited slowly and mechanically is much harder to recall accurately than one read with rhythm and feeling.) In addition, mechanically spoken words do not prompt the child to respond with speech that has emotional tone to it.

As children with NDRC achieve greater differentiation in their thinking, the stage of intense neediness and nonstop, fragmented talkativeness described earlier often passes. The children become calmer, less driven, and more capable of organized thought. Their emotional signaling, as well as their use of words, appears more and more adaptive.

Self-Motivated Opportunities for Differentiation

When a child is highly motivated—for example, when he is extremely interested in getting a certain kind of food or going outside—one has an excellent opportu-

nity to open and close many symbolic circles with him. The child who keeps trying to open the door because he wants to go out and is angry that he cannot may,
in the midst of all his crying and shouting, open and close 20 circles. Although one
should not deliberately frustrate the child, one should recognize that frustration
arising from a difference of opinion is an excellent motivator that occurs naturally
in the course of the day. In many such situations, the parent or teacher wishes to
cut short the power struggle or redirect the child ("maybe…but why don't you
look at your book instead?") because he is being so angry and demanding. Instead,
one should stretch out the periods of negotiation. It is great for a child to be demanding as long as he is verbally opening and closing circles of communication.
Extend these periods of motivated interaction and provide clear and direct feedback: "I want to go out!" "Not now." "Now!" "Not now—later," and so on. Simply
playing an interactive game, or a turn-taking game involving some impersonal
cognitive task, will not resonate at nearly the same level of emotional depth as an
extended conversation when the child is in a self-motivated state. The goal is not
simply to teach the child words but to offer him the opportunity to develop a sense
of himself as a person. This sense comes from deeply felt emotions and needs.

"Why" and "How" Questions

Children with NDRC cannot respond easily to "why?" and "how?" questions because these involve abstractions. If one asks, "Why did the puppet bite the cat?"
the child will look blank: she does not understand what "why" means. A parent or
clinician who is unaware of the sequence in which children learn concepts, or who
does not understand that children with NDRC take a much longer time than most
children to master basic concepts, may give up on interactive communication and
allow the child to march to her own drummer. Alternatively, the adult may over-
structure the dialogue by asking the child to label this or that body part or to name
items portrayed in a picture. Such tasks are fine for limited periods to help children
master specific words, but they will not help a child develop more differentiated
and abstract modes of thinking. Instead, one must use awareness of the sequence
by which children learn abstract concepts to engage the child in increasingly abstract symbolic dialogues. For example, children can handle "what" questions before "how" questions, and "how" questions before "why" questions. One must
experiment with simplifying one's questions until the child can close the circle of
communication. For example, consider the following exchange:

> Adult: Why do you want to go outside now?
> Child: I want to!
> Adult: But why?
> Child: Outside now!
> Adult: What is outside that you want?
> Child: Bicycle! Want ride bicycle!

Here, the adult realizes that the child cannot understand "why" and switches to a simpler "what" question, which allows the child to answer. The adult could end the discussion by rephrasing the child's answer in "why" form: "Oh, the reason why you want to go outside is to ride your bicycle!" After many such discussions, the child will eventually comprehend the meaning of "why."

Children have to master a great deal of differentiated thinking before they can answer a high-level "why" question with a high-level "because" answer. (A low-level "because" answer might be, for example, "Because that's the way it is." A higher-level answer would involve some cause-and-effect thinking: "John has to sit in this chair because he's big, and it's a big chair.") For children with NDRC, the ability to respond to such questions is a high achievement. The achievement is especially significant when the child's "because" answer comes in response to a personal question, such as one related to how the child is feeling or why he wants to do a certain thing.

Parents and clinicians must beware of scripting the child's dialogue by asking leading questions that require her only to fill in a word or two, or by talking about something for which she has already memorized pat phrases. (For example, an adult does not facilitate the child's ability to abstract by saying, "After one comes _____; and after two comes _____.") If the child is not surprising the adult with her comments, the adult is scripting the conversation too much.

Shifting From Concrete to Abstract Modes of Thought

Children with NDRC often find it especially difficult to move from concrete to abstract thinking, in part because they do not easily generalize from one experience to other, similar experiences. Learning that the answer to "Why do you want to go outside?" is "To play" will not enable them to figure out the answers to other "why" questions. Parents, teachers, and therapists frustrated by the child's slow progress may be tempted to create an illusion of progress by helping him master some rote-learned statements. They may justify this approach by saying, "I don't want to confuse him with too many new questions." However, the same principle that got the child to this level must continue: promote the spontaneous, child-initiated opening and closing of symbolic circles of communication. The more slowly the child is progressing toward abstraction and generalization, the more—not less—spontaneous, active, symbolic interaction he needs.

The adult needs to be ingenious in setting up opportunities for the child to initiate symbolic interaction and close circles. One can help a child elaborate her communication by moving from the general to the specific, always taking advantage of high states of motivation. For example, if a child is rolling a car toward a building, the adult can first enter the play gesturally by moving a second car alongside the child's and then ask, "What's going to happen?" If the child remains silent in the face of this most general elaboration, the adult should move to the next level: offering alternatives. "Should we go to the garage or the house over here?" In many cases, with such concrete alternatives, the child will say "Garage" or "House" or indicate her choice by pointing. If she remains silent, one simplifies the elaboration even further, while still being careful not to tell the child what to do. Instead of oversimplifying by saying, "Okay, we're going to the garage," one might say, "Okay, the cars are going into my mouth." The child may find this silly and say, "No, the garage!" or simply laugh. Either way, a nice symbolic circle has been closed. If the child continues to be unresponsive, the challenge is to come up with another set of gestures and ideas that build on hers, perhaps using simpler concepts and words.

Sometimes, parents and therapists become discouraged because although the child is learning more and more words, he still cannot answer simple questions like "What did you do at school today?" Yet consider that to answer such a question, the child has to have a symbolic sense of himself, not just in the here and now but in the immediate past. He must be able to form a mental image of himself in a space (the school) other than his immediate setting. In short, answering this simple question requires the child to be able to represent himself across time and across space. These abilities develop slowly, especially for children with NDRC. We can conceptualize the process of learning to use symbols as a gradual one comprising several early steps:

1. Using symbols in the here and now to seek immediate satisfaction of concrete needs (e.g., "Outside!" "Juice!")
2. Using symbols to meet needs other than immediate satisfaction (e.g., "Mom, come!" "What that?")
3. Using symbols to communicate about an object or activity of interest in a way that suggests emotions like curiosity or cooperation (e.g., pointing to a flower and saying, "Flower!" with a look of curiosity and pleasure that the child wishes to share)
4. Using symbols to communicate a wide variety of emotions in a way that indicates the child's flexibility and appreciation of the interactive, complex nature of these emotions (e.g., after a trip to the circus, a child puts on a silly hat, smiles proudly, and says, "Me clown!")

As the child progresses through these, and eventually more advanced, patterns of symbolic emotional interaction, she also progresses in her ability to build bridges between ideas. This process, again, comprises several early steps:

1. Expressing isolated ideas in the here and now (e.g., labeling objects, such as "table")
2. Connecting two or more ideas in the here and now (e.g., "Drink juice!")
3. Connecting two or more ideas in the here and now that involve various levels of causality (e.g., the child begins answering first "what," then "how," then "why" questions; statements like "I want to go outside because I do" eventually

yield to statements like "I want to go outside because it's sunny and I like to ride my bike when it's nice out.")

4. Connecting two or more ideas that require symbolizing oneself across time and space (e.g., "I want to play house with Sally at school tomorrow because I didn't get to do it today.")

These early steps form the foundation for more advanced modes of abstract thought in both the social-emotional and impersonal realms. Again, the developmentally delayed child must be provided with more, not less, interactive communication experience in order to reach his potential in mastering these steps. Parents, clinicians, and teachers must figure out ways to work around the child's auditory processing impairments, such as choosing simple words and dealing with clearly felt emotions or needs. They must create experiences in which the child wishes to initiate and maintain interactions, gradually challenge him to stretch out the continuous flow of symbolic interactions, and challenge him to use his emerging symbolic capacities in changing situations and contexts.

Parents, therapists, and teachers who are trying to help a child shift from concrete to abstract thought will find it helpful to remember that her processing difficulties do not imply a difficulty with central reasoning or creativity. She may have trouble understanding "why" or "how" questions, and she may be able to respond only to three-word, rather than six- or ten-word, sentences. However, such difficulties may well result from her processing problems rather from than any true deficiency in reasoning. The same child may well be able to create complicated spatial relationships in drawings or block-building projects, thus providing evidence of her creativity and central reasoning capacity. Consider how an accomplished physicist who speaks only a few words of English might discuss her theories with English-speaking colleagues. The physicists might have to use simple words, along with gestures and nonverbal media such as diagrams, to negotiate complex, sophisticated mathematical concepts. Similarly, a developmentally delayed child may be able to comprehend far more than her language delays allow her to show. She may, for example, understand the concepts "up" and "down" perfectly well even though she cannot understand the words that signify these concepts. By using hand gestures to illustrate "up" and "down" while saying, "This is *up* and this is *down*," an adult may be able to get a dialogue going with the child about these concepts. The same approach of using gestures combined with very simple words can be used to hold dialogues about complex concepts of size and even volume.

Shifting From Rigid to More Flexible Ways of Thinking and Relating

As a child with delays in relating and communicating begins to differentiate and logically connect ideas, one can expect him to enter a stage in which he generalizes too quickly and in a very concrete way. For example, when one father told his son, "I don't like candy," the son commented, "Oh, so children like candy and adults don't." This child made such statements frequently, prompting the father to lecture him on the illogic of his thinking. The child's therapist suggested that the father instead provide spontaneous, challenging feedback that would help his son "fine-tune" his logic. For example, he could say, with a grin, "But Mrs. Green, our neighbor, likes candy." Although the boy was temporarily confused by such responses, he slowly learned to think more flexibly.

Even a child's obsessive, ritualistic tendencies can provide the creative parent, therapist, or teacher with opportunities to enter into a spontaneous dialogue that will promote greater flexibility. For example, one boy became preoccupied with the "ing" sound at the end of words. Instead of ignoring this or fighting it, his parents and therapist said, "Do you love the 'ing' sound?" They joined him in thinking of "ing" words and making up "ing" songs, thus engaging him in a continuous flow of symbolic interaction around a topic that had initially been a solitary obsession. Another child repeatedly insisted that he was a certain cartoon character and told other people that they were certain characters or things. Instead of directly challenging these creative but fixed ideas, his parents and therapist used them to engage him in opening and closing symbolic and presymbolic circles. In this way, they gradually helped him think in a more flexible, differentiated manner.

A similar attitude is helpful when a child regresses, as many children with these disorders do, from a verbal, symbolic level of functioning to the level of disengagement. Instead of getting upset or assuming that a change of approach is needed, parents and therapist should see each regression as a communication and a chance to help the child learn what it is like to move back up the ladder—that is, to begin using gestures and words again. Children with large regressive ranges need to learn how to move in both directions.

Children with NDRC also tend toward rigidity in the affective realm. They attempt to avoid feeling anger and other strong emotions. One way in which they do this is by substituting rigid behavior and thoughts for feelings. Others in the child's world need to become comfortable responding with gentle "curve balls" that violate the child's rigid expectations. This will help the child become simultaneously more flexible and more direct in expressing anger and other emotions. Becoming secure in experiencing and expressing anger seems to be a critical step in the overall process of increasing affective flexibility. Consider the experience of one 4-year-old who was behaving provocatively after his therapist's vacation. He tuned out at any direct mention of vacations or feelings. One day, after he had kept the therapist waiting while he played in the waiting room, the therapist said, "You kept me waiting!" The boy looked at him, and the therapist said, "I guess I kept you waiting for 2 weeks." The boy smiled, took a doctor doll and started throwing it, and gave the therapist his first warm look since the therapist's return.

As these children become more organized at the gestural level, their affect system begins developing along a path that is very unusual for children with pervasive developmental disorder or autism spectrum problems: their affect begins to appear more and more normal. Children with NDRC are known for having idiosyncratic, mechanical affects. As one works interactively with them, however, their affects do not develop along an alternate pathway. Although they continue to have unique cognitive and sensory processing difficulties, their affect starts getting closer and closer to what we ordinarily expect. Of course, the degree of progress in this direction depends on the therapeutic work and on the parents' ability to interact successfully with their children, but even in cases in which this work is not completely successful, the children's affective experiences and expressions tend to become broader, deeper, and more differentiated.

Individual Differences ("I"): Different Ways of Understanding and Responding to the World

In order to help children master the foundations for relating, communicating, and thinking outlined in the prior section, it is essential to understand the child's unique way of processing sensory and motor patterns. This enables the clinician and caregivers to tailor learning interactions (i.e., interactions that facilitate mastery of the functional emotional developmental capacities) to the child's unique nervous system. Because children with autism spectrum disorders and other disorders of relating and communicating evidence many differences in the way they react to and process sensations and motor responses, the success of a program will often depend on its ability to tailor interactions to the child's unique qualities.

What is the best way to characterize each child's unique features? In technical terms we can talk about genetics and phenotypes. Yet how do the genes express themselves? Even before we are born, many environmental and genetic forces are at play in how our central nervous systems and physical bodies develop. How does what happens as our bodies develop before we are born express itself? After we are born and our bodies begin to mature, we are subjected to all sorts of influences that nurture, inhibit, and otherwise contribute to the variations that make us uniquely human. How do the early physical differences that are part of maturation and our biology express themselves?

To help understand the answers to these questions, we have identified a number of ways through which human beings process information and organize actions that express the uniqueness of each person's biology. By focusing on these specific processing areas, we can uncover the unique signature of each child—the special way in which that child engages the world in terms of understanding the information coming in and planning the response that goes out. In children with autism, challenges in the areas described in the following sections are often prominent, although children with other special needs and even typically developing children (and many adults) often evidence these differences to one degree or another.

Auditory Processing

Auditory processing is the way in which we receive information and comprehend it, and *language* is the way we express information. Auditory processing has to do with registering information through the ears, decoding what is heard—actually hearing different sounds and discriminating between them (e.g., high pitch or low pitch)—and making sense of the sounds in terms of the words and ideas being conveyed by another person. Language is the ability to express thoughts, ideas, and responses to others.

The most prominent processing challenges we see in children with autism, other special needs, and learning disabilities are differences in auditory processing and language. Sometimes a child has difficulty processing the information coming in. He just cannot make sense of it. Other times, he cannot express what is going on in his own mind. Sometimes, children with autism have troubles both in receiving information and getting it out to those around them.

Motor Planning and Sequencing

Motor planning and sequencing are the terms we use to describe how we act on our ideas or what we hear and see. We see this ability beginning in a little baby who is trying to turn to see where the voice is coming from. Although it appears that the baby is having an automatic response to a sound, there are actually quite a number of steps to it—a sequence that must be carried out to reach the baby's goal of looking for the voice. First, she must process the sound and be interested in it. Then she has to organize her muscles to move her body in such a way that it will turn toward the sound. Next, she has to physically turn her body, coordinating and sequencing the muscle movements so that she goes in the desired direction. Finally, she has to look for the voice and actually recognize that she has located the face it comes from.

Later on, when a child is just 16 months old, he can develop an even more complex motor planning and sequencing action by taking his mother by the hand, walking her to the refrigerator, and pointing to the food he wants. This, too, requires many complex actions sequenced in a row, but with the addition of sequencing and using emotions to get what is desired.

This type of motor planning and sequencing is also the underpinning for a later ability called *executive functioning,* or the ability to execute a series of actions leading to a specific goal. It is, for example, the 7- or 8-year-old's ability to solve problems and to stay on task, following through until the problem is solved. This is difficult for many children, not only those with autism and special needs but also for those with attentional learning problems. It can also be difficult for children who have no challenges at all. We all vary considerably in our ability to use this skill.

Visuospatial Processing

Visuospatial processing is the ability to make sense of and understand what we are seeing. In a young child, this can be the ability to size up a new house and figure out how to get from one room to another and back to mother. Children with difficulties in this processing area can sometimes "get lost" in a new place, get panicked and scared, and cry for mother to come find them. Older children might use this ability to build a house out of blocks or to set up a farm with a house, a barn, and all the animals in their places. A child with challenges in this area might just roll a toy car in and out of a garage repetitively. In general, visuospatial processing has to do with understanding how things go together and come apart, finding things that are hidden, finding one's way around in a physical space, and understanding the relationships between physical objects.

Sensory Modulation

The last processing area that helps describe a child's unique biology is the ability to modulate or regulate sensation as it is coming in. For example, we know that many children with special needs are overly sensitive to sensations such as sound and touch, such that light touch that is ordinarily very pleasurable to a child might feel like someone was abrading a scratch on his skin. With sounds, the ordinary human voice can feel like loud screeching to some children, even though the speaker is using a soft tone. We need to understand how children listen differently, experience touch differently, and even experience different sights. Bright lights, lots of color and movement, or even sunlight can be very overwhelming to some children.

By the same token, many children can be underreactive to certain types of sounds, touch, or sights. For example, some children hardly register that you are there when you talk to them, or they hardly register being touched. Such children may either retreat because they are not in touch with their worlds or they may seek out extra sensations—becoming daredevils. Children who are underreactive to sensation may run around trying to bang into people or trying to get extra sensory input because they crave and need it. They may be underreactive to pain, in which case they seem impervious when they fall or bang into things. Underreactive children are not actually impervious to the pain, however; they just do not register it quite as intensely as other children.

Working With Individual Differences: Tailoring Interactions to the Child's Unique Profile

Why is understanding a child's way of experiencing and modulating sensation so important? Well, for example, if the child is very overreactive to sound, we need to deal with that child in ways that are very different from those we might use for an underreactive child. Otherwise, we run the risk of overwhelming the child with sounds and having that child shut down, avoid, or move away from us rather than engage in a reciprocal interaction. We need to soothe and help regulate an overreactive child so we can pull her into a relationship with us. For the underreactive child, we need to do just the opposite. We have to energize up to pull that child in, using loud or compelling noises and extra touching—the very sensations that could drive an overreactive child further and further away into her own world.

If a child is stronger in visuospatial processing than auditory processing, we need to use that visuospatial strength to pull him into a relationship and engage him.

Basically, we try to *tailor our interactions with the child to that child's unique profile of biological differences.* In that way, we can use that unique profile to help the child master the fundamental milestones of attending, relating, communicating, and thinking. For example, a child with motor planning and sequencing differences can easily get lost in repetitive motions because she cannot plan meaningful actions. Yet as we help her become more interactive, she will not need to involve herself in the repetitive motions. The more interactive she becomes, the less she will involve herself in the meaningless motions. She can begin planning meaningful actions, which is part of what being interactive with another person means— the ability to initiate and respond to a series of interactions in a back-and-forth rhythm and sequence.

We identify the child's unique biology and processing capacities and use those to help him climb the ladder of mastering his functional emotional milestones. As we help him master these milestones—the ability to engage and relate, be purposeful, problem solve, and use ideas—we also help the child master the challenges of his unique biology. For a child who cannot plan actions, as we help him learn to solve problems, he also improves his ability to plan actions. As we help this child with motor planning and sequencing challenges use his ideas, he becomes able to use an idea to help plan what he wants to do.

It works the same with other processing differences. As a child who is very sensory overreactive learns to interact with others, she can begin regulating her environment. Instead of escaping, avoiding, and shutting down when the room is too noisy, she learns to point in such a way as to convey, "Be quiet." She might learn to go to the teacher and point to indicate that she has to go out of the room because it is overwhelming to her. Once she learns to use ideas, she can think, "Whew, I'm overloaded!" Now, instead of being ruled by her processing differences, she can be purposeful and intentional, controlling her world rather than just being overwhelmed by it.

Each of the functional emotional capacities has to be mastered to help us also master our unique biology and turn a potential problem into a strength. The child who is hyperreactive can become very intuitive, empathic, and sensitive to other people's needs rather than be overloaded. The child who is good visually but weaker auditorily can become a great artist or architect because he can use those visual skills. The potential can either be the source of a problem or an unusual gift depending on the child's capacities and how we work with them.

Relationships ("R"): Caregiver and Family Patterns

A clinician working with a developmentally delayed child can assume that each parent will have strong reactions to the child's disabilities. The child's difficulties, and the parents' response to them, will have a profound impact on the marital relationship and on the overall family dynamics. Uncovering and addressing the parents' feelings and patterns of response is a critical part of the therapeutic process.

Many parents feel depressed and withdraw from their children; others deny their sadness and disappointment and become perfectionistic and controlling. Some vacillate between depressed, withdrawn states and overly controlling interactions. Certain fantasies and feelings are common. Parents may feel guilty and wonder, "What did I do to make my child this way?" They may feel angry and disappointed and think, "This is unfair. I've worked too hard for this to be true." A parent may feel anger toward the child, toward his or her spouse, or toward clinicians and service providers.

In some parents, the signs of expectable feelings like anger, sadness, and disappointment are subtle. One mother, a professional educator, went through all the appropriate moves with her developmentally delayed daughter. She tried hard to read her daughter's signals, to be constructive and supportive. Her approach was well thought out, well organized, and appropriate. Yet she lacked a certain spirit, a gleam in her eye, and an emotional range in her voice: she seemed preoccupied and mechanical. The clinician commented that she seemed to be working very hard to be a good partner for her child, and added that he imagined she would like to be able to enjoy it more. By phrasing his comment in a supportive rather than a critical way, he enabled the mother to share her sadness and disappointment. She began to cry and to describe how it felt to have a child who did not respond to her:

> At first, when she wouldn't look at me or smile at me, I would get mad at her and want to shake her. Then I began wondering what I did wrong, and what my husband did wrong. I found myself vacillating between trying very hard and then giving up and just feeding her and making sure she was comfortable. I couldn't bear the pain of looking into her eyes and not getting a twinkle back. Then I think

I began doing what I'm doing now—trying to interact with her, but without any enthusiasm or zest. It's too painful; I can't want too much from her, because I know she can't provide it. I think it's best for me not to try to get too excited or too happy when she does look at me, because I'll only be disappointed next time.

As we worked with this mother, encouraging her to verbalize her feelings about her relationship with her daughter, she began to relate her pain to the feelings she had had as a child when her own parents were unresponsive to her. She also connected it with feelings about her marriage. Her husband was preoccupied with his work and did not have a gleam in his eye for her. She realized that all her life, she had been a "good soldier," carrying on bravely in the face of her disappointment at not getting the emotional responses she wished for from others. As she pursued this self-exploration in sessions alone with the therapist, this mother also began regular Floortime with her daughter. She developed new skills in opening and closing circles of communication, focusing not just on her choice of words but also on the range of emotion and animation in her face. By simultaneously engaging in self-exploration and working on the mechanics of her interaction with her daughter, the mother enabled herself to take a chance and begin experiencing some joy, particularly when her daughter looked at her with a little grin. As she unfroze her own emotions, just as her daughter was beginning to experiment with new emotions, chemistry began to evolve between the two. The mother's emotional signaling became warmer and richer, and the daughter moved in the same direction.

It is often necessary, as it was with this family, to establish a process in which improved mechanics of interaction help the child become more engaged while self-exploratory therapy helps the parent become more excited and sincere in relating to the child. The parents' reinvestment in the child captures some of the hope and expectation they felt at the child's birth. The therapist bolsters these feelings by giving the parents new tools that enable them to open and close circles and to experiment with more spontaneous affect. This is a slow process, but one that is absolutely essential for working with children who have severe developmental delays.

Some parents seem neither sad nor mechanical, instead behaving in angry, controlling ways toward their developmentally delayed children. One father regularly yelled at his son, ordering him to smile. He was a successful businessman, and this aggressive approach worked well when he was confronting adults who were highly competent. He could see, however, that yelling only caused his son to become more aimless and withdrawn. When he was able to identify and verbalize his pain and disappointment in having a delayed child, he was able to relax and approach his son more gently. Whatever a parent's overt reaction—depressed, angry, controlling, or idealizing—underneath is likely a struggle with expectable feelings of disappointment that the child does not provide the range of cues that most parents rely on and secretly wish for when they have a child. All human beings seek some degree of engagement, warmth, and intimacy from other human beings. Parents often expect their children to provide this; it is not uncommon for parents to expect a child to make up for the neglect they experienced during their own childhoods. Because of these high expectations, parental disappointment is not unusual even when a child's development is optimal. When development takes an unusual course, disappointment is likely to be massive and overwhelming but defended against. It is a feeling the therapist must address.

Each parent's relationships with other family members will be deeply affected by the parent's reaction to the delayed child. A mother who feels deprived by her child's unresponsiveness may expect more from her husband; a father may expect more from his wife. As a result of these new expectations, an equilibrium that worked earlier in the marriage may no longer suffice. Each partner may begin focusing on the perceived flaws of the other. Older siblings will have their own ways of reacting to the delayed child and to changes in the family. Marital therapy, family therapy, or both may need to be part of the treatment plan.

Specific Therapeutic Interventions: Speech and Language Therapy, Occupational and Physical Therapy, Early Childhood Education, and Special Education

Children with NDRC require a team of professionals that can help them attain and strengthen core developmental capacities. Each professional, however, in each discipline utilized in the child's program needs to implement his or her specific goals in the context of the DIR model outline in the prior sections. In particular, it is critical for each therapist and educator to work on helping the child master each of the functional emotional developmental capacities in the context of the child's individual differences as they work on particular language, motor, or sensory capacities. The speech pathologist or occupational therapist, therefore, will be most helpful when supporting relationships and the continuous flow of back-and-forth gesturing and signaling while focusing on a particular motor or language capacity. Similarly, educators will be most helpful when working on these fundamentals in the context of broad educational goals.

Professionals from each discipline will have unique goals. Occupational therapists develop strategies to foster fine motor and gross motor capacities and to normalize sensory reactivity, sensory processing, and sensory integration. In some cases, an occupational therapist and a physical therapist will work as a team: the occupational therapist focuses on fine motor skills and selected functional aspects of gross motor skills while the physical therapist works on more severe aspects of the child's motor delay.

Speech pathologists work on a child's comprehension of communication and his ability to generate communication. A speech pathologist might address familiar problems, such as a child's inability to make a certain sound, or more complicated ones, such as a child's difficulty comprehending the sequence of certain words and sounds. Speech pathologists have moved toward using more free and spontaneous interaction as a vehicle for teaching communication skills, and their framework has broadened to include not just verbal skills but all aspects of communication.

Educators have a long tradition of figuring out strategies to assist children in developing sensory, motor, and conceptual abilities. A teacher may, for example, use a series of semistructured tasks to teach fine motor skills or concepts like "hot" and "cold" or "more than" and "less than." In preschool early intervention programs, a child typically spends some time in group activities, some time with a speech pathologist, and some time with an occupational therapist, a physical therapist, or both. These specialists often consult with the educators in order to integrate principles of speech, language, and occupational therapy into the child's educational routine.

It is important for teachers and other professionals to understand that regardless of the specific task they are trying to teach, the real learning opportunities lie in the interaction processes that take place between professional and child. Some speech and occupational therapists spend too much time on mechanical, "do as I say" exercises. Instead, they should consider dividing each session into two halves, one more traditional and didactic but at least partly interactive, the other more spontaneous and following the child's initiative. In school settings as well, concrete exercises and tasks should be considered occasions for interaction, and the interactions that take place around specific tasks should be evaluated regularly to ensure that they promote, rather than undermine, the child's mastery of core developmental competencies. Even seemingly informal, noneducational contacts, such as discussion of where children should hang their coats and where they should sit in the classroom, can and should be used to help them open and close many circles of gestural and, where possible, symbolic communication.

Parents are the true integrators of all that relates to their child. They need not only to benefit from the insights of all professionals who work with their child but also to provide these professionals with feedback about what works and does not work at home. They need to keep the professionals apprised of the emotional climate that prevails in the family. Treatment team meetings, as well as discussions between individual team members, must be held regularly throughout treatment.

Long-Term Educational Planning

Most communities need to rethink the ways in which they organize education and intervention programs for children with NDRC (as well as for children with other disabilities). Many programs share certain weaknesses that undermine their effectiveness:

1. *Minimal mental health treatment.* Typical programs, generally part-day for preschoolers and full-day for older children, include special education, occupational therapy, and speech therapy but do not sufficiently address the fundamental emotional and social capacities the child needs in order to develop a sense of personhood.

2. *Insufficient family involvement.* In many programs, parents or caregivers meet only sporadically with teachers or social workers. As we have discussed earlier, caregivers and professionals must work closely together to optimally support the child's developmental progress.

3. *Insufficient opportunity for children to interact with more communicative peers.* In most programs, children with disabilities are grouped with others who share similar difficulties. In a classroom consisting of eight withdrawn and aimless children, very little spontaneous interaction can occur. If one child does spurt ahead in her ability to open and close gestural circles, she will likely obtain little socially or emotionally relevant feedback from her peers; because her new ability is precarious, she may well give up her overtures to classmates when these go unanswered.

4. *Inappropriate groupings of children.* In programs that serve children with a wide variety of disabilities, an aggressive, intrusive child may be placed in the same class with a passive, frightened, withdrawn child. The resulting peer-to-peer interaction and feedback will be maladaptive for both.

5. *Unreliable evaluation procedures.* Too often, standardized tests are employed in a manner inappropriate for infants and children with unusual developmental patterns. The result is a misleading assessment of a child's potential, which can easily become a self-fulfilling prophecy. Cross-sectional assessments of delayed children do not appear to be useful in predicting how well and how quickly they will progress. A far more accurate picture of a child's potential emerges from the slope of his learning curve after a comprehensive intervention program has been in place for 6–12 months. Only after a child has been pulled into, or pulled back into, interactive relationships can one obtain a true picture of her learning potential. No infant or child can learn in isolation, even when that isolation has resulted in part from his own information-processing difficulties. When it is time to evaluate the child's progress, the treatment team should focus on how to improve his learning process and should be cautious about making negative predictions, because these can undermine teaching and learning.

In order to help children with NDRC reach their full potential, an educational program should facilitate the children's mastery of the core developmental capacities outlined in the DIR model. We offer several recommendations for the design of such programs:

1. The program must focus during part of each day on the interaction patterns between the infant or child and her parents. This work must take into account the child's individual processing differences, the parents' personalities, and the family dynamics. It can be carried out by educators, speech pathologists, occupational therapists, and mental health professionals. If the personality organization of one or both parents, the core emotional capacities of the child, or both are contributing significantly to the child's problems, the participation of a mental health professional is especially important.

2. A professional needs to consult with the parents at least weekly to assist with family dynamics and interaction patterns at home. Periodic home visits should involve both parents and, as needed, other family members and caregivers.

3. The child should spend part of each day in a small peer group; educators working with the group should be well equipped to help its members master core developmental competencies as well as specific age-appropriate skills and concepts. A combination of interactive play, semistructured activities, and selected structured activities is usually appropriate for these goals.

4. The composition of the group should be approximately one or two children with developmental delays for each five nondelayed children of similar age or developmental level. Children with NDRC require peers who can, with appropriate help from their teachers, respond in age-appropriate ways to the delayed child's emerging interactive gestures.

5. Teachers must have interest and training in mobilizing peer interactions, particularly between delayed children and their nondelayed peers. Instead of ordering children to interact with one another, the teacher must know how to create opportunities for them to interact of their own volition.

   For example, suppose a child with developmental delays is sitting at a table making craft projects with three nondelayed peers. Jane wants the scissors, which are laying nearest to Harold, the child with NDRC. She asks her teacher to get the scissors for her. To facilitate the opening and closing of communication circles between them, the teacher says, "They aren't near me, they're near Harold. Can you ask him?" Jane, discouraged by prior attempts to ask Harold for things, looks at the teacher as if to say, "This is going to be hard." The teacher says, "I'll bet you Harold can pass you the scissors, if you figure out just the right way to ask him." Jane says, "Harold, give me the scissors." Harold does not respond. The teacher says, "I think you'll have to get him to look at you first, in order for there to be a chance that he'll respond to your request." Jane focuses her eyes on Harold's and says, "Harold," three times. He slowly looks at her, and she says, "Can you give me the scissors?" but he still does not respond. The teacher says, "If you show him with your hands, as well as your words, what you want, maybe you'll stand a better chance." As Jane does this,

Harold gives her a big smile and gives her the scissors. Jane has learned a lesson that is useful in all communication: always get the person's attention first, and when he does not understand what you are saying in one way, try adding on extra communicative gestures. Harold has also benefited enormously: he has opened and closed several circles with a peer in a spontaneous manner, even though the peer was getting some coaching.

In another situation, suppose Harold is watching Jane and two of her friends eagerly putting on crowns and pretending to be princesses. The teacher wants to get Harold involved but does not want to insist that Jane patronize Harold by saying something to him. Nor does she want to command Harold, "Go put on a crown," thus making him do something that lacks spontaneity. Instead, the teacher plays the role of instigator-provocateur. She says to the girls, "Who's going to be the king?" Jane replies, "Oh, Laura can be the king." The teacher says, "No, she's already a princess." Jane says, "Well, how about Sally?" The teacher: "Well, Sally you already have as the other princess, and you're the queen." When Jane does not respond, the teacher prompts further: "I think, if possible, it might be nice to have a boy be the king, because that's kind of a boy's role." Jane finally says, "Well, are you saying Harold should be the king?" The teacher: "Well, that's up to you, but I think he'd be a perfect king. The question is, can you get him to want to be the king?" With this instigation, the girls take on the project of getting Harold to want to be king. They ask him directly, but he looks confused. Then each of the girls puts her crown on herself, points to it, and gestures to Harold as if to ask if he would like the crown for himself. He smiles, nods, and begins interacting in a simple way. This episode illustrates the principle that, instead of pressuring a delayed child to interact in ways he might not yet understand or feel comfortable with, a teacher should creatively put pressure on the other children to pull him into interactions that will allow him to experience natural social situations. As a child such as Harold begins to enjoy gesturing and interacting, he will obtain feedback more easily from Jane and other nondelayed peers than he would in a group of children who are as delayed as he is.

6. Program staff should help parents understand that developmentally delayed children need more, not less, time playing with peers at home. Four or five play dates per week is not too many. Playing with peers his own age or younger who are very interactive will help the child abstract the rules of social interaction. Unfortunately, many children lack such opportunities and end up feeling clumsy and alienated when they are older.

7. Special education programs should not be isolated from mainstream educational settings. If professionals such as speech pathologists, occupational therapists, and special education teachers are located in a special school or teach only in a special program within a larger school, a child who moves to a main-

stream educational setting will lose these professionals and their expertise. Instead, we recommend designating certain educational settings as integrated settings. Children with NDRC would be in small classrooms where a majority of their peers are progressing adaptively in most areas. Both groups of children would have the advantage of the expertise provided by specialists. The nondelayed children would in no way be undermined in their learning by the availability of this expertise: because all children have subtle variations in processing capabilities and styles, the presence of the specialists would undoubtedly benefit all. The nondelayed children would also gain experience relating to types of peers they do not ordinarily interact with, experience that would deepen and broaden their sense of humanity and enhance—not compromise—their cognitive, emotional, and social growth.

8. As children progress to higher grade levels, the same principle of combining a few developmentally delayed children in a class with many nondelayed children must hold (sharing art, music, and recess is not sufficient). Teachers must continue to work creatively to make interactive experiences enriching for both groups. As a delayed child becomes more socially interactive and more emotionally secure, very specific learning disabilities may become evident, and teachers may be able to approach these much as they would with any child. Even children with profound learning disabilities, however, should never be placed only with children who share the same disabilities, because this undermines the child's ability to reach his full potential for normative peer interactions.

Case Illustrations

Brad

Brad was brought to me (S.G.) when he was 4½ years old because he was self-absorbed and had delayed speech development compounded by impulse control problems, including hitting his parents and being moody and unresponsive to questions and comments. He was not yet toilet trained and would throw tantrums lasting a half-hour or longer. Brad's parents worried that his tantrums interfered with his playing with other children, with whom he would not interact; at best he would parallel play. He could say only a few words clearly—most of his vocalizations were garbled sounds—so it was hard to tell how much he understood of what anyone was saying. Earlier evaluations had shown that, in addition to his severe articulation difficulty and delayed speech, Brad had decreased muscle tone and motor planning problems, although he could walk and jump.

The medical evaluation was negative in terms of metabolic and chromosome studies and pediatric well-baby evaluations. Furthermore, Brad showed signs of unusual cognitive abilities. He knew his alphabet, seemed to remember stories, and occasionally would spontaneously say phrases like "played wagon," or "in there," but he could not hold an interactive conversation. He enjoyed wrestling, tickling, and other forms of light roughhousing but did not like having his hair brushed. He could hold a pencil and draw a circle but could not draw a square or triangle.

According to his mother, Brad's early development was characterized by the fact that "he didn't cry much. He seemed happy, he smiled, slept through the night, and was very observant." She added that he liked to touch things and that "he would study first and then engage." She thought he was attentive but only partially related during his first year and very passive in terms of two-way communication in the second half of that year. He would respond—if she handed him a rattle, he would look at her and take it—but he rarely initiated or followed through in an activity.

In Brad's second year, his parents recognized that he had problems. Although he made sounds, he was not using any words, and he could be unclear when indicating his needs and desires. He might look at what he wanted or cry in a scattered way, but he more often seemed self-absorbed. During his second year and into his third, Brad periodically wanted to be with mother all the time. He would cling to her and was fearful of being with other people. Only in the past 6 months could he stay alone with father. Father reported that he had felt "removed" from the family during Brad's second and third years; he was preoccupied with work and did not feel very involved with his son.

At age 2 years, Brad started banging his head but responded to physical restraint. When around other children, he would occasionally hug and stroke them but did not interact with them verbally or through symbolic play.

Brad had had a number of evaluations, all of which gave him a diagnosis of an autism spectrum disorder. One evaluation stated autism; another pervasive development disorder not otherwise specified.

During the first visit, I observed the parents playing with Brad. Mother took a puppet and bit Brad on the nose with it, and he copied her by biting her back. Yet when she asked him some questions, he seemed to ignore her and tune out. Despite the imitative gesturing, there was no spontaneous exchange of gestures, words, or emotional expressions. Father started to tickle Brad, which caused him to smile a little, but then he became passive and turned away from father to explore how the toys worked. There was very little reciprocity between father and son, on either a symbolic or gestural level. Both parents seemed to want to be close to Brad, and he was intermittently engaged with them, but only on a simple gestural level, with smiles and looks and an occasional word. There were no complex gestures or interactive use of symbols and representations.

Brad seemed to be functioning as a 1½- to 2-year-old at his highest levels, and he had some splinter skills. At his lowest level of functioning, Brad would be self-absorbed, indifferent to his parents' communications, or avoidant in favor of exploring the toys. At the same time, he showed a capacity to concentrate, particularly when trying to figure out how the toys worked. He also showed a bit of warmth through faint smiles or looks of recognition.

The pregnancy and delivery had been unremarkable—mother reported that Brad moved vigorously in utero—although he was delivered via C-section. He weighed 8 lb at birth, breathed and cried immediately, and had 9/9 Apgars. He took a bottle well and went home with mother.

An earlier psychological test evaluation of Brad at age 3 years showed "delay in his development, with uneven skills." At that time, he was functioning at a 2-year-old level and sometimes up to 2½ in terms of some of the nonverbal form board tasks. However, his social development seemed to be at the 18-month-old level. He had a precocious interest in letters, numbers, and colors. The psychologist also noted Brad's irritability, difficulty with transitions, and inappropriate—or lack of—relatedness to other people.

A number of professionals had verbally indicated to Brad's parents that they thought he was "borderline retarded, or educably retarded." In addition to his autism spectrum disorder, they concluded that he had considerable behavioral and emotional difficulties and that his social and emotional behavior lagged even further behind than his cognitive and language performance.

At our next meeting, I observed more of the parent–child interaction patterns. Father moved in much too quickly, not letting Brad develop his own gestures or take the symbolic or gestural initiative. When Brad was functioning in his higher range, such as beginning some pretend play with a car, father would move in and take charge of the play. Mother showed less energy than father in playing with Brad. She often seemed preoccupied and depressed. At other times, she would become fragmented and overload him. Brad vacillated between being "spacey" when mother was not generating enough energy to pull him in and being whiny when she got too active and animated. Besides whining and crying, Brad would become disorganized, without generating much interaction. Mother felt overwhelmed and guilty. She recognized that she went back and forth between a depressive preoccupation and an anxious helplessness, which was consistent with her relationship history.

Father, a busy economist, knew that he was frustrated and angry and that he and Brad had the same problems. Father had been a slow developer, but he said, "Unlike Brad, I got it together." He had warmth and empathy for his son but did not know what to do with his impatience and anger and his feeling that Brad had "let [him] down." As he talked, father revealed an aspiration that Brad could be much better coordinated and a better athlete than father had been.

As both parents became aware of the feelings behind their styles of interaction, they wanted to learn to read Brad's signals more clearly and play with him more constructively. We developed a program to help Brad that would further elaborate some of the evaluative and diagnostic issues. The parents were to try engaging Brad at four levels. First, they would get his attention and maintain a pleasurable connectedness by following his lead in an activity he was enjoying. Then they would try to open and close gestural communication circles—starting with simple ones and moving on to more complex ones. I suggested that they not worry about his advanced interest in letters and numbers, or about any symbolic interactions, but let the symbolic part of the play emerge spontaneously. They would empathize verbally with what Brad was doing and follow his lead and respect his initiative while closing circles. When he ignored them, they would pull him back in and encourage him to build on their responses. Each of the parents would do this for at least a half-hour each day; mother, if she had time, would do this two or three times a day.

We also consulted the speech pathologist who was working with Brad three times a week on his pronunciation, receptive language, and ability to carry out instructions. The consultation included helping her make more use of spontaneous play and interaction in her sessions, so that Brad would get a sense of his own efficacy and intentionality. The speech pathologist revealed that Brad's speech capacity was uneven, ranging from the 1½-year-old range in terms of intermittent reciprocity to scattered verbal skills in the 2- to 3-year-old range. He could occasionally put together two or three words or follow simple commands and could sometimes even follow a two-sequence command such as, "Please get that block and put it here."

Brad also began twice-a-week visits to a play therapist, who would follow Brad's lead and help him symbolize his emotions as well as interact in a more organized gestural way. The play therapy was organized along the four levels described earlier; Brad's parents also would be involved, to help them improve their interactions at home.

The parents were anxious not only in regard to Brad but also in their marital relationship. There was often obvious tension between them as they expressed their different opinions about the best way to work with their son; each felt let down by the other. I suggested weekly psychiatric sessions in which they could discuss their problems and get more help in dealing with Brad's troubling behavior, such as his withdrawal and perseveration. (Although I did not observe perseverative behavior in our sessions, the parents reported that Brad perseverated at home, and we discussed techniques for making the perseverations interactive.)

In summary, we developed a comprehensive approach that included daily work with the parents and regular sessions with a child psychiatrist, speech therapist, and play therapist. In addition, Brad received an occupational therapy evaluation for his low motor tone, motor planning problems that were suggested by his developmental history, fine motor lags, and indications of sensory reactivity difficulties. Weekly occupational therapy was added to his program.

From the beginning of the program, Brad showed consistent improvement, at first primarily in terms of connectedness. When he came to see me 4 months after the program was instituted, he had a gleam in his eye and was much more affectively involved with his parents. Despite not having seen me for 4 months, he gave me a knowing look instead of ignoring me as he had done before. He could now interact with mother using four to five gestural sequences in a row and could add symbolic make-believe to these sequences. For example, he might take out a car he particularly liked and have a doll sit in the car. The doll would then get out and be bathed. As he gestured to give the dirty doll a bath, he might look at mother with a faint grin and say, "Dirty." "Yes, dirty," mother would reply. "Now we have to clean him up." After four or five of these elements, Brad would switch to another activity. While playing with mother, he might smile at me as well and make other gestures and expressions.

When Brad played with father, father chose more aggressive dramas with soldiers and shooting. Brad focused on what father was doing and could interrelate a series of gestures and ideas with him. Father was warmer, more supportive, and more contingent on this visit; he had practiced at home and previewed this play with the play therapist. Father began this sequence somewhat impatiently, as he had in the earlier visit, but this time Brad smiled at him, and father relaxed. He let Brad take the gun from him, and Brad smiled faintly and said, "Boom, boom. Boom, boom." Father returned the "boom, boom," and then they exchanged three or four gestures and words and made "booming" noises back and forth.

Brad was related almost the entire time with mother, father, and me. He could organize a series of five or six gestures in a row, closing circles and giving them the feel of a normal social interaction, and the symbols or ideas in his play were natural and coordinated with the gestures. He had a warm, likeable quality, and showed excellent concentration.

However, Brad's progress seemed to level off over the next 6 months. His symbolic comprehension did not seem to increase. When mother or father asked him
simple questions during play time, he could follow their gestures but could only
close simple symbolic circles. For example, they might ask, "Does the car want to
go here or there?" and he would move the car in one direction or the other. The
more they structured it, the easier it was for Brad to close a circle. Yet if they asked
him, "What does the car do next?" he would look puzzled and tune out a bit or
become random in his behavior. It was also hard for him to shift from pretend to
a reality-based conversation, such as when asked, "What do you want for lunch?"
and he found it even harder to close circles in a reality-based conversation. (When
familiar with the routine, he could respond to certain structured tasks with his
speech pathologist and occupational therapist.) After a while, the parents became
demoralized, wondering whether he was in fact "retarded" and whether he was capable of significant gains.

I closely examined the parents' interactions with Brad; it appeared that they
were not giving him much practice in taking the lead. Although they were engaging him and closing gestural circles, they were subtly structuring the experiences
for him. In their eagerness to have him close multiple circles, their desire for him
to "perform well," they were giving him practice only in answering yes or no questions. I pointed out how this was a kind of overcontrol and that Brad was not able
to get a sense of what he could do. For example, when he seemed puzzled about
what to do with the car, rather than asking, "Do you want to move it here or
there?" they could be patient and gesture back with another car, asking, "Where
car go?" With this kind of play, Brad eventually said, "Car go there," pointing to a
chair and making the car go up the chair. When the chair became a garage, he was
showing signs of greater sophistication in his play.

Over the next 4 months, Brad's abilities improved greatly. He began closing
quite complex circles, showing a continuing sense of "being connected and with-
it." On his next visit, he looked at me, smiled, and interacted with appropriate gestures and words. He spontaneously told me about school and a teacher named
"Teed." When he did not understand a question that I asked him about school, he
would answer randomly but still looked and gestured with intention. We talked
about the kind of toys he liked to play with—he said he liked "soldiers and
trucks"—and he chose ones to play with. As he was trying to put a soldier in a
truck, he said, "The soldier's too big for the truck."

This kind of play was now characteristic of Brad's interactions with his parents.
They were supporting him in taking more of the lead. At school, he was solidly at
the prekindergarten level. The parents reported that at home, Brad was much easier to engage; they were having little conversations and exchanging lots of gestures
with him. He would still have tantrums and bite and kick when he was frustrated;
however, they were not so intimidated by his tantrums now. They were setting
more effective limits, using gestures, words, and physical restraint as needed.

Brad's progress continued. In follow-up sessions, he showed greater elaboration in his play, using representational modes that were intimately connected with
his gestures. For example, in one session he asked mother to "get monster house."
Mother got it and held it up. "Okay," said Brad. Mother asked, "What's happening?" and Brad replied, "They are climbing up." "What next?" mother asked.
"Look for hotel," Brad answered. He then played out monsters trying to scare people in the hotel—his first elaborate make-believe drama.

However, the parents admitted that they were still frustrated; they wished Brad could hold conversations about school or solve simple problems, such as what he wanted for dinner. They felt they had to structure their interactions with him too much. We discussed spending 20 minutes a day on problem-solving or reality-based conversations. Just as they did in pretend play, they would help Brad with cues, but only the minimal amount he needed in order to have an exchange. They would become more demanding in terms of setting at least half the agenda when talking about school or a television program, and so forth.

Over the next several months, Brad improved in this area as well, and the parents began using problem-solving time to discuss his "temper tantrums." For the first time, he began using words and pretend play to deal with feelings and talked about feeling mad and "wanting to be boss." The parents were delighted but also frightened by this development. Now that Brad could use words in this way, they worried that he would be "mad at them" most of the time. They relaxed a bit once they realized that this advance would actually make Brad less frustrated; even if he were mad, their empathy and engagement with him would show him how much they loved him. The parents examined how they each had dealt with anger as children (both had their own issues, which are not explored here).

Many children with developmental delays have an especially hard time with angry feelings. The ability to represent anger and deal with it constructively is a critical milestone in logically relating to the world. If children are comfortable with anger, they do not need to use regressive modes of fragmentation, such as withdrawal and avoidance, as much. Yet, they first need to develop the representational capacities and circle-closing gestural interactions that will allow them to deal constructively with anger. Therefore, at a certain point in the treatment, helping the child to verbalize angry feelings through pretend play is very important. It builds on the respect for the child's assertiveness and helps him or her develop in terms of the necessary gestures and representations.

As Brad's progress continued, the speech pathologist and play therapist wondered if they should reduce the frequency of their sessions. I urged them to continue at their current schedule until Brad was functioning completely at age level in all areas—a goal they had not even considered when the work began. There is a tendency in cases like this for parents and therapists to work less aggressively when a child is making progress in order to give the child "more time to play with friends and peers." This tendency often reflects an unconscious wish to be satisfied with a lesser goal for the child. If the parents are motivated, they can usually find time for play with other children on weekends and after special programs. If the work is done skillfully, with empathy and warmth, truly following the child's lead, the child will find the sessions rewarding as opposed to tiring.

As his progress continued, Brad began using his new skills in interactions with other children. In school, his teacher observed spontaneous use of verbal interaction and pretend play with other children in typical ways—tea parties, cars crashing, soldiers fighting. When the play became too aggressive, Brad would withdraw a bit and parallel play while observing from a safe distance, but he could recover and rejoin the others.

He became close to one little boy who became a "friend." He talked about this boy at home and invited him over for play sessions, in which they would giggle and laugh, run around and jump, and do pretend play with trucks, cars, and soldiers. This was a major breakthrough for Brad, who had never had a "close friend" nor shown the capacity for pleasure with a child his own age. His friend also had some uneven development and learning delays but was somewhat more socially advanced than Brad. Brad used the relationship to improve his own social interactive skills and learned how to share, how to experience joy and pleasure, and even how to defend himself when his friend wanted a toy that Brad wanted to play with. He learned how to say, "Me first."

Brad's progress was most evident in his sessions about 2 years after the start of the program, when he was a little more than 6 years old. His parents began letting up on their Floortime, not realizing that the source of his progress was their own work with him on the floor. With my encouragement, they regrouped and resumed their support. In one session, Brad played with mother and she tried to give him "the mean dolls." He said, "I don't want meany. I don't want those." Dad joined in, saying, "Maybe the policeman should come over and do something with the bad guys." The parents seemed to be relaxed and to be enjoying the play.

As mother tried to take the lead, Brad showed for the first time an ability to compete with her and take over the rhythm. Mother asked, "What's happening here?" trying to distract Brad from what he was doing. He looked at her and said, "Come here." He directed her to the drama he was developing with trucks taking rocks from one place to another. Then father took the truck from his son and put it in his face intrusively (as parents relax, they sometimes revert to old patterns). Brad, showing his greater assertiveness, grabbed the truck back and said, "Look, the truck is going bang-bang," turning the truck into a gun and shooting at father. He then made the father be the bad guy and sent him to the other side of the room, thereby getting father out of his face and taking charge of the drama.

Brad then built a fort out of the pillows, and he and father shot at each other across the room. Brad giggled and seemed pleased at the elaboration of his drama and at his ability to control father. Later, he made two girl dolls go down a slide. He said that the little one was a girl and the big one was a "lady" and that they were sliding down a slide. He made the slide a part of the house and talked about which doll was bigger than the other. Then one of the dolls got injured and had to be fixed up by the doctor.

Playing with me during this session, Brad was very relaxed, with good intentional gestures and a with-it quality. He related to me almost like a child of his own age would. A theme of "putting on masks" emerged, one for me and one for him. He showed me how to put on the mask (which was of a popular robot-type toy). Then he said, "Let's fight the monsters together." He kept coming back to me with my mask, asking me to join him in the fight between the two groups of robots. He was very interested in figuring out how the robots worked, asking if a robot could do this or that. During this play, he was also able to engage in chitchat; I asked about a friend at school, and he would try to answer and then drift back into the pretend play after a minute or two. With my help, he refocused on the question. He vacillated between struggling to answer me and avoiding the question by returning to pretend play.

My sense was that Brad was warm, relaxed, related, and focused but could not yet fully differentiate his representational capacities. These capacities were quite elaborate and creative, and he had many islands of differentiation for emotional and logical thinking. However, his tendency to drift into pretend when it was too difficult for him to answer questions indicated that he could not solidly shift between reality and fantasy. In this way, he was in the 4½-year-old range, but in some of the elaborations of his play he was clearly in the 5- to 5½-year-old range. I empathetically asked him how he felt when he could not find a word or answer a question. With great difficulty, he told me that he sometimes got "mad," and he kicked the doll.

I talked with the parents about the challenges ahead. Stringing together numerous logical ideas into cohesive themes would help Brad hold a more normal conversation—a skill that usually develops between the ages of 3½ and 7 years. We wanted to maintain the elaborateness of his pretend dramas and help him articulate his feelings more, particularly the frustration and anger secondary to some of his articulation problems that had a mechanical and motor component to them. I stressed how important it was for the parents to empathize with Brad's frustration.

In a session when Brad was 6½, he showed another huge development. He walked in the door with a look of complete normalcy and a very eager and friendly sense about him. He smiled warmly and said, "Hello, Dr. Greenspan," clearly remembering me and seeming happy to visit an old friend. His parents began talking about some of their battles with him at home: Brad wanted to play with a certain popular toy that father did not like because it was too aggressive and "weird." I spontaneously turned to Brad (rather than organizing the pretend play sequences the way I usually did) and made the toy the focus of a family discussion. "I gather from your daddy that you like this toy," I said to Brad. "Yes," he answered. "Why?" I asked, and he replied, "I like to play with it because it is fun." "Can you?" "No, daddy doesn't let me." "How come?" "He thinks it's too scary." "Is daddy a scaredy-cat?" Brad began giggling and said, "No" with a broad smile and a knowing look— it was both fun and a little scary to make fun of his father. He was not quite ready to do it, although he enjoyed the idea that father was a scaredy-cat.

This exchange, which Brad would not have been able to have a few months earlier, suggested that he now had excellent abilities for holding logical conversations. He could build on my ideas without much cuing, and at home he could deal with a conflict situation in a logical, problem-solving discussion. This was a major milestone in terms of Brad's ability to be logical intellectually; in addition, the pleasure he showed in making fun of father suggested major gains in his capacity to be pleasurable and emotionally assertive. His articulation and the depth of his warmth had also dramatically improved.

However, both parents were still a bit patronizing and overstructured in their discussions and pretend play with him. (They would say, "Now, Brad, tell Dr. Greenspan A, B, or C.") I reminded them that Brad did not need them to cue him up anymore, that he could think for himself now, and it was important that they respect this ability. Their being patronizing and overstructured would hold back Brad's progress.

In this session, while Brad still played out elaborate fantasy dramas as he had before, he did not drift off. He could hold a conversation about school, friends, or a toy he liked for 5 or 10 minutes or more; he would only begin playing when we were done with the conversation.

He was also progressing well at school. He enjoyed playing with other children and continued to have a "best friend." He showed more of the characteristics of a 4- to 7-year-old child. He was increasingly comfortable using words for feelings, such as being mad or sad; he only had tantrums now when he was tired or in a real power struggle with his parents.

In summary, this is a case of a child who originally appeared to be operating only intermittently, in terms of shared attention and engagement and of having achieved two-way gestural communication with some irregular and splinter representational skills. Some maturational unevenness was contributing to these patterns, putting him anywhere from 1½–3 years behind his actual age. His problems included low motor tone and motor planning deficits, language articulation deficits, and receptive language deficits. The family's unfavorable interaction patterns added to the complexity of the case: father was overly intrusive, impatient, and angry at the child; and mother vacillated between being fragmented and being anxious, withdrawn, preoccupied, and depressed.

Therefore, there were both maturational and family interactive contributions to Brad's difficulties, which appeared in a number of developmental areas: emotional, social, language, and—to a lesser degree—motor. A comprehensive program focused on each of the factors contributing to his current level of development—the maturational side (through occupational and speech therapy), the family side (through family counseling), and the interactive side (through parent–child interactional help and Floortime work).

This case illustrates a comprehensive evaluation and intervention approach with a child who evidenced language, social relationship, and motor and sensory processing challenges. This case demonstrated a comprehensive DIR-based approach involving an intensive home program, appropriate therapies, and educational program—all working together to help Brad move forward and master successively higher levels of functional emotional developmental capacities. It also demonstrated how, at the same time, he was able to strengthen his different processing capacities that contribute to social and intellectual capacities.

It is important to emphasize that working with Brad's family and helping his caregivers understand their own personalities so they could implement an optimal program (i.e., so they could work around their own challenges) was a vital part of the approach. The DIR model summarizes this overall approach—to facilitate development (D), by focusing on individual processing differences (I), and tailoring learning relationships (R) to these individual differences in order to help the child climb his or her developmental ladder.

In terms of our classification approach—NDRC—this case illustrates the importance of having a framework to describe subtypes of relationship and communication problems within a broad developmental framework. Brad had received a diagnosis of an autism spectrum disorder before he was referred to us. The diagnosis, however, did not capture Brad's unique strengths and vulnerabilities. Children with autism spectrum disorder diagnoses vary enormously in terms of their presenting characteristics and capacities. In our new framework for classifying types of disorders of relating and communicating, Brad would be illustrative of a child meeting the criteria for Type I. His response to a comprehensive intervention approach and his progress was consistent with this initial impression. In the DIR model an attempt is made to include the child's response to an optimal intervention program as part of the diagnostic impression. In other words, the DIR model emphasizes a dynamic developmental framework for understanding a child's and a family's challenges.

On further follow-ups without continuing intervention, Brad has maintained his gains and moved fully into adolescence. He has warm and meaningful friendships with peers, a creative imagination, solid academic skills, and the expected family joys and challenges of a bright teenager. We have now been able to follow a large number of children who—like Brad—have done very well, into their adolescent years and beyond (Greenspan 2005; Greenspan and Wieder 2004).

Alan

Alan, a 3½-year-old boy, was brought to me (S.G.) by his parents because he had problems with relating to others, thinking and conversation, and with helping himself. The parents explained that he tended to "march to the beat of his own drummer." Alan knew numerous songs and had perfect pitch (music was a big part of his life), but if they asked him a question, he would just repeat it; he did not seem to understand how to answer.

They described him as "jittery"—he would "hop around a lot"—with an anxious, tense voice. He enjoyed being around other children, but his play was intrusive and tended to scare them; instead of engaging in pretend or interactive play, he might toss objects and occasionally hurt other children or take toys away from them without seeming to understand their feelings.

Alan played a bit more with mother, but he would try to keep an object—such as a ball—instead of sharing it with her or throwing it back and forth. She felt he tried to get her "irritated," but also that he could not tell the difference between her being angry at him, excited with him, or accepting of him. Sometimes he would giggle excitedly if she gave him an angry look.

Mother said that Alan and his father did not have much of a relationship; father responded that his wife kept him and Alan apart because she wanted to control everything. "She thinks she knows best," he said.

The parents had noticed that Alan's fine motor development and coordination were poor when he was about 3 years old. He had a neurologic evaluation, which led to an occupational therapy evaluation that revealed some decrease of muscle tone in the upper extremities and some problems with motor planning; he was now receiving occupational therapy once a week to improve his fine motor skills. His occupational therapist reported that he was also very sensory overreactive, especially to touch and sound.

While the parents gave me the history, I watched Alan play. He looked serious, but he engaged me: he looked at me, pointed at toys, looked at me again for permission to go into the closet. I nodded to him that he could go. He made occasional comments such as "What's this?" and "What's that?" and he seemed interested in trucks. At one point he put the whale puppet on his hand, and I asked him, "Does the whale talk?" He toyed with the whale, almost making it talk back at me, and then put it down. He seemed to be struggling to understand what the whale could pretend to do.

Mother said that Alan had trouble answering "why" or "how" questions. He had some conversational abilities, but they seemed below the 3-year-old level. Mother added that Alan ate and slept well and would cuddle with both her and father at times, although he seemed to prefer her. Father repeated, "That's because she keeps us apart." He felt that mother was controlling and overprotective. "I'm angry at her, but I tend to give in," he said. He felt that there was a lot of "guerilla warfare" in the family.

Mother seemed to be worried, anxious, and protective. She worked half-time and had babysitters for Alan who changed about every 6 months. She felt that father tended to be too passive and avoided conflict. Father disagreed, feeling that she overreacted to his "occasional depression," although he admitted that he would pull away when she did not seem to welcome his overtures. There was a lot of marital tension around whether mother was controlling and rejecting or father was passive and avoidant. They each agreed that they had some of these tendencies; it was a question of who was reacting to whom.

Alan had been adopted when he was 8 months old; at that time he was not very reactive or responsive. Although his sleeping and eating patterns were good, he did not seem to respond to sights, sounds, or the parents' emotional gestures. He was late in sitting up and crawling, although he started walking between 13 and 14 months. "Now he runs like a whirlwind," mother said, and he had learned to skip and hop 6 months earlier. However, his motor planning was slow in terms of complex, planned movements, which had led the parents to the evaluations. His fine motor ability was also low in terms of activities like holding a pencil, writing, drawing, and tying shoelaces.

Alan gradually came out of his nonreactive state during his first year; by 12 months he was engaged with them and could smile warmly, but he was very passive. Intermittently, however, he overreacted to selected sounds. Only lately had he begun initiating hugs, for example, although he had been receptive to their hugs.

After he learned to walk, Alan seemed to be in "perpetual motion," mother said. His behavior became intentional. He would play intently with cars and trucks and was warm when approached; at other times he would wander around the room, fidgeting and exploring many different objects. Toward the middle of his second year, he began pulling other children's hair, and also mother's and father's hair. Sometimes when he got frustrated he would lie on the floor and bang his head. Alan's speech was delayed, but he did start to vocalize many different sounds toward the end of his second year. He started using words at 2½ and had just started putting words together into sentences a few months before this evaluation.

Alan had had no serious medical illnesses; he had been adopted from South America and mother did not know his genetic history. Mother revealed, reluctantly, that she was worried because one of his evaluators diagnosed pervasive developmental disorder not otherwise specified, and his teacher had suggested that Alan had "autistic features." His tendency to move around aimlessly and seem unrelated worried her in this regard.

Playing with mother, Alan could relate and engage intermittently and have partial gestural and verbal communication. Mother was quite attentive and contingent and responded to Alan's overtures gesturally and symbolically. As they played with toy cars and trucks, mother empathized with his pleasure in movement. They also played with the doll house, making some soldiers go to the top of the house, some to the bottom of the house, and some jump off the roof. Alan occasionally used a few words like "jumping" and "falling" and looked serious, expressing a narrow range of emotion and periodically becoming self-absorbed. Mother was tense and occasionally overcontrolling but could also be supportive and gentle.

When it was father's turn to play with Alan, he said to him, "Look here, I've found a globe." Alan ignored him and went to mother, and father then became passive and silent. He admitted that he was confused when Alan ignored him. He kept trying to interest Alan in different toys, but he had a serious, passive expression and not much wooing power. Alan would look at the toy for a second, then go back to mother, jumping in her lap or putting the truck he was holding on her knee.

Alan appeared to have a history of motor planning problems and uneven motor development. He was passive and did not take much initiative but had partially progressed through some of the core developmental processes, such as the early stages of sharing attention and engaging and two-way gestural communication. He had trouble with very complex gestures and with fully engaging at the level of symbolic differentiation in the stage he had reached and had only partially engaged in full representational elaboration in terms of developing themes and make-believe (i.e., he had not yet mastered the use of emotional ideas and emotional thinking—although these elements were in place). To handle aggression and frustration, he tended to withdraw and become aimless or avoidant. However, during most of the time in my office, Alan was partially related and showed some gestural and verbal communication, especially with mother.

At the end of this first session, it seemed clear that Alan had a pattern of uneven development and was lagging in social and emotional functioning as well as in aspects of cognitive and language functioning. I suggested the following next steps:

1. A speech evaluation in addition to the occupational therapy evaluation Alan had already completed
2. Floortime, in which the parents would help Alan expand to very complex gestural modes in the hope that this would enable him to enter more into the symbolic level of emotional ideas and begin pretend play
3. Increasing his access to peers, with mother or another adult serving as an intermediary to inhibit aggressive acting out

Alan was already in a special education developmental disabilities preschool program because of his uneven motor development and lack of age-appropriate language development as well as his emotional and social behavior difficulties. We consulted with his school about instituting the same kind of Floortime the parents would be doing. I stressed the importance of father doing daily Floortime and not letting his feelings about mother make him passive or avoidant. I referred them to a couples' therapist to work on their relationship, especially on the tendency each had to view the other as the culpable one. Perhaps if father could deal with his avoidant pattern, and mother could deal with her overcontrolling, anxious, and fragmented style, they could learn to work better as a team. They seemed committed to each other and wanted to work together to help Alan.

The parents returned a few months later, reporting that they had worked hard at carrying out my suggestions. They had done daily Floortime to help Alan relate to them more fully and use his existing language to decide what he wanted to eat or what games he wanted to play. I observed greater relatedness and more continuous back-and-forth gesturing as well as more purposeful use of words and phrases.

In a follow-up meeting, the parents reported that they were following the recommendations of the occupational and speech therapists. In their Floortime, they were also working on reality-based problem-solving discussions in which they helped Alan close a logical circle of communication using words. Father had become very involved with Alan, and mother was helping Alan increase the gestural complexity of his play. She had noticed some spontaneous emergence of symbolic play, an area in which he had not been fully involved. (This may have accounted, in part, for his tendency toward more primitive, aggressive modes of interacting and for some of his inability to deal with peers.)

When Alan came in 3 months later, he engaged me much more warmly than he had on his first visit. He said, "Hello" with a smile on his face and immediately asked, "Where's the Halloween toy?" I took it out of the closet, and he looked at me and started playing with it. I asked him if he liked it, and he said, "Yes," but then tuned me out and played with the toy. I had to work to keep him engaged; if I did, he opened and closed circles, stayed related, and talked to me in sentences. I asked him if there was anything he wanted to tell me about, and he said, "I went to an amusement park." I asked him what was there, and he replied, "A Ferris wheel." Mother said, "He's making that up," and I said that I thought it was a pretty good answer, whether Alan was making it up or not.

As he played, I wondered out loud why he liked certain toys more than others, and he said, "Because I like them!" While this was a low-level response to a "why" questions, his intonation suggested a comprehension of the "why" kind of question. His play tended to be somewhat fragmented; he used the toys he saw in front of him rather than trying to find others. However, he did begin some pretend play: he put an animal on a truck and talked about the wolf biting the little girl doll.

This time, Alan played with father first and told him that he was "going to turn the truck into an airplane." When Alan made the truck fly, father first tried to follow his lead but then slipped into passivity and silence rather than building on the themes. I encouraged father to relax and be more active with him and not worry about taking over. As the session went on, he relaxed and had better pretend play with Alan. There was a sense of relatedness, and Alan was clearly closer to his father this time; he did not run away to mother. Toward the end of the session, they had a nice sequence in which Alan turned the truck into an airplane and flew it onto mother's lap but then flew it back into a sort of hangar that father had made with his hands. When father wondered out loud if the airplane needed a place to rest, Alan smiled broadly. It was clear that he could incorporate mother into the play while keeping a focus on father.

While he played with mother, Alan wanted to know if a certain object was a machine and tried to plug it in. When he discovered it was a tape-recorder, he wanted to sing "Happy Birthday" onto the tape. Mother asked him if that was his favorite song, and he answered, "Yes, Happy Birthday." Then mother asked about the presents he wanted for his birthday, and he was able to tell her. Alan seemed to thoroughly enjoy being with mother, and she seemed more relaxed.

The parents' current concern was that when Alan was around a lot of noise he became "hyper." He had said to a very noisy child in his preschool program, "It hurts my ears." Mother reported that he also had trouble with other people's anger; he covered his face if either parent got angry with him and would cry if mother raised her voice too much. Mother also thought that Alan tended to perseverate during play—repeating game movements or using prepackaged sequences instead of innovating. We talked about the play partner adding innovative twists (i.e., putting a doll in front of a moving toy car) and helping Alan discuss his feelings about noise. They could create play sequences in which one animal or doll was noisy, then Alan could put into words how the noise made him feel. Similarly, they could talk about people's anger through pretend play and some reality-based discussions, because Alan was now verbal enough to do this.

The parents worried that innovating during play would overwhelm Alan. I suggested they move slowly out of a particular pattern, allowing him to innovate. His lack of innovative play was more likely a result of his anxiety about being assertive than directly due to organicity. I also noted that his uneven motor development and word retrieval problems led him to seek the security of repetition. I urged father not to "spoon-feed" Alan as much during play; he could be more challenging. Mother would work on consolidating her great rhythm and warmth and on diminishing her controlling style by encouraging Alan to challenge her a bit more.

Alan was becoming more involved in make-believe and fantasy in his play with mother. Yet because he sometimes preferred to play with girl dolls and could shy away from aggressive play, mother was worried about his "gender identity"—despite the fact that Alan was quite assertive and masculine in his style and orientation. As mother talked about her conflicts with assertive, aggressive men, such as her brother (her husband was, as noted earlier, very passive), it was clear that she was projecting these conflicts onto Alan. She wanted him to be assertive and confident but was also frightened as themes of power and assertiveness began to emerge in his play, and she exaggerated his interests in the body, girls, and girl dolls.

While empathizing with mother's concerns and their connection to her experience with her brother, I stressed the importance of the parents accurately reading Alan's communications and empathizing with him, helping him elaborate emotional ideas; their ability to do these things would help him move fully into the stage of representational differentiation and emotional thinking. The parents needed to know their own inclinations and fears. Mother was able to see how she might be anxious about the very thing she wished for—that Alan be a competent and assertive male. Now that Alan was starting to differentiate his emotional ideas, we talked about helping him label and discuss his feelings more, both in rational dialogue and pretend play modes.

In subsequent sessions, it was clear that both parents had been doing their homework as well as reflecting on their own feelings about Alan and how they interacted with him. They set up play times with other children and continued their own interactions with him. As Alan became more cooperative, during his visits with me he vacillated between new, more assertive and powerful themes in his play (such as being king of the jungle, or being a powerful gorilla who knocked down houses) and a fear of things being broken, such as arms being broken off dolls. I helped his parents to both support his power-oriented play and empathize with the scary feelings about things being broken.

Alan became more verbal and elaborative as he played out these themes in make-believe. For example, as he played with father during one session, he said, "Let's get more toys." He searched around assertively, like a big, tough guy, but then came across a broken doll and said with concern, "This one is broken." Then he immediately switched modes, saying, "I want lots of toys." He came across another broken doll and said, "I don't want this one. Let's put it away and hide it." Father asked, "Why do you want to hide it?" and Alan answered, "That's for a baby to play with. I don't want to play with things that are for babies." Father wondered why the broken things were only for babies and asked if Alan could fix them. "I'm not into fixing things," Alan stated. He then started playing with the Potato Head doll. Father talked for the Potato Head, asking how they should play. Alan started taking out other animals and said, "This is a duck. Look how funny it is." He made the toy act silly and then for the first time experimented by breaking the leg off another duck. "Oh, look! It's broken," he said, as part of his dialogue with Potato Head. He got a little nervous and went back to a more powerful posture by saying, "Let's forget the Potato Head and go on to the wolves."

Throughout the play, Alan was connecting islands of emotional ideas and playing out an important emotional drama. In keeping with his mother's concerns about his gender identification, he played with Barbie dolls during this session, but he picked out one with a missing leg. "She had one leg off and one leg on," he said. He eagerly searched for the missing leg, and mother was able to search with him instead of getting anxious. Alan eventually found the leg and fixed the doll, then picked out some cars and tried to hook them together. "They are not going to hook up," mother warned. Alan replied, "Where's the Scotch tape? Maybe we can hook them up using that." "They're still not going to hook up," said mother. Yet Alan found some tape and figured out a way to hook the cars together. He made a long train out of the cars and smiled broadly. Mother was surprised, and understood that his ability to hook the cars together reflected his competence and assertive orientation.

Around this time, father revealed that he was very afraid of violence—this was related to his passive orientation—and was worried that Alan would hurt himself. Mother continued to deal with her projections about Alan's masculinity but was becoming increasingly aware of her own conflicts. For example, she was able to help him with his curiosity about a pregnant babysitter. Alan wondered about where children come from and whether "he could have a baby some day." Mother empathized with him about that and helped him ask the questions he wanted to ask about the babysitter.

In a later session, at age 4½ (after about 1 year of treatment), Alan came in with his parents and immediately began looking for toys. He had a serious expression but easily engaged me in organized conversation. He asked "how" and "why" questions and closed circles, talking about rational, day-to-day concerns as well as make-believe. For example, as he was examining the toys, I asked him which one he was interested in. "That one," he said, and then asked, "Mom, how does it work?" I asked him, "Why did you ask mom rather than figuring it out for yourself?" and he answered, "Because she has a big brain." I asked, "How about dad?" "Mom is smarter," Alan responded. "Are you saying dad is a dummy?" I asked. Then Alan laughed and began chanting, "Dumb daddy, dumb daddy," but then immediately became anxious and serious. He was still uncomfortable with making fun of father or competing openly with him. Nonetheless, this sequence illustrated his growing ability to make logical connections between complex thoughts and to communicate logically.

Alan began a pretend play sequence with mother in which she was a doctor who took care of him. He had a boo-boo on his knee and said, "You ran out of medicine—call CVS" (the pharmacy where they got medicine). Mother said, "Well, the medicine doesn't work." "Get some more," Alan demanded. "Still doesn't work," mother said. So Alan said, "Well, get me some more juice or maybe give me some lemonade. That's my favorite." Mother pretended to do that, and he said, "Now I'm better." Mother asked, "How did you get better? Was it just giving you the medicine or the juice?" Alan replied, "Well, I also have a special machine and it has lemonade in it and it gives me lemonade whenever I want it." He then took a toy and pretended it was the machine. Mother wondered how the machine worked, and Alan said, "Like magic." This drama was interesting in terms of his expectations of mother and the development of "magic" as an extension of these expectations.

Although Alan still favored mother over father, he now related much more warmly to father and their relationship was developing. With father, Alan's play was more inconsistent, and after a few minutes he announced, "I'm getting too bored." However, he brought father to the lemonade machine, and they tried to build an even better machine together. Intermittently, he went back to mother, saying that he was bored with playing and wanted to go outside.

Alan now seemed appropriately in the early phases of triangular issues. He was working out competition, rivalry, and self-sufficiency as well as his needs for care and nurturing. He had lots of "how" and "why" questions and easily elaborated fantasy and rational dialogue in his play. At times he would just add elements to his play that were available close by, but at other times his play seemed planned. In addition to a more elaborate capacity for fantasy, Alan was showing a more differentiated capacity for connecting up his emotional ideas. He was working on age-appropriate emotional ideas and was beginning to have best friends, whom he talked about. He said that sometimes he got upset if other kids were mean to him; mother reported that he never felt angry, only sad or upset. (It appeared that he needed more help with elaborating specific feelings in a representationally differentiated way, particularly anger and competitiveness.)

In other areas of development, Alan's teacher said that he still had unusual body movements, which became more intense when he was anxious. His fine motor skills were improving, and he could write his name. He played with both girls and boys and especially liked playing with active boys, but he had a favorite girl friend he liked to play with and invite to his house. His best friend at day care was a boy, and his best friend around the block was a girl—he once proudly said that she had hugged him. The teacher's only worry was that he seemed obsessed with drawing circles.

Mother was still concerned that, after lots of activity or work at drawing or coloring, he would get tired and put his head on the floor as if overwhelmed. But both mother and teacher were pleased that when Alan got angry now, he would say, "I'm mad" or "I hate you" but did not hit. He could not always find the word he wanted to use and was sometimes slow in constructing his sentences, but he was giggling more and showing more joy, and his sense of humor was improving.

Structurally, Alan was now functioning at age-appropriate levels. He could not only share attention, engage, and have two-way gestural communication but also use emotional ideas to elaborate his thoughts and categorize his ideas into patterns of emotional thinking. He could see the connections between different themes in his pretend play and organize rational dialogue. He had mild constrictions around competition, rivalry, and aggression, tending to feel hurt and sad rather than angry. He was struggling with his dependency on mother's nurturance and negotiating how to "build his own machine"; not only did he want it to give him the medicine, but he was discovering how to form a collaboration with the machine around father. Both of these were age-appropriate challenges.

In summary, Alan had constitutional contributions in terms of motor delay and motor planning problems, some early deprivation (in terms of being adopted from an orphanage at 8 months), and some ongoing environmental struggles with his parents—mother being anxious and somewhat fragmented, and father being passive and avoidant. Alan's problematic behavior reflected his inability to negotiate the stages of representational elaboration and differentiation. In the course of a year, he stabilized the early stages and became fully involved in more age-appropriate stages.

Therapeutic work continued to help Alan learn more about his feelings and conflicts; now he possessed the structural capacity to understand and work through these feelings, conflicts, and fears. He continued occupational therapy for his motor coordination and mild sensory overreactivity (i.e., to sound). Finally, the parents continued to work on their marriage.

Alan's case also illustrates the application of the DIR model of assessment and intervention to a child and family with challenges at a number of levels. In Alan's case, his social, emotional, and cognitive development was, in part, compromised due to early deprivation. Nonetheless, when he presented he demonstrated processing challenges (motor planning difficulties) that were quite similar to those we observe in children who have optimal family support. In such cases, it is difficult to know whether the processing challenges are due to biological variations or early deprivation. Nonetheless, in Alan's case, a combination of factors contributed to his pervasive developmental difficulties.

Even though cases such as Alan's leave questions regarding the source of the difficulties, the DIR model enables us to describe their functioning in terms of its various dimensions so that we can construct a comprehensive intervention program tailored to the child and the family's unique profile. As the description of the case illustrates, Alan made excellent progress with this type of comprehensive approach.

Like Brad, Alan would also illustrate a pattern consistent with the criteria for Type I in our new classification of NDRC. Clearly, Alan's case could also be thought of as a deprivation reaction, as well as having characteristics of an attachment disorder. However, when a child evidences difficulties in the fundamental capacities for relating, communicating, and thinking, we recommend using the category of *neurodevelopmental disorders of relating and communicating* to describe the child's pattern of functioning. The specific influencing factors in Alan's case of his early deprivation can then be described as an important contributing factor. Each child will typically evidence his own unique developmental pathway to the pervasive developmental challenges that characterize NDRC. Even children with optimal family support will evidence a wide range of biologically based processing profiles (e.g., one child will be hyperreactive to touch and sound, whereas another will be hyporeactive to touch and sound; one child will have relative strengths in visual memory, whereas another in auditory memory).

As Alan has moved into his adolescent years, he has continued to make progress with only periodic re-evaluations and family guidance. He has a tendency to be concerned with "people not being there for me and needing to do it myself" whenever he is under a great deal of stress, is having difficulty with a friendship, or is rebuffed by a young lady on whom he has a crush. Personally, however, he has some perspective on this internal picture and can relate it to his own past history. His prognosis is good for continuing progress.

Conclusion

In this chapter, we have outlined principles of intervention with children who have NDRC. Central to all our recommendations is the concept of helping each child develop a sense of his own personhood. This sense develops as the child learns to focus, concentrate, engage, initiate two-way interaction, use simple and complex gestures for shared social problem solving, use words and symbols, and build logical bridges between ideas. All therapeutic efforts must have the goal of facilitating the child's mastery of these core developmental competencies. The educational system must collaborate by making available—routinely and not as an exception—integrated classrooms and normative peer interactions that harness the developmentally delayed child's emerging social and emotional capacities.

References

American Psychiatric Association: Diagnostic and Statistical Manual of Mental Disorders, 4th Edition, Text Revision. Washington, DC, American Psychiatric Association, 2000

Bredekamp S, Copple C: Developmentally Appropriate Practices in Early Childhood Programs. Washington, DC, National Association for the Education of Young Children, 1997

Diagnostic Classification Task Force: Diagnostic Classification 0–3: Diagnostic Classification of Mental Health and Developmental Disorders of Infancy and Early Childhood. Arlington, VA, ZERO TO THREE: National Center for Clinical Infant Programs, 1994

Greenspan SI: Infancy and Early Childhood: The Practice of Clinical Assessment and Intervention With Emotional and Developmental Challenges. Madison, CT, International Universities Press, 1992

Greenspan SI: Engaging Autism. Cambridge, MA, DaCapo Press/Perseus Books, 2005

Greenspan SI, Shanker S: The First Idea: How Symbols, Language and Intelligence Evolved From Our Primate Ancestors to Modern Humans. Reading, MA, Perseus Books, 2004

Greenspan SI, Wieder S: Developmental patterns and outcomes in infants and children with disorders in relating and communicating: a chart review of 200 cases of children with autistic spectrum diagnoses. Journal of Developmental and Learning Disorders 1:87–141, 1997

Greenspan SI, Wieder S: The Child With Special Needs: Encouraging Intellectual and Emotional Growth. Reading, MA, Perseus Books, 1998

Greenspan SI, Wieder S: A functional developmental approach to autism spectrum disorders. J Assoc Pers Sev Handicaps 24:147–161, 1999

Greenspan SI, Wieder S: Reversing the core deficits of ASD: progress and new directions. Report Given on Panel #1, Interdisciplinary Council on Developmental and Learning Disorders 8th International Conference. Bethesda, MD, Interdisciplinary Council on Developmental and Learning Disorders, 2004

Interdisciplinary Council on Developmental and Learning Disorders Clinical Practice Guidelines Workgroup: Interdisciplinary Council on Developmental and Learning Disorders' Clinical Practice Guidelines: Redefining the Standards of Care for Infants, Children, and Families With Special Needs. Bethesda, MD, Interdisciplinary Council on Developmental and Learning Disorders, 2000

Interdisciplinary Council on Developmental and Learning Disorders Diagnostic Manual for Infancy and Early Childhood Workgroups: Interdisciplinary Council on Developmental and Learning Disorders Diagnostic Manual for Infancy and Early Childhood Mental Health Disorders, Developmental Disorders, Regulatory-Sensory Processing Disorders, Language Disorders, and Learning Challenges. Bethesda, MD, Interdisciplinary Council on Developmental and Learning Disorders, 2005

World Health Organization: International Statistical Classification of Diseases and Related Health Problems, 10th Revision. Geneva, World Health Organization, 1992

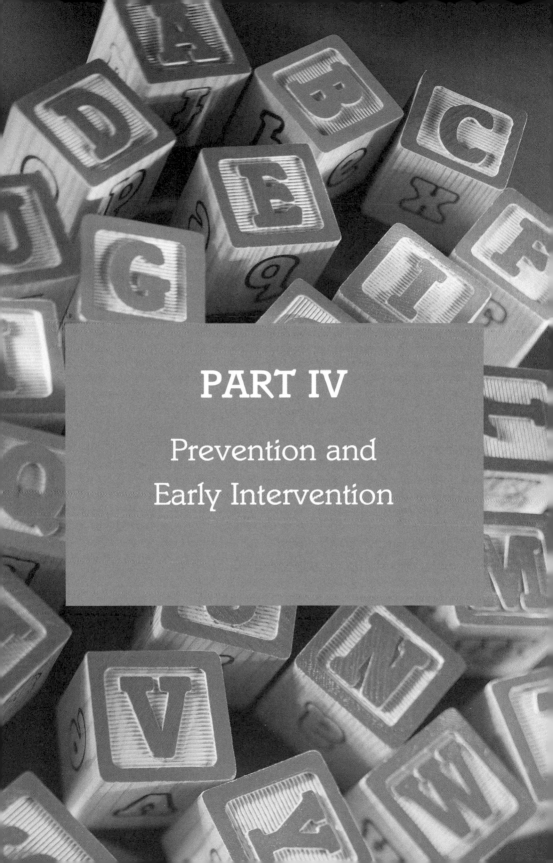

PART IV

Prevention and
Early Intervention

Introduction

One of the most important goals of infant and early childhood mental health services is prevention and early intervention. Understanding the developmental pathways leading to healthy emotional and intellectual growth, as well as to challenges, provides a framework to work with infants, young children, and their families at earlier and earlier ages—both to strengthen the fundamental building blocks of healthy development and to intervene to address emerging challenges before they become chronic (i.e., to help infants and young children and their families get back on a healthy developmental trajectory).

However, prevention and early intervention approaches have faced a major challenge in reaching the multiproblem and multirisk families that have appeared beyond the reach of most programs. These families often refuse to volunteer for or cooperate with such services. Another challenge has been to organize programs that are sufficiently comprehensive to help infants, young children, and families with all aspects of their development. This includes emotional and social functioning, language and cognitive capacities, and motor and sensory abilities as well as overall family and community functioning. Most prevention and early intervention programs have tended to focus on only one or another feature of human development, such as selected cognitive or motor skills or nutritional support, without fully dealing with the fact that all aspects of the child's and family's development are intimately interrelated.

Reaching the seemingly unreachable and providing comprehensive preventive and early intervention services for all infants, young children, and their families must therefore be the goal of modern approaches to prevention and early intervention. In Chapter 10 ("Infants in Multirisk Families: A Model for Developmentally Based Preventive Intervention"), we summarize the elements that are essential in such programs (Figure 10–1). We examine these elements in both Chapters 10 ("Infants in Multirisk Families") and 11 ("A Model for Comprehensive Prevention and Early Intervention Services for All Families").

Some families, like those described in Chapter 10 ("Infants in Multirisk Families"), require all elements on the service pyramid. Other families only require the first three levels on the pyramid, starting from its base of concrete services. In general, prevention and early intervention approaches must begin with the education of teenagers and young adults regarding all aspects of child and family development. It is somewhat paradoxical that our schools enthusiastically emphasize literature, science, and math, including human and animal biology, but place relatively little emphasis on human social, intellectual, and emotional growth and family functioning. Knowledge that all children and young adults will require for one of the most important aspects of life—raising families—is surprisingly underemphasized in our educational system. We try to prepare our children for work and a career but not for the other half of their lives.

In addition to educational programs during the school years, including college, prevention and intervention programs must embrace a very active component during the prenatal months, not only in terms of facilitating healthy prenatal development but also providing the knowledge and emotional support that will be needed to facilitate healthy development when the new baby is born. Hence, it is vital that prevention and early intervention approaches be integrated into well-baby care and all settings in which infants and young children and their families may find themselves. This may include direct educational opportunities for parents and other caregivers, programs at daycare centers, and special programs for families under stress or at risk for difficulties. Prevention and early intervention approaches should then continue throughout childhood as each new stage of development challenges parents and other caregivers and growing children in new ways, offering opportunities to benefit from educational guidance and, when needed, clinical intervention.

The next two chapters describe some of the nuts and bolts of how to implement the kind of comprehensive approach we have been discussing. In Chapter 10 ("Infants in Multirisk Families"), we explore how to work with families that have often been beyond the reach of most programs but may in fact require and use the largest share of human services. We present a model for working with infants in multirisk or multiproblem families. In Chapter 11 ("A Model for Comprehensive Prevention and Early Intervention Services for All Families"), we present a model for prevention and early intervention work with all infants, young children, and their families—ranging from those who are progressing in a healthy manner, but nonetheless could benefit from further strengthening of already emerging competencies—to those with a variety of challenges. The best way for the reader to use these two chapters together is to picture the framework for working with infants in multirisk families as providing the intensive and comprehensive model required when all elements, including basic family functioning, need to be addressed. Chapter 10 shows how only certain elements of this model may need to be applied to lesser challenges and elaborates the principles that can facilitate healthy emotional, social, and intellectual growth in all children.

10

Infants in Multirisk Families:
A Model for Developmentally
Based Preventive Intervention

In the previous chapter, we described how children with neurodevelopmental disorders of relating and communicating require a team of professionals who can each address different aspects of the child's development and who meet regularly to coordinate their services and assess the child's progress. A team approach is equally important—and even more complex—for what are sometimes called "multirisk" or "multiproblem" families. These terms refer to families who face a host of challenges that contribute to developmental difficulties in the children and that complicate the treatment of such difficulties. Although each family is unique, common problems include lack of basic resources such as food and affordable shelter, untreated psychiatric illnesses in one or both parents, maladaptive patterns of interaction among family members, and lack of connection to the traditional array of social services available in the community. To effectively address developmental deficits and challenges in such families, a truly comprehensive, coordinated program of services is essential.

This chapter is based on our book *Infants in Multirisk Families*, edited by Greenspan SI, Wieder S, Lieberman A, et al. Madison, CT, International Universities Press, 1987.

Recruiting and Engaging Families for a Preventive Intervention Program

In the mid-1970s, we developed a Clinical Infant Development Program (CIDP) for infants in multirisk families residing in Prince Georges County, Maryland. This program, which we operated into the 1980s, has been replicated and adapted by agencies in several other counties and cities in the United States. We recruited pregnant women who had already shown severe difficulties in fulfilling one of the primary maternal functions or both of the secondary maternal functions for an older child and who seemed likely to repeat the pattern with the new infant. (*Primary maternal functions* are the ability to provide physical care and protection, the ability to read an infant's signals of pleasure or displeasure, and the ability to provide sufficient emotional nurturing for a human attachment between mother and infant. *Secondary maternal functions* are the ability to discern a child's changing developmental needs during the first 2 years and the ability to respond promptly, effectively, and empathically to the child's signals.)

Because multirisk families tend to remain outside the traditional mental health system, rarely seeking appointments and generally distrusting service providers, we launched an extensive outreach effort to recruit mothers. We stationed clinicians at prenatal clinics, where they made presentations about the program to groups of women and approached individual mothers directly. We called on social service agencies, the courts, child protective services, state mental hospitals, community mental health agencies, and the police, asking them to send us their most difficult and challenging clients. We made it clear that no family would be turned away because of the severity of its problems. Soon calls started coming in from prenatal clinics regarding mothers who had missed appointments, appeared confused, or were not following medical guidance as well as from child protective service and court workers involved with families in which an older child was neglected and the mother was pregnant again.

Identifying potential participants was only the first step. In some cases, repeated visits and outreach were needed before mothers consented to sign up for the program. The key to recruiting and engaging the families was our staff's ability to deal with patterns of avoidance, rejection, and anger as well as illogical and antisocial behavior and substance abuse. We selected experienced clinicians who were not frightened by such behavior and who could sensitively but persistently pursue mothers while resisting the impulse to conclude, "she just doesn't want help," or "they told us they don't want us, we're just being a burden to them." In the early phases of working with a family, it was sometimes necessary for the clinician to make five or six home visits, knock on the door, hear someone walking around inside, make a few comments through the door, get no answer, and then return 3 days later to try again, until the person inside felt comfortable enough to open the door and let the clinician in. Even more difficult were mothers who eagerly embraced the program and then disappeared. In many cases, the clinician's continual outreach and offering of an interested ear eventually met with success. Sometimes, a year would pass before a consistent pattern of relatedness evolved.

Sixty-one women were eventually recruited. (An additional 29 women signed consent forms but immediately or shortly thereafter refused to participate in the program.) Evaluation of prospective participants was based on clinical interviews with the mother, clinical assessments of existing children, observations of maternal and child functioning, free-play observations at home and in our office, psychological testing of the mother, and the records or reports of other agencies.

The initial evaluations were conducted not in the traditional format of psychiatric interviews in an office setting but instead during the process of engaging and forming relationships with the mothers. We asked what help they needed and tried to be useful so that they would permit us to visit and observe again. Because so many were struggling with survival, we could always find ways to help with concrete services. While driving clients to health or social service agencies and while meeting with them in their homes, our clinicians could ask questions and make observations of general and maternal functioning. Once a relationship was established, clients were more likely to agree to formal interviews, testing, and observations in our office. Each contact with a client was recorded in narrative process form. Although the course each evaluation took varied somewhat from mother to mother, the information gathered, when summarized, resulted in a complete psychiatric evaluation and a clinical team consensus on the mother's risk level and diagnosis. (For details on the research protocols, validation procedures, and clinical rating scales used in the evaluations, see *Infants in Multirisk Families* [Greenspan et al. 1987]).

Based on the evaluation, 47 of the mothers recruited were considered at significant risk for failure to provide adequate mothering for the children they were carrying at the time of evaluation. Another 14 were determined to be at low risk. The low-risk mothers were assigned to Group A. The high-risk mothers were assigned to one of two groups, Group B or Group C. Families in Group B received clinical, developmental, and psychosocial assessments and feedback and were then referred to the community agency or agencies best suited to meet their needs. Group C families received the same assessments but were then offered the intervention resources of the CIDP. The index children of all three groups were systematically assessed at regular intervals with the identical research protocol (Greenspan et al. 1987).

The 47 high-risk mothers we worked with had anywhere from one to six children already born; lived in communities in Prince Georges County, Maryland, that range from urban to rural; and were mostly married or involved in an ongoing relationship with the fathers of their children. They ranged from 18 to 36 years old (median age 23.9), with 27 identifying themselves as black and 20 identifying themselves as white. More than half of the mothers had not graduated from high school. Only six mothers were employed; most depended on more than one individual or system to meet their own and their children's needs for food, clothing, shelter, and other necessities. Sources of support included families of origin, the fathers of their children, government programs, and nongovernment agencies such as churches or the Salvation Army.

We were extremely interested in understanding the histories of the mothers; we hoped to identify the antecedent factors that may have contributed to their high-risk status and maternal difficulties. We quickly learned, however, that traditional interview techniques would not yield the information we sought. We were reaching out to women who had not sought psychiatric services and were often suspicious or scared of "helping professionals." As described earlier, we began by offering the mothers help with immediate needs and gathered information gradually as we built a relationship with each mother. Because many of the mothers had great difficulty revealing aspects of their histories that were shrouded in secrecy or shame—such as early abandonment, family mental illness, abuse, or incest—such information often emerged only after a strong therapeutic relationship had developed, a process that in some cases took years.

We discovered that all the mothers had had difficult lives and many problems before their children were born and that their difficulties did not go away. The profile of the typical mother in our program revealed a woman who was born into a family experiencing psychiatric dysfunction, who displayed marked impairment in her own social and emotional development as a child, and who, as an adult, bore children whose functioning seemed already compromised in the earliest years of life. To capture, if only in a limited way, the degree to which multiple risk factors or antecedent variables came together for each participant, we constructed an index of misfortunes experienced by the women prior to their entry into the program. Each woman's score was obtained by counting the number of misfortunes, out of a list of 18, that she had experienced and dividing that number by 18 to derive a percentage. A score of 0 would indicate that the person had experienced none of the 18 misfortunes; a person with a score of 1 would have experienced all of them. The misfortunes, or antecedent variables, are listed in Table 10–1.

We found that the median value of the index for the high-risk women was 0.49. That is, half of the 47 high-risk women had experienced nine or more of the misfortunes before entering the program. Fifteen percent of them had experienced close to 12 of these events. In contrast, the median value of the index for the low-risk women (Group A) was 0.09—that is, the women in the low-risk group generally had experienced none of these misfortunes in their lives. The maximum value for the index in this group was 0.21, or 3.7 misfortunes. There was a moderate relationship between the index of misfortune and the rating of maternal functioning ($r=-0.34$, $P=0.01$) and also between the index and the participant's capacity to engage in a therapeutic relationship ($r=-0.34$, $P=0.01$). The fact that our index correlates, although moderately, with these two independent measures of psychiatric status at entry to the program leads us to believe that the index may

TABLE 10–1.	Maternal risk factors used to calculate index of misfortune

1. Psychiatric illness in family of origin
2. Psychiatric hospitalization
3. Physical neglect experienced before age 18
4. Physical abuse experienced before age 18
5. Sexual abuse experienced before age 18
6. Witnessing abuse of others before age 18
7. Physical abuse by mate
8. Physical abuse or neglect of own children
9. Disruption of significant relationship before age 12
10. Impaired functioning in family before age 18
11. Impaired functioning in peer group before age 18
12. Impaired functioning in school before age 18
13. Impaired functioning in family at or above age 18
14. Impaired functioning in peer group at or above age 18
15. Impaired functioning at work at or above age 18
16. Chronic antisocial behavior
17. Expulsion from school
18. Chronic violation of rules at home or school before age 15

have some predictive utility. (For a full statistical presentation of the demographics and antecedent variables that characterized our participants, see Greenspan et al. 1987).

Essential Components of Preventive Intervention

Because the families we recruited had not found it possible to use the standard, often fragmented array of social services in their communities, the CDIP combined, either directly or through collaboration with other agencies, services seldom found in a single organization. Our approach had three major components:

1. We had to support basic survival and help clients meet concrete needs. This meant searching for apartments with participants who were facing eviction, making clinic appointments and providing transportation so mothers would keep them, and delivering emergency food and diapers. It also meant working in collaboration with other agencies and authorities on behalf of the families.

2. We had to develop some regularity and continuity in our contacts with the mothers in order to build trust and a healing relationship. We needed to con-

sider the nature of each mother's pathology and the impact of her past relationships as we persisted in our outreach in the face of avoidance that, in many cases, lasted for months.

3. We had to develop specific clinical techniques and patterns of care suited to the highly varied constitutional capacities of the babies. The infants in the program ranged from the very vulnerable—for example, those with unique tactile or auditory sensitivities—to the very resilient. We set up an Infant Center to provide, at one site, part-time or full-day therapeutic day care for the infant, outreach to the parent, and training and supervision of program staff. As our contacts with the mothers stabilized and attachments formed between the mothers and program staff, we began working to bring the mothers to higher developmental levels by helping them relate to their children's individual vulnerabilities, strengths, and emerging capacities for human interaction, from early two-way interchanges to later representational elaboration.

Staffing the CIDP: The Team Approach

CIDP staff were called "primary clinicians" and "infant specialists" in order to reflect our program's difference from traditional services and to avoid the stigma or fear our families might attach to traditional titles such as "therapist." Mothers in the program were referred to as "participants" rather than "patients" or "clients." This practice reflected our decision not to formally diagnose mothers or require them to identify a problem or need as a condition of joining the CIDP.

We realized that a team approach would be needed to provide effective help to our families. The sheer number of things to be done, agencies to involve, and children present in the families of our mothers required the energies of more than one person. Furthermore, the emotional stress of working with these families was difficult for one clinician to tolerate alone. By assigning at least two staff to each family, we ensured that staff could support each other in the face of multiple rejections as we pursued participants. Once a family began to engage, if the mother was angry with one team member, or if one team member became too overwhelmed and despairing to be effective, the second team member could take over for a time. We found that composing teams of people with different skills and professions facilitated this process: some mothers, for example, felt more comfortable with a nurse than with a social worker. Finally, and most important, a flexible team was needed to give equal attention to the infant, the mother, and the entire family. We found that the mothers, most of whom had never had adequate nurturing themselves, tended to compete with their infants for the attention of program staff. With a team approach, the mother could work through painful issues of her own in sessions with one clinician, while an infant specialist conducted less emotional sessions focused on the baby. In these sessions, the infant specialist could help the mother recognize and understand her baby's unique capacities and learn to interact with him in ways that furthered his healthy development. If, as sometimes happened, the mother was unable to focus on her infant and the clinician was still in the process of helping her with her patterns of avoidance, the infant specialist could provide the baby with crucial experiences until the mother was more available. If a mother happened to feel most comfortable with her baby and the infant specialist, the more intense therapeutic process emerged between mother and infant specialist; in such cases, the clinician was available to focus on the baby. For other cases, reaching both mother and infant proved so difficult that the additional services of the Infant Center were needed.

Our staff consisted of social workers, psychologists, nurses, educators, and paraprofessionals. As the program progressed, it became apparent that an ability to tolerate the stresses of the work was more important than background in a particular discipline. Successful staff members learned in the course of our program about subtle individual differences in infants and how these expressed themselves in infant–caregiver patterns of interaction. An especially sensitive infant who found his mother's voice noxious, for example, required a staff member who could both coach the mother to try different ways of holding, touching, and vocalizing with the infant and empathize with the mother's feelings of defectiveness, rejection, and anger. Several years of prior experience in some form of outreach or community-based service seemed to be a prerequisite for effectiveness. The only two staff members (out of 16) to leave the CIDP because of difficulties in doing the work had come from academic settings in which their authority derived in part from that of the institution. These clinicians found it especially challenging to function "outside," where they had to represent themselves without institutional backing and where a teaching posture was less effective.

For staff, it was the continual supervision and conferences as well as the team approach that relieved the stress of working in the CIDP. At some stages, just as much time was spent in supervision and support as in direct contacts with program participants. We needed a highly experienced clinical supervisory staff who could pay close attention to the impact of the work on both participants and staff. Each clinician had a weekly session with an individual supervisor. Team meetings, which periodically included the CIDP psychologist and developmental clinician in addition to the team members and supervisor, were held biweekly. Where needed, interagency meetings were held regularly. Finally, all members of the clinical staff, administrative supervisors, and program directors participated in a weekly case conference, which permitted the regular review of all families following each assessment interval. The critical underlying task in all these meetings was dealing with the reactions, or countertransference, stirred up by the difficult work with participants.

Limited caseloads were another element of support for staff. Typically, each clinician could carry only five or six intensive cases in Group C while following about the same number of cases in Group B, the community-referral group. (The Group B cases at first presented a source of conflict, as staff struggled over just how much help the CIDP should be offering this group. As time went on, clinicians welcomed the lower levels of intervention involved in these cases, despite the difficulty of keeping them engaged, simply because they required less effort than the families receiving comprehensive services.) Caseloads were determined primarily by the amount of effort needed to work with families rather than by an arbitrary number. Fortunately, even the most difficult cases usually stabilized around the infant's first birthday, at which time we would sense a consolidation of our efforts and a shift to easier stages of intervention. As some families achieved stability, clinicians could take on new participants; thus, during the program's first years, caseloads increased slowly as the stage of work with each participant was assessed.

Some of the traditional patient–therapist boundaries were lacking between CIDP participants and clinicians, who needed the capacity to tolerate a certain degree of merging out of which differentiation could grow. This intimacy took very concrete forms, as clinicians joined in participants' struggle for survival, experienced their fears and fury, and became the nurturing figures who slowly helped to create some order in their lives and those of their children, a necessary foundation for growth and development.

The Service Pyramid

As we increased our understanding of the developmental challenges facing young children and their families and the kinds of intervention needed to address these challenges, we also acquired a basis for conceptualizing therapeutic intervention at both the service system level and the clinical level.

The developmental, individual-differences, relationship-based (DIR) model provides the rationale for comprehensive intervention approaches, as opposed to approaches focused on isolated symptoms or behaviors. The CIDP was designed to achieve the same goals as the other interventions we have described in this book: to enable the infant to progress developmentally—that is, to master the capacities of attention and self-regulation, engagement and attachment, purposeful two-way communication, problem-solving communication and an emerging sense of self, symbolization, and building logical connections between symbols. Like the interventions described in earlier chapters, our work with the CIDP families addressed the infant's inborn processing tendencies, the family's dynamics and social context, and the interactions experienced by the infant.

Because the CIDP families faced such a multitude of problems, however, a more complex and wide-ranging array of interventions was necessary to support the mastery of each developmental level. We found it useful to visualize preventive services as a pyramid, with the services that support the earliest developmental stage at the base (see Figure 10–1).

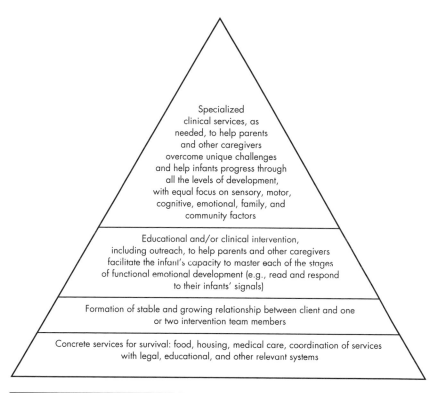

FIGURE 10–1. The service pyramid.

The service pyramid depicts an overall framework for services. Note that the third level up from the bottom of the pyramid refers to facilitating the infant's capacity to master each of the six core developmental capacities.

Level 1: Shared Attention and Regulation

For a baby to achieve self-regulation and develop interest in the world, she must have an environment that is protective and that permits her to engage the world in a comforting and self-regulating manner. This implies that the baby and her parents must have adequate nutrition, shelter, medical care, and basic safety. At the base of our service pyramid, therefore, are interventions that help pregnant mothers and their families with basic survival. Service system planning at this level must be based not on the easiest, but on the most difficult case—that is, on the multi-problem family that does not make itself available to the traditional service system.

In addition to all the social services (including, where needed, child protective services, the legal system, the educational system, and the health and mental health systems) working in an integrated manner, two pivotal components are needed to support basic security and self-regulation. The first is active and skillful outreach programs with staff who can make daily home visits where needed. The second is a project headquarters, such as our Infant Center, to which the most vulnerable families, often with severe psychopathology in the caregivers, can come every day. Here, other adults are available to meet the infant's need for physical care and protection and to support the infant in developing the capacity to attend and self-regulate. At the same site, staff can engage and support the caregiver. Daily visits to a center like this can help a family avoid the need for foster care. An extensive, well-integrated service system can make it possible for a family to attain the strength to stay together and to avoid later patterns that can lead to debilitating psychological, social, and intellectual difficulties and even to institutionalization of children.

Level 2: Engagement and Relating

When basic survival needs are met, parents can become more available for a relationship with their new infant. Just above the base of the pyramid are services necessary to support the family's capacity to provide a loving, satisfying attachment. All the services supporting level 1 are needed, as well as skilled psychotherapy for the parents. Program staff should, along with offering help with practical issues such as food and housing, make themselves available regularly and consistently to enable a trusting relationship with parents to develop. When parent and clinician have a warm and trusting enough relationship to meet regularly, they can begin working toward the next developmental level.

Level 3: Two-Way Intentional Affective Signaling and Communication

At the third level, staff must use specific clinical approaches to help parents read their infant's signals and engage in emotionally attuned reciprocal communication. Many parents, in order to recognize both cognitive and emotional signals in their infants, must first learn to recognize such signals in themselves. Thus, the opportunity to establish a warm relationship with a skilled clinician, in the context of which the capacity for self-observation can develop, is essential. This relationship must be able to tolerate negative feelings, such as disappointment or anger, without interruption of its reliability and regularity.

Some parents cannot achieve a self-observing capacity at an emotional level. Even for such parents, simple support combined with educative approaches can teach the ability to read their infant's signals cognitively. The optimal goal, however, is to teach both cognitive and affective observation of and response to signals, because this capacity is necessary to support all further stages of development. Infant specialists, nurses, and if necessary, skilled homemakers can facilitate the development of this capacity.

Level 4: Long Chains of Coregulated Emotional Signaling and Shared Social Problem Solving

Parents must now be able to maintain the self-observing function over a wide range of affective experience and complicated behavioral patterns. In working with a woman who had an underlying thought disorder, for example, we observed that she was capable of maintaining a self-observing function and reality orientation during simple communication. Once emotions became complicated, however (e.g., a mixture of love and aggression), she became overwhelmed, and her self-observing capacity and ability to read signals deteriorated. In such a case, the parent must be helped to strengthen her self-observing capacity and to tolerate highly complex emotions, such as ambivalence. The service system must now make available a new level on the pyramid: a specialized clinical team that helps parents learn to observe and understand their own and their child's feelings and communications. In addition, a trained clinician-educator can work with the child, either individually or in a toddlers' group, to help the child deal with complex emotions and social interactions. If the child has sensory, motor, or language lags, remedial occupational therapy or special education services are needed.

Level 5: Creating Representations (or Ideas)

At the next level of the pyramid are services to support the child's emerging capacity for *symbolization*, or the use of ideas to label feelings and guide behavior. The service system must now support the parents' own capacity for symbolization. In many cases, we have found that if we can help the parents represent their own experiences in *words, fantasies,* and *rich mental imagery*, they can then interact with their growing child in this mode. Parents who cannot do this often maintain a concrete way of relating that undermines the natural development of symbolic capacities in their toddlers and young children.

At level 5 of the service pyramid, a therapeutic relationship with the parents must unfold for a long enough time to help the parents develop the capacity for mental imagery, if they never had that capacity before. If the parents' capacity for symbolization is constricted by intrapsychic conflicts or characterological limitations, therapy can help them "liberate" or expand their representational capacity, at least where their relationship with their toddler is concerned. This effort requires sophisticated therapeutic work in which the parents' own fantasies are permitted to emerge. In their relationship with the therapist, the parents are encouraged to observe their own way of handling fantasy and mental imagery and are coached to recognize signs of this emerging capacity in their children. If necessary, while the parents are working to develop their own representational capacity, direct therapy with the toddler in a free-play setting can allow the child to begin to symbolize a variety of emotions through pretend play.

Level 6: Building Bridges Between Ideas: Logical Thinking

The capacity for differentiation, organization, and connection of ideas takes us to the top level of the pyramid. Here, the task is not simply to help parents develop and elaborate mental imagery but also to help them develop a reality orientation—that is, to help them differentiate ideas and imagery that pertain to the outside world from those that pertain to their inner life. With this ability, they can begin to facilitate a similar reality orientation in their young children. The capacity to distinguish reality from fantasy enables parents to make pivotal judgments about when to set limits and point out the reality of a situation and when to support the make-believe play of their children. Healthy, competent parents make these often-subtle distinctions intuitively. For example, a parent with a well-developed capacity for symbolization and symbolic differentiation knows that if her toddler is having one doll hit another, this is make-believe play dramatizing feelings, altogether different than if the toddler were himself hitting another child.

When parents have characterological constrictions, severe intrapsychic conflicts, or tendencies toward fragmentation, intensive therapeutic work may be required. Establishing or stabilizing ego functions such as reality testing, impulse regulation, mood stabilization, and the capacity for attending and concentrating can lay the foundation for establishing these same functions in the child. Preschool programs and one-on-one therapy can provide opportunities for children to practice and strengthen their new capacities.

We have outlined the six steps of a developmentally based pyramid of services for preventive intervention with multirisk families. In cases where financial or other crises are interfering with a family's otherwise healthy capacity to promote their children's achievement of the core developmental capacities, the concrete services and service coordination at the base of the pyramid may be enough. For most of the families we worked with, however, this was not so. Once the family's immediate crises were alleviated and a relationship between program staff and parents began to develop, the more specialized and sophisticated services at higher levels of the pyramid were needed.

In our experience, we have found that the kinds of interactive experiences a family needs to support each level of development can usually be provided through a program that integrates the existing network of community-based social services. However, our experience with the CIDP families demonstrated that the most challenging families often require intensive daily care and, depending on their level on the pyramid, highly specific clinical interventions. An outreach program and an Infant Center are needed to augment more traditional program approaches for such families.

It is worth emphasizing again that strengthening a family sometimes involves working directly with the youngster. If the parents are unavailable during important stages of the child's early development because of their own psychopathology or other circumstances, direct work with the child can help him become a "stronger team member" in the family. The child can then help his parents help him. For example, an 8-month-old infant who sends his emotional signals in a weak manner, or who has a withdrawn mother who does not read his signals, can be taught by an infant specialist to send stronger signals. As the mother gets stronger feedback from her infant, she may be drawn out of her depression to some degree, allowing her to engage more.

Dimensions and Levels of Helping Relationships

Our experience engaging and developing working relationships with these challenging families helped us to recognize and delineate what we believe are the most basic elements of any helping relationship. We conceptualize four parallel dimensions of such a relationship: regularity and stability, emotional depth, process of communication, and thematic content of communication. Each dimension can be evaluated at any point in the relationship.

Considering each dimension separately focuses attention on the very earliest stages of human services intervention: capturing a prospective client's interest, establishing a regular pattern of contact, facilitating the development of an emotional relationship, promoting purposeful two-way communication, and helping the client tolerate discomfort without fleeing. Too often, human services professionals and programs neglect these early stages. To use the example of psychotherapy, consider how much must be accomplished by therapist and client before they can begin doing what is typically considered "therapy." First, a prospective client must have some interest in the service offered. Ideally, the client begins to feel emotionally invested in both the therapist and the program of therapy and engages in an organized, purposeful exchange of signals with the therapist, in the process learning to tolerate whatever uncomfortable feelings are stirred up by the exchanges. At higher levels, the therapeutic relationship provides a context in which the client can observe her behavioral and emotional patterns, relinquish maladaptive patterns, and embrace new ways of functioning. It is only at these higher levels that specific therapeutic techniques, such as psychoanalytic treatment or cognitive-behavioral approaches, begin to vary, each taking its own route to helping the patient alter old patterns.

We believe the four dimensions offer a means for understanding and evaluating the progress of relationships not only between psychotherapists and their clients but also between visiting baby nurses and new parents, between teachers and the parents or guardians of their pupils, between doctors and their patients, between public health workers and individuals at risk of disease, and indeed between any helping professional and a person he or she attempts to assist. (In fact, the dimensions appear to characterize the development of *any* relationship between two people. As we describe the dimensions, we use examples from everyday social interactions as well as from human service situations.)

The First Dimension: Regularity and Stability

In models of service in which prospective clients voluntarily present themselves with a request for help or to enroll in a program, regularity and stability are often assumed. Even when self-referred clients seek help, however, regularity and stability are sometimes disrupted. Clients who feel ambivalent about seeking help may cancel appointments or fail to show up early in the process. Later, when the client–worker relationship stirs up unpleasant feelings that clients have heretofore succeeded in avoiding, they may respond by canceling meetings or by emotionally withdrawing from the worker during encounters.

In any situation in which a helping professional interacts, or attempts to interact, with someone who needs assistance, it is possible to evaluate the regularity and stability of meetings. Where home visiting is involved, for example, a client or prospective client demonstrates her initial interest simply by opening the door and making herself available for a conversation. At this earliest level, one would expect a mother to be able to engage in a simple conversation about occurrences in daily life or about her infant's physical health or feeding patterns. Even at this stage, one can distinguish between a person who will only occasionally appear for a scheduled appointment or let a home visitor in and one who meets regularly. Also vividly apparent is the difference between a client who appears alert, interested, and engaged with the worker and one who falls asleep or withdraws into a state of self-absorption.

Several stages or levels in the establishment of regularity and stability in the helping relationship can be identified:

1. The initial meeting, for example, to discuss needs or for any other purpose
2. The attempt to arrange follow-up meetings
3. Meeting according to some pattern, however unpredictable it may be at times
4. Meeting regularly according to schedule, with occasional disruptions such as a cancellation following a difficult conversation
5. Meeting regularly with minimal disruptions

Progress from one level to the next is not necessarily smooth or linear: client and worker may go back and forth between levels. Some relationships never move beyond level 1 or level 2. Think of the experience of getting to know a new neighbor. One might invite the newcomer over for coffee as a gesture of welcome, or simply exchange introductions upon encountering him by chance. The two of you might never say more than a polite "hi" after this initial exchange. In an alternative scenario, you might arrange to get together again, discover you enjoy each other's company, and continue to socialize frequently, in the process becoming close friends. If your new neighbor happens to be very shy or guarded, you stand a better chance of getting to know him if you respect his need to go slowly in forming this new connection. You may need to persist, gently and not too intrusively, and to tolerate some awkward silences or stilted conversation before discovering some topic that he feels comfortable discussing. Similarly, for a client–worker relationship to move toward regularity and stability, the helping professional must adopt a stance that supports such movement. A delicate balance of patience and persistence is called for. An outreach worker may, for example, knock on a prospective client's door on several occasions without succeeding in meeting him or her face to face. Perhaps the knock is met with silence on the first several attempts, or the prospective client turns out the lights and hides in a back room. On a later occasion, perhaps the worker is rewarded with a glimpse of someone peeking out a window. Finally, the person inside may feel safe enough and curious enough to open the door. A willingness to meet prospective clients on their own turf, to persist in inquiring what they perceive their most urgent needs to be, and to tolerate their expressions of disinterest, suspicion, or even hostility, are prerequisites for engaging them in a relationship that has the potential to progress toward regularity and stability.

Madeline

Madeline, a depressed young mother of four children, initially told the CIDP clinician to visit her because she liked "a little company sometimes," but rarely could she be found. For months, Madeline moved from place to place with her children, desperately seeking refuge but antagonizing those who took her in. The clinician and infant specialist pursued her with food, diapers, and offers of transportation. Although Madeline never called or informed the staff of her next move, she would be angry if they did not come to see her. There was no regularity in Madeline's life, nor could there be any in the helping relationships at this stage.

Only after 8 months of persistent pursuit did some regularity begin to be established. Madeline grew less frightened and more able to tolerate predictable contacts with the clinician (step 3). These contacts focused mostly on day-to-day survival and helping Madeline acquire some life skills. Madeline never acknowledged that she needed therapy and was not yet able to talk about her life, but she was willing to be with the therapist in order to be nurtured. As regularity of contact stabilized (step 4) and Madeline developed a stronger attachment to the clinician, she began to reveal some of her history.

Suzanne

Suzanne was a bright, articulate woman who married at 17 and proceeded to have one child after another, staying within the confines of a small apartment while her husband negotiated the outside world. She was referred to us after a severe marital crisis that precipitated a brief stay in a women's shelter before she reconciled with her husband. The CIDP clinician offered concrete help to Suzanne, as well as the opportunity to discuss her concerns. Suzanne never refused and never expressed any suspiciousness, allowing the clinician to schedule meeting after meeting (step 2). On the day of each visit, however, Suzanne would take 20–30 minutes to answer the door. If the clinician called before coming, or from a phone booth because there was no answer at the door, the phone would ring 20–30 times before Suzanne answered.

Once Suzanne finally answered the door, she would graciously invite the clinician to come in and sit down but would then excuse herself and disappear into a back room for half an hour or more. When she finally appeared, Suzanne would ask the clinician questions about the clinician's own past and about problems of the clinician's children. Suzanne would refuse to discuss her own concerns; even the mildest comment by the clinician regarding Suzanne's behavior or feelings was met with denial and even longer waits at the door or on the phone.

The clinician persisted, however, responding sensitively on Suzanne's terms. Soon, Suzanne started to call for rides and accepted our referrals for her children. She started to answer the door in 10 or 15 minutes and took less time to adapt to the clinician's presence in her home. Yet cancellations and interruptions were still frequent, and for every two or three contacts, one was missed (step 3). If Suzanne saw the infant specialist one week, she would not meet with the clinician during the same week. Eventually, Suzanne could meet regularly and twice weekly (step 4). By this time, she had formed a strong emotional bond with the treatment team.

Anita

Another young mother, Anita, was unable to establish regularity and stability despite months of persistence by CIDP staff. Anita had been abused as a child and had lived in several foster homes by the time she reached adolescence and began to have children of her own. When we met her, she was again pregnant, lived in her boyfriend's truck, and had two children in foster care. Anita seemed to accept our help at first, meeting with us sporadically before her baby was born and for a few months afterward (steps 1 and 2). We attempted to arrange stable housing and to coordinate efforts with other agencies. Anita, however, remained distant and unrevealing. Once her son was born, she could not contain streams of projections regarding his "badness, orneriness" and all the "evil" he was doing her. When he turned away, she shook and jostled him in frustration. Despite our many efforts to maintain contact and offer help, Anita fled from address to address. Unlike Madeline, she left no trail to pursue.

Almost 2 years after her son's birth, Anita walked into our Infant Center and asked us to assess him. She would not say why, nor would she reveal her whereabouts. After the assessment, we shared some concerns regarding the severe developmental delays he evidenced and urged her to return so that we could do a more complete evaluation and offer help to her and her son. She did not return. We contacted everyone who had been involved with her case but could not find her again.

As these vignettes illustrate, maintaining even a minimal degree of interest and regularity in a social service relationship is an achievement for many clients that should not be underestimated. Because of their early experiences, fears, and psychological disturbances, many people in need of help cannot make even this level of commitment. Programs that assume that all clients can be responsible for coming regularly for treatment, labeling those who fail to do so "unmotivated" or "untreatable," will fail many clients. Similarly, programs that ignore the first steps in establishing a relationship and instead attempt to engage the patient at higher levels of the therapeutic process, such as discussion of complex feelings, are building a house on a very shaky foundation.

The Second Dimension: Emotional Depth of the Relationship

A client's relationship with a helping professional tends to develop in the following stages:

1. *The client or prospective client is interested only in the concrete services that the worker or program can provide.* At this stage, the client shows little interest in the helping professional as an individual, and it may matter little which worker offers the services. (This stance is common among clients who continually have to meet with different workers to obtain social services.) After repeated contacts with a single worker, however, the client may begin to respond emotionally. He may ask for help and feel dependent on the worker, or feel angry and attack the worker for failing to do more, or vacillate between these two stances. The nature of a client's emotional responses to the helping professional will suggest what kind of relationships that client has experienced during his life. For example, suppose a parent habitually approaches his child's new teachers with a guarded, suspicious attitude and is quick to anger if he perceives they are displeased with his child. One might hypothesize that this man's prior experiences with authority figures, or with relationships involving criticism or evaluation, had been painful in some way.

2. *The client begins to show signs of emotional interest in the helping professional.* Perhaps she smiles and looks joyful when the worker arrives. She may tell the worker about a new friendship she has made outside the program, perhaps indicating that she has similar feelings toward the worker. At this stage, the client may perceive the helping professional as someone she feels good with, like a sister or a friend. She may make highly personalized statements, including negative ones (e.g., "You hurt my feelings"), which give evidence of emotional relatedness.

3. *The client engages in purposeful two-way exchanges with the helping professional, using the relationship to communicate in a logical manner.* She may ask for advice or discuss concrete matters such as how to pay bills, purchase food, obtain financial assistance from the government, or diaper a baby. Even the person who sits quietly and passively for most of the meeting but at the end looks up and

asks about the time and date of the next meeting has made a logical, purposeful communication. This stage should be distinguished from higher levels of the relationship, at which more sensitive, private matters and complex feeling states such as love, empathy, and jealousy may be discussed.

4. *The client's relationship with the helping professional is stable enough that the client can experience uncomfortable and scary feelings without fleeing or seriously disrupting the relationship.* Although minor upsets, including missed appointments, may occur at this stage, the overall relationship and the emotional connection survive. For example, suppose a male patient, after several appointments with the same doctor, comes to trust the doctor enough to reveal a secret: a year ago he visited a prostitute, and he fears he may be at risk for AIDS. The doctor schedules an HIV test, but the patient, now feeling abashed at the thought of having shared his shameful secret and fearing that the doctor may judge or reject him, fails to show up for the test. His relationship with his doctor is stable enough, however, that he calls back a week later and makes a new appointment, which he succeeds in keeping. Negative feelings such as anger, remorse, suspiciousness, and feelings of being exploited are the most potentially disruptive to a helping relationship; however, for many clients, feelings of intimacy, warmth, or sexual longing are the most frightening.

5. *The client feels secure in being "known" by the helping professional.* Because she can now allow the worker to know her full range of feelings and characteristics, both positive and negative, the relationship now involves many emotions, allowing the client to compare her current feelings and interactions with other experiences and to work through maladaptive patterns. At this level, one can observe satisfaction and often affection in the relationship, along with a sense of accomplishment in a task jointly well done.

At its higher levels, the dimension of emotional depth may overlap with the higher process levels described later. In evaluating emotional depth, however, one focuses on the depth of feeling and degree of differentiation that characterize the relationship between client and helping professional. At the highest level, the client can acknowledge the depth and meaning of the relationship. One can get a feel for this dimension by considering the steps in the development of a close friendship. On his first day of college, for example, a freshman meets many fellow students, in the process learning their names and perhaps a few facts about each one. He is unlikely to feel a strong bond with any one classmate, but unless he has severe difficulties relating to others, as the weeks pass he will develop stronger and more complex feelings toward certain individuals. Their feelings and behavior will increasingly hold meaning for him and have the ability to affect his emotional state. If an experience of hurt feelings or other painful emotions disrupts one of his new friendships, it may have progressed to the level at which the two friends can discuss their conflict and continue the relationship. One or more of his friendships may develop to the highest level, at which he feels secure in having the full range of his feelings and qualities known by his friend.

The Third Dimension: Process of Communication

In evaluating the third dimension, one considers the structure, rather than the content, of communications between client and worker. The dimension of process also encompasses aspects of the first two dimensions, regularity and affective investment in the relationship.

We have observed that the structure of communications between client and helping professional, or between any two people, can reach nine stages or levels:

1. *Attention.* One must capture someone's attention before attempting further communication, and that person must be capable of at least briefly focusing attention if further interaction is to occur. (At a party, for example, one is unlikely to attempt conversation with a stranger who has not yet glanced in one's direction.)

2. *Engagement.* Is there some degree of warmth and connectedness between the two people? For example, does a mother greet her home visitor with a warm smile and relaxed physical stance, or does she stare at the visitor with a flat expression or avert her gaze despite an obvious awareness of the visitor's presence?

3. *Purposeful, two-way gestural communication.* From the middle of the first year of life, individuals rely on gestures to communicate. One can evaluate whether two people are using gestures to open and close circles of communication. If the first person smiles, does the other respond with a smile or greeting, and does the first person respond in turn? If so, the two have closed a circle. Consider the case of strangers riding an elevator together. Their interaction is generally minimal, but one frequently observes at least an exchange of slight smiles or nods. Two people who have yet to close a circle cannot proceed to higher levels of communication; a worker and client who have not succeeded in closing circles cannot proceed toward any collaborative work.

4. *Verbal communication.* At this level, we see more complex interactions involving the opening and closing of many circles of communication and the use of words to communicate and to get one's needs met. At this stage in the interaction between client and worker, discussion of practical needs, such as food and housing, and provision of concrete services are often involved. However, communication begins to include verbal support and sharing of information. If our hypothetical elevator riders reach this level, they may carry on a conversation about the weather or other neutral topics that reveal little about the speakers themselves.

5. *Symbolic communication.* Can a client, or any partner in communication, use words or drawing or other media to express feelings and ideas? This level of communication requires that both parties have at least a rudimentary capacity for communicating with words or other symbols. Perhaps a client says, "I wanted my wife to take care of the baby and I got angry. Then I felt scared and ran out and got drunk and came back and beat her up." Two people have clearly reached the level of symbolic communication when their conversation begins to include discussion of their feelings. This level can be divided into three sublevels: a) using symbols to describe only actions, rather than intentions or feelings (e.g., "I hit him."); b) using symbols to describe only a physical state (e.g., "My belly hurts," "My muscles feel like they're about to explode."); and c) using symbols to describe intentions or feelings (e.g., "I want to do it now," "I feel sad.") Describing an intention involves stating what one wants to do, rather than simply what one is doing.

6. *Building logical bridges between ideas.* At this level, a person does not merely report ideas or feelings but can elaborate on these. She can perceive and describe the logical connections between two or more ideas. Instead of simply reporting, "I was mad," a person can say, "I may have gotten mad and so I withdrew from my boyfriend. I can see why this might have made him feel sad and perhaps discouraged." Here we see a capacity to perceive the interactions between different feelings—in this case, the interactions between one person's feelings and another's.

7. *Multicause and triangular thinking.* Does communication include exploration of multiple reasons for a feeling, comparison of different feelings, and evidence that the parties understand triadic interactions between feeling states? A person who can communicate the idea, "I feel left out because Sharon likes Teresa better than me" is functioning at this level of the process dimension.

8. *Gray-area and comparative thinking.* Does communication include descriptions of gradations among differentiated feeling states? At this level, a person says things like, "When he said that, I wasn't just a little bit mad anymore— I was furious!" The communication also may involve comparisons between different feelings, relationships, and so on.

9. *Thinking from a stable sense of self and an internal standard.* People functioning at this level can reflect on and discuss feelings in relation to a stable, internalized sense of identity. For example, a client might say to his therapist, "I felt so hurt and rejected when Mary turned down my invitation. I don't get it—it's not like me to feel so upset about something like that."

By attending to the process dimension, a helping professional can evaluate whether he and his client are communicating at the level required to achieve the particular goals of the intervention or program. Suppose, for example, that a social service agency offers classes to prepare clients to get a job and function well enough in the workplace to keep the job. A participant who is so distractible that she cannot attend and focus in class will need help with her distractibility first. This may seem obvious, but in many classroom situations, an instructor simply lectures on and on without evaluating whether students are actually taking in the information. A counselor or therapist who has not considered the process dimension may persist in trying to explore feelings, or the connections between feelings, with a client who has not yet mastered symbolic communication and can only report events and behaviors, not internal states. By asking himself at what process level he and the client are actually functioning, the therapist can avoid giving up in frustration and instead reframe the task as first developing a relationship with the client through simpler two-way gestural and verbal exchanges and then helping the client develop the capacity for symbolic communication.

The Fourth Dimension: Content of Communication

Which emotional themes predominate in communications between client and the helping professional as their relationship develops? During the journey from infancy to old age, certain themes predominate at each stage of life. The client–worker relationship, with its inevitable power imbalance and echoes of early relationships with parents, teachers, and other authority figures, cannot help but evoke core developmental themes. One can arrange possible themes in a hierarchy, beginning with those that characterize infancy and childhood:

1. Dependency/safety/security
2. Autonomy/independence
3. Curiosity/exploration/expansiveness
4. Power/grandiosity
5. Competition/rivalry/intrigue
6. Containment/control
7. Collaboration/cooperation
8. Experimentation
9. Self-awareness/consolidation of identity

One can observe the interactions and listen to the conversation between two people and ask, which of these themes seems to predominate at this moment? Of course, a relationship of any duration and complexity will involve fluctuation among themes, including a revisiting, at times, of themes that predominated earlier in the relationship. When a new mother first opens her door to the visiting baby nurse sent by the hospital where she gave birth, their initial glances and exchanges are likely to involve the theme of dependency and security, although neither may state this explicitly. The mother is wondering: can I trust this nurse with my baby? Will she think I'm a bad mother because my house is messy and my baby is crying? Is it safe to let her see how overwhelmed I feel right now? The nurse, if she is sensitive to these unspoken concerns, will attempt to convey her acceptance and understanding as well as her confidence in her ability to evaluate the baby's health. If she wins the mother's trust, on a future visit the pair may progress to the theme of autonomy and independence, with the mother feeling free to explain why she has made some parenting choices different from those the nurse recommends.

By understanding the dimension of thematic content, a helping professional can avoid moving too fast or leaping ahead to themes that cannot yet be explored with a particular client. For example, in the CIDP we encountered some participants who expressed great enthusiasm about the program upon enrolling but then disappeared almost immediately. With such participants, it was easy to make the mistake of assuming that the theme of collaboration and cooperation already predominated in our relationship. In truth, the earlier themes, beginning with dependency and safety, had not been negotiated, as became evident when the clients fled. In some cases, persistent but sensitive pursuit enabled the client to return and begin to establish a sense of safety with one or more members of the treatment team.

The Value of the Four Dimensions

The four dimensions just described define where the helping relationship begins, what the subsequent tasks of the client and professional must be, and when their work is complete. Unlike assessment of individual client variables relevant to the particular service being offered—symptoms of psychopathology, ego strength, educational level, parenting style, awareness of children's nutritional needs, or any other characteristic of the client as an individual—assessment of the relationship dimensions directly defines what work needs to be done. Profiling a client according to the levels she has attained on each dimension suggests which intervention approaches—outreach, home-based treatment or instruction, provision of services at a clinic, school, or other central location, and so on—may be most effective at a particular stage. Because use of the dimensions allows helping professionals to recognize the steps most basic to a worker–client relationship and to appreciate even small improvements, it may help workers to feel more sanguine about the abilities and "motivation" of many people needing help.

An appreciation of the multiple steps involved in each relationship dimension also enables helping professionals to work patiently toward gradual progress. Many agencies and third-party payers require systematic documentation of goals and progress. Understanding the complex steps involved in the four components of relationship-building enables one to document both the goals and the progress more clearly. What at times may appear to the untrained eye as merely a "holding pattern" may in fact represent the mastery of critical steps in a relationship leading toward substantial overall progress. For research and program evaluation, clients' progress in each dimension can be rated and compared with predictions of treatment outcomes.

Understanding the dimensions also enables helping individuals to appreciate the value of their own work. It is easy to become demoralized or, at minimum, discouraged, if one has no way of comprehending the important steps toward progress that one is a part of. Repeatedly, we observed in our work with multiproblem families and their babies that these important dimensions of the helping relationship took a long time to master, sometimes a year or two or even three, but we were able to show that they had a substantial long-term positive impact on the lives of the families. For example, many of the mothers who had been neglecting or abusing their infants learned how to be nurturing and supportive. Equally important, when they had their next babies, many began that new relationship being extraordinarily warm and nurturing and appropriately interactive. We were initially surprised to see how fundamental the changes were for many of our participants. When we examined their progress through the steps of the relationship dimensions outlined earlier, however, we could understand why the changes were substantial and enduring. For an outline of the four dimensions and the steps involved in each, see Table 10–2.

A Case of Double Vulnerability: Louise and Robbie[1]

The case of Louise and her infant son, Robbie, provides a vivid illustration of the principles of intervention described in this chapter. Louise and Robbie both needed our treatment team's help to negotiate the very earliest developmental levels: self-regulation and attachment.

Louise was an attractive African-American woman in her mid-20s who had a 6-year-old daughter and was 5 months pregnant when she entered our program, which she learned about at her prenatal clinic. Louise had had a chaotic childhood marked by abandonment, psychological rejection, and physical abuse. Records from a mental health center she had contacted a few years before starting the CIDP indicated she had been diagnosed with "schizoid personality with paranoid features and periodic transient psychotic states." Louise's initial hostility and intense suspiciousness toward the clinician, combined with the disorganization of her thinking under stress and her difficulties with impulse control, made us consider very seriously the possibility that this diagnosis was accurate. This worrisome

---

[1]The team that provided the clinical services and worked on the initial case report included Delise Williams, Robert Nover, Joan Castellan, Stanley Greenspan, and Alicia Lieberman.

TABLE 10–2.   Dimensions and levels of helping relationships

Dimension 1: Regularity and stability

1.   Initial meeting

2.   Attempt to arrange follow-up meetings

3.   Meeting according to some pattern, however unpredictable at times

4.   Meeting regularly according to schedule, with occasional disruptions

5.   Meeting regularly with minimal disruptions

Dimension 2: Emotional depth of the relationship

1.   Client interested only in concrete services

2.   Client shows signs of emotional interest in helping professional

3.   Client engages in purposeful two-way exchanges with helping professional

4.   Client can experience uncomfortable feelings in helping relationship without fleeing or seriously disrupting relationship

5.   Client feels secure in being "known" by helping professional

Dimension 3: Process of communication

1.   Attention

2.   Engagement

3.   Purposeful, two-way gestural communication

4.   Verbal communication

5.   Symbolic communication

6.   Building logical bridges between ideas

7.   Multicause and triangular thinking

8.   Gray-area and comparative thinking

9.   Thinking from a stable sense of self and an internal standard

Dimension 4: Thematic content of communication

1.   Dependency/safety/security

2.   Autonomy/independence

3.   Curiosity/exploration/expansiveness

4.   Power/grandiosity

5.   Competition/rivalry/intrigue

6.   Containment/control

7.   Collaboration/cooperation

8.   Experimentation

9.   Self-awareness/consolidation of identity

---

picture was compounded by Louise's overt ambivalence, first toward the pregnancy and later toward her child; by her anger that her baby's birth interfered with her working; and by her warnings to the treatment team that she became depressed when she stayed at home and spent "too much time" with her children. In the context of Louise's own experience of rejection and abuse as a child, these feelings conveyed to us Louise's fears that she could not nurture her child, and her fears became our concerns.

The First Stage of Treatment: The Prenatal Period

Louise told us that she was joining the program to help us in our stated goal of better understanding parent–infant relationships. She did not mention any problems or concerns of her own. However, the clinician immediately suspected that Louise did have difficulties, based on her flat affect, suspicious glances, fleeting eye contact, constantly fidgeting hands, evasiveness in answering questions, and halting yet sarcastic speech.

The beginnings of our intervention were not promising. Louise failed to keep appointment after appointment. On some occasions, she was clearly at home but refused to open the door to our clinician. Yet she phoned us regularly, often calling after a missed appointment to request another one, which she then failed to keep. We interpreted this pattern as an expression of her simultaneous wish for contact and fear of closeness. She seemed to be testing whether the clinician's interest would persist in the face of her elusiveness.

The clinician's interest did persist, and long phone conversations eventually gave way to appointments that were kept. This shift occurred about 6 weeks before Louise's due date, perhaps indicating that as the delivery approached, Louise felt more keenly the need for support.

In these initial sessions, Louise was frequently angry and withdrawn. She sullenly refused to speak about the pregnancy and showed no joyous anticipation of the new baby. She was most communicative when expressing anger, which she did in long tirades. She raged against her baby's father for his failure to provide emotional and financial support. She complained bitterly about the indifference of welfare caseworkers. Although her anger often seemed justified, Louise gave the impression of struggling with global, barely controlled rage. At such times, the clinician sympathized with the intensity of Louise's feelings and tried to provide boundaries for her anger by making suggestions about concrete steps that Louise could take to feel more in control of the situation. Louise often turned her anger toward the clinician, either challenging every question she asked or refusing to be drawn into conversation.

Occasionally, however, Louise showed signs of a greater ability to experience and communicate warmth and engagement. She told the clinician that it felt good to have such a reliable visitor. She showed a surprising ability to respond to the clinician's cautious attempts at emotional exploration, and she expressed a wish to understand her feelings better. At one point, she even volunteered that the events in her past had "made it hard to trust people now, and that is bad." These rare moments of reflection gave us hope that Louise could be helped to have better mastery of the feelings that so troubled her.

The main task of these prenatal sessions was to establish regularity and stability and to facilitate the development of a therapeutic relationship that would eventually permit emotional exploration. The clinician absorbed Louise's angry outbursts, encouraged the verbal expression of disappointment and anger Louise felt in her, and kept appearing, week after week, regardless of Louise's behavior. The surprise and relief often evident on Louise's face when she saw the clinician at the door were an eloquent testimony to the absence of such sustained relationships in her past.

Slowly, Louise began to confide the many fears that plagued her. She was afraid to use the bus, because she considered buses to be dangerous places where she could be attacked. The darkness terrified her because she thought that menacing figures lurked there. She needed a nightlight to fall asleep, but she never slept well because she saw unidentified "things" moving in her room, and she feared being attacked by them. Louise was afraid that these experiences meant she was "crazy." The clinician assured Louise that she could learn to deal with her fears. Perhaps most important, the clinician kept coming to visit, providing Louise with concrete proof that the emerging information would not scare her away.

Robbie's Birth and After: Infant, Mother, and Their Interaction

Robbie's delivery presented no medical complications. He was of average height and weight, and his scores on the Apgar scale and other indices of newborn functioning were in the normal range. However, it quickly became apparent that this baby would make difficult demands even on a mother with unconflicted nurturing resources. Although Robbie was a cuddly baby, he easily became irritable and was difficult to console. His own attempts at self-soothing (for example, by taking a hand to his mouth) were mostly unsuccessful. He exhibited muscle tension, tremors, and startles, although these were not severe enough to be a cause for worry in their own right. He showed poor orientation to faces and voices. A month after birth, his orientation had deteriorated further—a reversal from the expectation that a baby will orient better with increased maturity—and he had become more physically tense and less cuddly. We began to observe gaze aversion. Such deterioration in an infant's capacity for regulation and interest in the world is, in most cases, an extremely worrisome early sign.

The interaction between Robbie and his mother was far from optimal, and we hypothesized that this was an important factor in Robbie's failure to become better organized. Louise had difficulty looking at her baby and held him in a wooden posture, with a striking lack of accommodation to the baby's body. These qualities seemed to be mirrored in Robbie's behavior.

Given Louise's suspiciousness and already intense ambivalence, we feared that she would interpret the baby's behavior as a rejection of her as a mother, setting up a dangerous cycle in which the mother's pain and anger led to rejection of and withdrawal from the child. This appraisal led us to formulate a treatment plan in which the clinician would engage Louise in psychotherapy and an infant specialist would work directly with Robbie. We adopted this strategy because we thought that Louise's own primitive neediness was of such proportions that she would feel rejected and jealous if she had to share a single therapist's attention with her baby. Having her own therapist would help Louise feel she had value in her own right and would provide her with the experiences necessary to help her become the clinician's ally on behalf of her child; meanwhile, the infant specialist could provide Robbie with specially designed patterns of care and relaxed interpersonal experiences until the mother became able to do so, thus helping him to achieve developmental milestones despite his mother's difficulties.

Over the next few months, we gradually discovered that the periods of greatest detachment between Robbie and his mother occurred when Louise was feeling exploited or rejected by "Big Robert," the baby's father. At such times, Louise could become downright neglectful. Although she once remarked that she disliked the baby's name, she emphatically denied any connection between her feelings toward Big Robert and her ability to care for Robbie. The clinician had to postpone exploration of this very sensitive, yet central issue. (Big Robert never responded to our invitation, through Louise, to participate in the program. He visited Robbie at Louise's home once a week at most and less often when his relations with Louise were stormy.)

In-Home Intervention With Robbie: The First 4 Months

While Louise began, in her own therapy, to speak of her fears of rejection, the infant specialist began working directly with Robbie during home visits. In attempting to reverse Robbie's persistent gaze aversion, she noticed that although he avoided eye contact with people, he gazed at inanimate objects for long periods. Capitalizing on this tendency, she drew a face on a piece of paper that she wore as a mask, enticing Robbie to follow her with his eyes as she slowly moved her head up and down in front of him. After several such trials, she lowered the mask and greeted Robbie with eye contact while smiling and talking to him. At first, Robbie shifted his gaze; slowly, he was able to sustain eye contact for a few seconds. As this game was played again and again, with much animation and in various forms—such as playing peekaboo in different contexts and with different masks—Robbie started responding more and more. He appeared to find the human face first interesting and later, we surmise, pleasurable. It is worth noting that the infant specialist's affective expression could be enlarged only gradually, because Robbie started out finding all human affective exchange so frightening.

Vocalization—another area in which Robbie lagged severely—was encouraged in the most natural of ways: by making simple but playful sounds until Robbie could imitate them, then elaborating on the original sound by adding new vowels and consonants. Talking warmly to the baby, greeting him on arrival, and saying good-bye on departure—in short, relating to him as a person who was a legitimate partner in social speech—were also part of the infant specialist's approach.

Finally, Robbie's stiff muscle tone, uncomfortable posture, lack of cuddliness, and difficulty with cross-sensory and sensory-motor integration were addressed through interactive floor games. Activities included playfully rolling Robbie on the floor, rhythmically extending and flexing his arms and legs while singing or making rhythmic sounds, playing pat-a-cake and other games that encourage midline reach, and playing games like "This Little Pig Went to Market" to entice Robbie to reach for his toes and play with his feet. The specialist placed her attractive toys just out of Robbie's reach, to encourage reaching and holding, which seemed to be restricted by the tightness of the muscles in his shoulder girdle and upper arms and by the fact that his hands tended to fist when he reached or brought the hands to midline. When Robbie seemed tired after all these activities, he was encouraged to cuddle in the arms of the infant specialist, who sang a lullaby until his body relaxed or he fell asleep. When Robbie's disorganized body motion prevented him from falling asleep, he was swaddled, enabling him to relax and nod off.

Note that these interventions were never mechanical: they were unobtrusively built into affectionate exchanges with Robbie. The goal was not global stimulation per se, but rather to encourage internal regulation and interest in the world, specifically in interaction with human partners, in order to build the basis for human attachments.

Every attempt was made to encourage Louise to participate in these sessions and to take over the infant specialist's role. Her reaction varied according to her mood. Sometimes, she looked on with interest and entered into the games, showing considerable ability to be in tune with Robbie. At other times, she simply stared out the window with a sullen expression. Occasionally, she made a comment that reflected some longing to have had in her own childhood the kind of attention Robbie was now receiving. The infant specialist felt worried and discouraged, recognizing that Louise was limited in what she could offer her son.

All this time, Robbie's health and nutritional status were carefully monitored. Staff spent many hours advocating for Louise and Robbie to ensure that they received food from the Women, Infants, and Children (WIC) supplemental food program. Appointments were made for Robbie at a well-baby clinic, and staff drove mother and baby to appointments when no other transportation was available.

The Therapeutic Infant Center

A formal 4-month developmental assessment suggested that more intensive intervention was needed to get Robbie on track developmentally. With Louise's agreement, we arranged for Robbie to spend at least part of each week at our Infant Center, where the infant specialist could work with him and other staff could care for him in ways that reinforced the specialist's work. Louise sometimes met him at the center at the end of her workday; she spent some time finding out how he had spent the day, chatting with other mothers and with staff, and watching what were, for her, novel ways of interacting with children. This plan remained in effect throughout treatment, with modifications and interruptions that mirrored the changes in Louise's life. When no babysitter was available (Louise worked long hours at two part-time jobs), Robbie might spend the whole day at the Center for weeks at a time. When Louise was angry with her clinician, she sometimes "took revenge" by not bringing Robbie in for a few days. During a few months when Robbie had a babysitter who was especially nurturing and responsive, we ourselves reduced his hours at the center. As Robbie grew older, we added a new task to help him negotiate the fourth developmental level: problem-solving communication and an emerging sense of self. We worked on reading Robbie's changing affective signals, providing purposeful feedback, and facilitating his persistence.

Louise's Treatment: Ongoing Course

When Louise requested the clinician's help in finding an affordable apartment so she could move out of her foster father's home, the two women began spending many hours driving to look at prospective apartments. The car provided a physical proximity that seemed to promote intimacy without arousing fear. It was in the car, talking about the pressures of finding a place to live, that Louise voiced her wish to be taken care of and her simultaneous fear of getting too close. She illustrated these tendencies by talking of the many men who had given her money, food, and clothes, and how she had used them until "they got too close," at which time she abruptly told them to leave. Exploration of what "getting close" meant revealed Louise's fear that people would become too involved in her "business." She was reluctant to elaborate on this term, but we gradually learned that it referred to secrets involving a psychiatric hospitalization, involvement with prostitution, and an episode of venereal disease. We surmised that these events represented for Louise proof of the dreaded "badness" that she attributed to herself, her deep shame about aspects of her feelings and wishes, and her fear that discovery of these feelings by others would lead once again to abandonment and rejection. Although at times she was able to explore these feelings and withstand the pain they elicited, Louise often turned to intense rage as her most potent defense. On these occasions, Louise often repeated a simple sentence, as though trying to encase in words, and thus get control of, her disorganizing anger.

The clinician started with very structured interventions aimed at clarifying and providing labels for feelings. What did Louise feel, toward whom, for what reasons? As Louise herself became more skillful in these tasks, the clinician could move on to show her the common element between the different situations that elicited certain feelings. In this way, Louise gradually became aware of her tendency to set up chaotic external circumstances to escape inner turmoil, of how she used rage as a defense against feelings of helplessness, and of how she tried to fend off rejection by rejecting others first. Ultimately, Louise also became aware of her deeply rooted perception of herself as "evil." The prevailing theme in the sessions was a constant reworking of her fear that people would leave her once she exposed her worst side, that is, her rage.

This process was filled with turmoil. At many moments, we wondered whether Louise had learned more about herself than she could tolerate. However, as this material emerged and the implications for the therapeutic relationship were explored (i.e., Louise's fear of hurting the clinician or being rejected by her), Louise's bond with the clinician invariably seemed to become more stable. The therapeutic relationship seemed to provide the support Louise needed in order to begin identifying patterns in her life. During this time, an unexpected avenue emerged to explore painful feelings: the daily soap operas, which Louise watched avidly, often leaving the television on during sessions. The clinician used Louise's identification with certain characters to explore her feelings in greater depth and also to show her that these feelings were experienced by many people and were not a sign that Louise was "strange," "crazy," or "stupid," adjectives that recurred in her attempts to clarify for herself who she was.

We noted a marked parallel between Louise's relationship with the clinician and her ability to care for and engage her son. As Louise began to make use of the clinician as a partner in a stable relationship, as well as an auxiliary ego and a figure for identification, she became more reflective and started to discuss her plans for the future instead of implementing them impulsively. She began to imitate the clinician's style of dress. With Robbie, she began to express genuine pleasure in his relatedness to her and to others. She showed more patience and tenderness toward him, responded far more promptly and effectively when he was distressed, cuddled him more often, and spoke to him playfully and lovingly for longer periods of time. We believe that her emerging capacity to establish an enduring relationship with the clinician was directly responsible for her progress in nurturing and interacting with Robbie more consistently.

A Crisis

This progress was interrupted by Louise's reaction when, at Thanksgiving and again at Christmas, the clinician declined invitations to dinner at Louise's home. Old feelings of loss, rejection, and abandonment were triggered, and Louise retreated to her previous sullen guardedness. The clinician's attempts to address Louise's disappointment in her met with denial. Louise's behavior with Robbie illustrated how deeply the child was still enmeshed in his mother's internal conflicts. She threatened to abandon him ("You will find him on your doorstep," she told the clinician). On meeting Robbie one day after a long separation, she stared at him from a distance, as if seething with rage, and brushed aside his hand when he persistently tried to make contact with her. She did not, however, quit the program, and she continued to keep her appointments. Robbie's 8-month assessment revealed that he had made impressive strides: with the exception of vocalizations, which had increased but were still below age level, the major areas of cognitive and sensorimotor function were adequate. Most important, Robbie now engaged in organized and sustained social interactions. Far from averting his gaze from his mother, he now sought her out by looking and smiling at her, cooing to her, and grabbing her hand. Louise repeatedly ignored these overtures, but Robbie showed impressive persistence, finally eliciting a response from her after a great many attempts.

The clinician attempted to show Louise how her feelings of anger and rejection spilled over into her relationship with Robbie, but all such attempts were met by a blank stare and a refusal to discuss any negative feelings Louise might have toward her child. As though to underscore her determination to escape the feelings that threatened to overwhelm her, Louise moved abruptly from her cozy apartment to a noisy, overcrowded household. Instead of being the only child in the home of a caring and affectionate babysitter, Robbie, at 9 months, was now cared for by whomever was available. The infant specialist soon noticed that his activity level was increasing and his attention span was declining. He became less available for play, and his vocalizations decreased. We decided to increase Robbie's hours at the Infant Center to 4 days a week, 4–6 hours a day.

Louise's Treatment Continues: Addressing Themes of Loss and Separation

Louise's flight to a chaotic household was addressed by the clinician as an attempt to escape from the feelings of disorganization that she experienced when she perceived that others abandoned or rejected her. While persistently denying this connection, Louise implicitly confirmed it by beginning to talk about her inability to sustain long-term relationships. She then spontaneously began to talk about her 6-year-old daughter, Terry. Although Louise often demonstrated an ability to respond appropriately and with empathy to Terry, she said that she sometimes treated Terry in ways that she did not like—ignoring her, scolding her, or responding abruptly to her approaches. She spoke regretfully about Terry's becoming an adult and leaving her. It was important for the clinician to listen to Louise's discussion of this core theme in the context of her less conflicted relationship with her daughter. As Louise began to acknowledge her fears of being left, the clinician sensed that the time was right to point out to Louise how she often retreated from her children in order to forestall the future pain of separation.

Louise began spending more time with both Terry and Robbie. She also began speaking directly about her fondness for the clinician and asked for some sort of guarantee that their relationship would continue. The clinician responded by expressing empathy for Louise's desire for reassurance now that she was taking the risk of showing love and concern for her children. Here again, a further deepening of Louise's relationship with the clinician allowed her to become more psychologically available to her children. Louise seemed to have reached a new level of development, in which experiencing and expressing warmth were less frightening and fears of loss could be verbalized, rather than avoided through preemptive action. Her progress was vividly reflected at Robbie's 12-month assessment. She began the semistructured play session by picking up the play telephone and saying, "Robbie, are you there?" This simple action eloquently expressed Louise's core conflict: reaching out, coupled with fear that Robbie might not be there to respond. Robbie was very much there, turning to his mother repeatedly, giving her toys, and returning for a hug after exploring at a distance from her. This time, Louise was able both to allow her son to explore and to welcome him back when he returned. This interactive pattern showed clearly the beginnings of an organized pattern of reciprocal behavior as well as initiative and originality.

During the following 6 months, Louise began spontaneously to link her everchaotic relationship with Robbie's father to her feelings toward her biological mother, who had placed her with another family when she was 6 months old. She noted a resemblance between her sense of unsatisfied need for Big Robert and her own mother's unavailability. She could not yet see, however, how she triggered her boyfriend's absences through her paroxysms of rage; she could only see herself as a victim of abandonment. Her inability to see herself in an active role interfered with her ability to empathize with Robbie's feelings when she was unavailable to him. (She had an easier time imaging the feelings of her daughter, who was less identified in Louise's mind with her boyfriend.) Despite this limitation, however, Louise's ongoing therapeutic work enabled her to see herself, for the first time, as a mother responsible for the well-being of her children. She now spoke of how her actions would affect her children. She anticipated Robbie's discomfort on being left with a new babysitter.

At his 18-month evaluation, Robbie again showed steady improvement. Mother and child were clearly able to address core conflicts adaptively through play. In one videotaped sequence, Louise chases Robbie, who runs away; she catches him, and both laugh. Louise then teases Robbie by going out of the room and closing the door, but she immediately knocks to signal that she is still there (i.e., this is only a "pretend" desertion); Robbie attempts to open the door, and his mother returns. Louise then leaves again. This time, Robbie does not seek her out but hides instead, under the table. Louise seeks him out, but he flails at her. She laughs and hugs him. We interpreted this sequence as a symbolic enacting of Louise's central conflict, the theme of abandonment and rejection. Whereas earlier in the treatment, this theme was acted out through actual neglect and all-too-real threats of abandonment, it was now expressed through a richly organized symbolic game. We also saw an integration, rather than a splitting off, of the theme. In contrast to earlier one-sided attempts by one partner to woo the other, Louise and Robbie were now taking turns pursuing each other. Finally, we saw a new ability on the part of each partner to recover from rejection and reach out anew, instead of withdrawing or becoming disorganized. Their ability to deal with this central conflict at an emerging symbolic level was truly impressive.

A second indication of Louise's progress in addressing her core conflict was her handling of the clinician's announcement, when Robbie was 18 months old, of her own pregnancy and plans for maternity leave. Louise's strong bond and identification with the clinician, who was now to become a mother herself, seemed to permit Louise to strengthen her own identity as a mother. Whereas she had previously been reluctant to "share" her therapy time with Robbie by departing from her own issues during sessions, she began using some sessions to ask for advice about child-rearing issues, such as how best to respond to Robbie's tantrums. She showed a more active interest in how Robbie spent his day at the Infant Center and even proposed that she and the staff each keep a baby diary to keep each other informed of day-to-day occurrences in his routine. In anticipation of the clinician's absence, she started cultivating a relationship with Infant Center staff and became more involved with Robbie's infant specialist. In these adaptive maneuvers, Louise showed a new ability to reach out to others, instead of fleeing and becoming disorganized at the prospect of loss and separation.

As the clinician's pregnancy progressed, Louise became more solicitous toward her. She also spoke openly of her longing for the clinician's eventual return, repeatedly shortening her estimation of the length of her absence, reducing it from an original 8 months to "2 or 3 weeks." Gradually, Louise became aware that these behaviors signaled her sadness at the clinician's anticipated absence and her wish for a speedy reunion. She then started writing down how she felt about loneliness and what friendship meant to her, and she showed these writings to the clinician. At no time did she relapse into the angry outbursts and sudden withdrawal that had characterized her earlier responses to separation and perceived rejection. During the clinician's absence, Louise kept on good terms with Infant Center staff. She phoned the clinician every week, but limited her calls to asking how she and the new baby were and kept each call appropriately brief. Although this was a poignant illustration of Louise's enduring need for a concrete presence, it also showed her new ability to take the lead in establishing contact and to subordinate her own needs to someone else's.

When the clinician returned, the therapeutic relationship was reestablished with minimal difficulty. Louise's pattern of introspective self-examination continued, and many traumatic early memories emerged. As Louise vividly recalled these memories and shared them with the clinician, she stopped having "hallucinations" at night, slept better, and seldom needed a nightlight. When she did have trouble sleeping, she now considered what feelings might be troubling her until she arrived at some understanding that was comforting for her. She found a new freedom of movement: not only did she begin using the bus system, but she learned to drive and bought a car, which she used for errands and to take her children on family outings. Clearly, Louise had learned to use introspection, instead of acting out, as a means to protect herself against becoming overwhelmed and disorganized by her feelings.

As Louise's participation in our program drew to an end, she continued to make strides in her relationship with her children. She still withdrew from Robbie on occasion, but far less than she used to. She continued to have some difficulty controlling and regulating her anger, but she now acknowledged that this difficulty lay within herself rather than in her children, and she actively attempted to find ways of protecting her children from her anger.

The case of Louise and Robbie illustrates the fruitfulness of the comprehensive assessment and treatment planning approach we have described in this book. It also vividly illustrates the need for a dual approach in cases where both parent and child exhibit severe developmental lags. Intervention with only one party would likely have limited value, because the vulnerability in the other party would persist, preventing the two from building the kind of relationship that can promote developmental progress.

Reference

Greenspan SI, Wieder S, Lieberman A, et al: Infants in Multirisk Families: Case Studies in Preventive Intervention. Clinical Infant Reports, No. 3. New York, International Universities Press, 1987

11

A Model for Comprehensive Prevention and Early Intervention Services for All Families

In Chapter 10 ("Infants in Multirisk Families: A Model for Developmentally Based Preventive Intervention"), we described a comprehensive prevention and early intervention program for multirisk or multiproblem families. The majority of individuals and families in our society will not require such a variety and intensity of services, and many will never require the services at the base of the service pyramid (see Figure 11–1). However, all families and our society as a whole will benefit if parents, parents-to-be, educators, and other adults who work with children have a thorough, comprehensive understanding of how children develop as well as access to information and coaching (and, where needed, specialized clinical services) to help them interact with children in ways that will best promote healthy emotional, social, and intellectual development. The developmental, individual-differences, relationship-based (DIR) model can serve as a basis for efforts to ensure that this knowledge becomes more widespread.

Such information and coaching can be offered in myriad settings and formats, including pediatricians' offices, parent training and support groups, training and continuing education programs for teachers and other professionals who work with children, childbirth and parenting preparation programs for expectant parents, human development classes from elementary school onward, and so forth. Parents, teachers, and other professionals who have gained a comprehensive understanding of human emotional, social, and intellectual development and learned to interact with children in ways that promote healthy development will be able

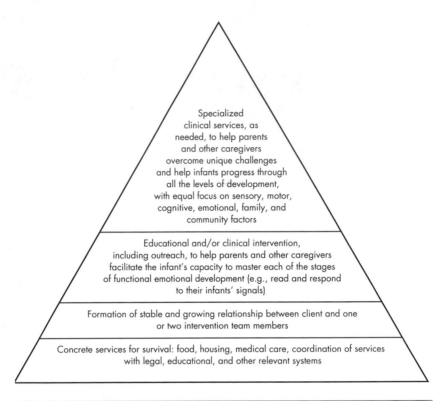

FIGURE 11–1.   The service pyramid.

The service pyramid depicts an overall framework for services. Note that the third level up from the bottom of the pyramid refers to facilitating the infant's capacity to master each of the six core developmental capacities.

to prevent many potential developmental problems. They will also be in a position to quickly recognize when a child's biologically based processing differences or fundamental difficulties with relating and communicating are severe enough to warrant referral for specialized clinical or educational services.

We first describe the kinds of information that prevention programs should provide to parents, parents-to-be, and professionals who work with children. We then describe how this information can be adapted as part of more intensive prevention and early intervention programs for children and families who face various developmental challenges and may require specialized assessment and intervention services but who do not fall into the "multirisk" or "multiproblem" category. To enable readers to use this chapter on its own, we repeat some information that appears in Chapter 10 ("Infants in Multirisk Families: A Model for Developmentally Based Preventive Intervention") and elsewhere in this volume.

Understanding and Assessing the Stages of Development

Historically, researchers, clinicians, and educators have thought of development in very isolated ways. For motor development, we had a timetable for sitting up, walking, and so on. In language development, we identified age ranges for making the first sound, speaking the first words, combining two words, and so on. In cognitive development, we identified when a child searches for a hidden object, when a child can stack blocks in a certain way, and so forth. In social and emotional development, we knew when a child learns to greet others, when a child begins playing with peers, when a child will do some pretending. We identified separate lines of development, considering each area separately as though they functioned independently of one another. For the child, however, all these lines of development are intertwined. The child does not somehow isolate his motor skills from his language skills. He does not say, "Well, I'm a 4-year-old motor wise, only a 2-year-old language wise, and only an 8-month-old socially and emotionally." The child integrates all these functions, much as the members of a basketball team play as an integrated unit. To evaluate a team's effectiveness, one cannot consider each player's skills and performance separately. It is the way in which the members play together that determines whether the team wins or loses.

As indicated earlier, we have developed a framework for understanding how the human "mental team" functions together (including language, motor, sensory, cognitive, social, and emotional functioning). As discussed in some detail throughout the text, we identify six functional emotional developmental capacities that characterize the levels at which this "mental team" functions. This framework enables us to specify which capacities are missing or evidence compromise. The six levels are

- *Level 1: Shared attention and regulation.* During the first few months of life, parents and other key caregivers help the infant calmly regulate himself while he becomes interested in and takes pleasure in the sights, sounds, tastes, and touches the caregivers offer.
- *Level 2: Engagement and relating.* Between 3 and 6 months of age, the baby grows in her ability to engage in intimate, loving relationships with parents or other primary caregivers. She derives more and more feelings of warmth and pleasure from these relationships.
- *Level 3: Two-way intentional affective signaling and communication.* By 9 months, the toddler is well into this stage. He and his caregivers engage in back-and-forth emotional signaling involving gestures, smiles, smirks, nods, and so forth. With the caregivers' help, he will eventually be able to string together longer and longer chains of emotional expressions, sounds, and actions.
- *Level 4: Long chains of coregulated emotional signaling and shared social problem solving.* By 1–1½ years, the child can take her mother by the hand, walk her to

the refrigerator, bang on the door, and point to the orange juice after she opens the door. The child is starting to figure out that problems get solved through many interrelated steps, and that the world—including her physical surroundings, her own personality, and the personalities of her caregivers—is made up of patterns.

- *Level 5: Creating representations (or ideas).* The child now begins to use emotionally meaningful ideas in language (e.g., "Me hungry, juice please") or in pretend play (e.g., feeding and hugging dolls).
- *Level 6: Building bridges between ideas: logical thinking.* This ability emerges in more elaborate pretend play, in debates with parents over bedtime or cookies, and in the conversations that ensue when a parent asks a child his opinion about something.

Each of these levels, or *core developmental capacities*, builds on those the child has already attained. For each of the six levels, we can identify the particular motor skills, language skills, and visuospatial processing skills that are needed to support the child's mastery of that level. This gives us an integrated picture of development. In assessing a particular child and his difficulties, we determine which levels he has mastered and which he has negotiated incompletely or not at all. We then determine how motor and sensory processing differences and family and community interactions have worked together to create the child's difficulties with one or more levels. Armed with this information, we can determine how best to intervene to help the child get on track developmentally.

Note that all six core developmental capacities grow out of the child's experience of intimate relationships with his parents or other primary caregivers during infancy and into the first 3–4 years of life. Despite considerable evidence for the importance of early experience, some argue that later experiences are equally important. However, they are not distinguishing the six core capacities, which enable children to relate, read social cues, and think, from specific attitudes, values, and academic skills that are acquired throughout life. Others argue that genes are more important than experience in shaping personality and behavior. However, much of the research on identical twins, which is the basis for many claims that behavior is genetically determined, is flawed. Because identical twins share similar physical and temperamental characteristics, their caregivers tend to respond to them more similarly than would caregivers of nonidentical twins. Because typical caregivers tend to respond similarly to physical and temperamental characteristics, these observations may tend to hold even when identical twins are reared in different households. Near-identical interaction patterns, rather than identical genes, may account for the similarities exhibited by these twins. Psychosocial and biological patterns operate together, like a "dance," in human development. They each influence each other, and therefore we advocate a biopsychosocial model.

To determine whether a child is on track developmentally and to understand how the child's inborn processing style affects her ability to master the six functional emotional capacities, a parent, teacher, or clinician can gather information in several ways. One can directly observe a child exhibiting the functional emotional capacities and directly observe evidence of the child's processing style. Is it easy to capture the child's attention? Does the child engage warmly and readily? Does she clearly hear one's words but seem to have difficulty understanding what she hears? One can also ask the parents questions about the child's development, her response to various sensations. For example, "Does your infant look at or turn toward interesting sounds?" "Are you able to help your infant or child calm down when she's agitated?" "Can your preschooler describe her feelings to explain why she is doing something or wants something, e.g., 'Why do you want the juice?' 'Because I'm thirsty'?" "Does your child enjoy being touched or touching different things?" "Can your child be calm when experiencing different smells?" Those who prefer a more formal way of assessing a child can use our Functional Emotional Growth Chart (see Table 11–1 and Figure 11–2) and ask the caregivers to complete the Social-Emotional Growth Chart Parent (Caregiver) Questionnaire, which has been field-tested and shown to be reliable and valid (Greenspan 2004). For those who wish to have a clinical observational tool for formal assessment, we have devised that as well (Greenspan et al. 2001).

Determining How and Where to Intervene

However one gathers the information, the goal of doing so is to help each child and family to develop relationships that are tailored to the unique nervous system of the child and that will help him move forward developmentally—that is, to move on to higher, age-appropriate functional emotional capacities. To tailor interactions to the child to help him master the next levels up, families need various levels of support from the educator, clinical intervention team, or other service provider. Some families will only need information and minimal coaching and be capable of developing growth-promoting interactions on their own. These families can be offered developmentally based information and coaching as part of well-baby visits to the pediatrician. They are also good candidates for parent-oriented literature and self-help books. Useful information can be provided through public information campaigns using television, radio, the Internet, and other media. Some families will need just a little more ongoing help of the kind that can be provided in parenting classes, at daycare centers, or in other community-based settings. Still other families will need more intensive, ongoing support and relationships in order to implement parent–child interactions that support their children's developmental progress. The "multiproblem" or "multirisk" families described in Chapter 10 ("Infants in Multirisk Families: A Model for Developmentally Based Preventive Intervention") fall into this category.

TABLE 11–1. The functional emotional developmental levels from infancy to adulthood

Developmental level	Level of organizing and representing
Shared attention and regulation	Experiencing affective interest in sights, sounds, touch, movement, and other sensory experiences; also begin initial experiences of modulating affects (i.e., calming down)
Engagement and relating	Pleasurable affects characterize relationships; experiencing growing feelings of intimacy
Two-way intentional affective signaling and communication	Using a range of affects in back-and-forth affective signaling to convey intentions (e.g., reading and responding to affective signals)
Long chains of coregulated emotional signaling and shared social problem solving	Organizing affective interactions into action or behavioral patterns to express wishes and needs and to solve problems (e.g., showing someone what one wants with a pattern of actions rather than words or pictures): *Fragmented level:* Little islands of intentional problem-solving behavior *Polarized level:* Organized patterns of behavior expressing only one or another feeling states (e.g., organized aggression and impulsivity or organized clinging; needy, dependent behavior; or organized fearful patterns) *Integrated level:* Different emotional patterns—dependency, assertiveness, pleasure, etc.—organized into integrated, problem-solving affective interactions such as flirting, seeking closeness, and then getting help to find a needed object
Creating representations (or ideas)	Using words and actions together (ideas are acted out in action, but words are also used to signify the action) Using somatic or physical words to convey feeling state ("My muscles are exploding," "Head is aching") Putting desires or feelings into actions (e.g., hugging, hitting, biting) Using action words instead of actions to convey intent ("Hit you!") Conveying feelings as real rather than as signals ("I'm mad," "Hungry," or "Need a hug" as compared with "I feel mad," "I feel hungry," or "I feel like I need a hug"). In the first instance, the feeling state demands action and is very close to action; in the second, it is more a signal for something going on inside that leads to a consideration of many possible thoughts and/or actions Expressing global feeling states ("I feel awful," "I feel OK," etc.) Expressing polarized feeling states (feelings tend to be characterized as all good or all bad)

TABLE 11–1. The functional emotional developmental levels from infancy to adulthood *(continued)*

Developmental level	Level of organizing and representing
Building bridges between ideas: logical thinking	Expressing differentiated feelings (gradually there are increasingly subtle descriptions of feeling states, such as loneliness, sadness, annoyance, anger, delight, and happiness) Creating connections between differentiated feeling states ("I feel angry when you are mad at me")
Triangular thinking	Expressing triadic interactions among feeling states ("I feel left out because Susie likes Janet better than me")
Relativistic thinking	Expressing shades and gradations among differentiated feeling states (ability to describe degrees of feelings around anger, love, excitement, love, disappointment—"I feel a little annoyed")
Internalized sense of self (the world inside me)	Reflecting on feelings in relationship to an internalized sense of self ("It's not like me to feel so angry," or "I shouldn't feel this jealous")
Extended representational capacity	Expanding reflective feeling descriptors into new realms, including sexuality, romance, closer and more intimate peer relationships, school, community, culture, and emerging sense of identity ("I have such an intense crush on that new boy that I know it's silly; I don't even know him") Using feelings to anticipate and judge (including probablizing) future possibilities in light of current and past experience ("I don't think I would be able to really fall in love with him because he likes to flirt with everyone and that has always made me feel neglected and sad")
Adult	Expanding feeling states to include reflections and anticipatory judgment regarding new levels and types of feelings associated with the stages of adulthood, including the following: Ability to experience intimacy (serious long-term relationships) Ability to function independently from, and yet remain close to and internalize many of the positive features of, one's nuclear family Ability to nurture and empathize with one's children without overidentifying with them Ability to broaden one's nurturing and empathetic capacities beyond one's family and into the larger community Ability to experience and reflect on the new feelings of intimacy, mastery, pride, competition, disappointment, and loss associated with the family, career, and intrapersonal changes of midlife and the aging process

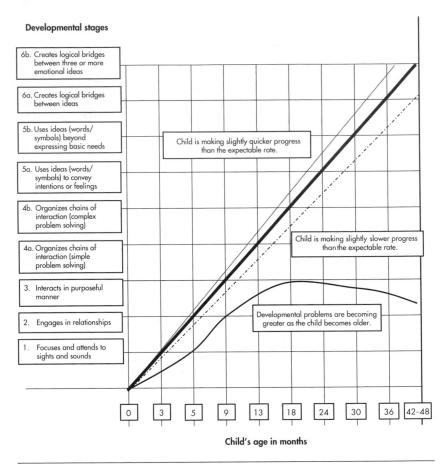

FIGURE 11–2.   Social-emotional developmental growth chart.

How can clinicians, educators, social service agency staff, and others who wish to help families promote their children's healthy development determine which level of intervention a particular family will require? Recall our model, "Dimensions and Levels of Helping Relationships," described in Chapter 10 ("Infants in Multirisk Families"). One can use this model to assess the relationship between client (or potential client) and worker on four dimensions: 1) regularity and stability, 2) emotional depth, 3) process of communication, and 4) content of communication.

Regularity and Stability

Is the parent or caregiver capable of enough basic trust and relatedness to keep pediatrician appointments, meet as needed with an educator or clinician, or attend a parenting workshop? Is the family's life too chaotic, because of multiple crises or unmet needs, to allow regularity and stability of contact?

Several stages or levels in the establishment of regularity and stability in the helping relationship can be identified:

1. The initial meeting, for example, to discuss needs or for any other purpose
2. The attempt to arrange follow-up meetings
3. Meeting according to some pattern, however unpredictable it may be at times
4. Meeting regularly according to schedule, with occasional disruptions such as a cancellation following a difficult conversation
5. Meeting regularly with minimal disruptions

Progress from one level to the next is not necessarily smooth or linear; client and worker may go back and forth between levels. Some relationships never move beyond level 1 or level 2.

Emotional Depth

What degree of emotional depth can the parent or caregiver tolerate in the relationship with a provider or potential provider of services? Does the parent need to keep emotional distance and express interest only in concrete services, or can he or she feel connected to the worker and tolerate a relationship that stirs up strong feelings?

The emotional connection between a client and a helping professional tends to develop in the following stages:

1. The client or prospective client is interested only in the concrete services that the worker or program can provide.
2. The client begins to show signs of emotional interest in the helping professional.
3. The client engages in purposeful two-way exchanges with the helping professional, using the relationship to communicate in a logical manner.
4. The client's relationship with the helping professional is stable enough that the client can experience uncomfortable and scary feelings without fleeing or seriously disrupting the relationship.
5. The client feels secure in being "known" by the helping professional.

Process of Communication

Which core developmental capacities does the parent exhibit in the context of interactions with the worker or potential service provider? Is it a challenge even to get and keep the parent's attention? Or does the parent quickly develop a warm connection, engage in emotionally meaningful back-and-forth communication, and exhibit the higher developmental levels in exchanges with the worker?

The communication process between client and helping professional, or between any two people, can reach nine stages or levels:

1. Attention
2. Engagement
3. Purposeful, two-way gestural communication
4. Verbal communication
5. Symbolic communication
6. Building logical bridges between ideas
7. Multicause and triangular thinking
8. Gray-area and comparative thinking
9. Thinking from a stable sense of self and an internal standard

Content of Communication

Is the parent or caregiver able to encompass a broad range of emotional themes, ranging from those characterizing early stages of development (dependency/security, autonomy/independence) to those associated with later stages and with mature adulthood (collaboration/cooperation, experimentation, self awareness/consolidation of identity)? Or do all encounters with the service provider seem to center on one or two themes?

One can arrange possible themes in a hierarchy, beginning with those that characterize infancy and childhood:

1. Dependency/safety/security
2. Autonomy/independence
3. Curiosity/exploration/expansiveness
4. Power/grandiosity
5. Competition/rivalry/intrigue
6. Containment/control
7. Collaboration/cooperation
8. Experimentation
9. Self-awareness/consolidation of identity

When considering how best to assist a particular family, one can consider where the parent or parents currently stand on each dimension to get a snapshot of the kind and depth of relationship that will be possible to have with the family. The families who need only information and minimal coaching will tend to be on the higher end of each dimension; those who need a bit more ongoing coaching or training will tend to be in the middle; and families like those described in Chapter 10 ("Infants in Multirisk Families"), who need intensive, ongoing, multifaceted services, will tend to be on the lower end. To determine how best to convey information about the kinds of interactions that will promote healthy development in a particular child, it is essential to assess what kind of relationship is possible with the child's parents or caregivers. It is important to emphasize that the goal is to help families progress in their relationship capacities and broaden the range of their experiences.

Floortime: Supporting the Six Core Developmental Capacities in All Infants and Young Children

So far, we have considered the process of determining what level of educational or clinical intervention a family needs and how and where the services can most effectively be offered. Yet what is it that we want parents, caregivers, and others who work with infants and children to know? What knowledge will enable adults to know how to interact with children in ways that most effectively help them move from early developmental levels to higher ones?

The cornerstone of our approach to prevention and early intervention is what we call "Floortime." This term is a sort of shorthand for a set of principles that guide the application of the DIR model in family relationships, therapeutic interactions, and educational settings. The most fundamental principle of Floortime is that of engaging an infant or child in interactions that mobilize his six core developmental capacities. To be successful, a developmentally based prevention program or early intervention—whether it involves only a brief exchange or two with the child's pediatrician, a 6-week parent training class offered in a community center, or a whole program of social services to assist struggling families—must result in parents or caregivers being able to engage a child in this way.

Technically, Floortime is a period of unstructured, spontaneous play or talk in which the adult follows the child's lead, tuning in as closely as possible to the child's interests and rhythms and attempting to respond in ways that support and amplify whatever themes the child seems to be expressing. With infants and very young children, the adult needs literally to get down on the floor with the child. With older children, one might be playing basketball, walking in the woods, talking on a couch, or sharing in some other activity. Regardless of the activity, the goal of Floortime is to build a warm, trusting relationship in which shared attention, interaction, and communication are occurring on the child's terms. A parent, educator, or therapist can engage a child in this way; a comprehensive therapeutic program may involve all three.

In a perfect world, parents and their children would engage in Floortime regularly and spontaneously. In our busy, work-oriented society, however, Floortime usually must be penciled into mom's or dad's day planner. It is important for parents to reserve at least 20–30 minutes or more for each Floortime session with each child. Often, children will need a number of Floortime sessions. Several 5-minute exchanges during the course of a day do not equal Floortime, because interaction, play, and dialogue have insufficient time to develop fully.

Following the Child's Lead

During Floortime, the parent gets down on the child's level, joining her in activities of her choosing and on her terms. Until the child is well into her school years, parent and child will often literally play on the floor. Playing eye-to-eye with the child generates an atmosphere of equality that encourages the child to engage with the parent, take initiative, and act more assertively. Interacting on the child's terms can also occur when the parent playfully makes funny faces at the child while changing her diaper, chats with her at the dinner table, or takes a long walk with her outside. Whatever the setting, the child's "home turf" is her interests, initiatives, and ideas. The child chooses the emotional tone of the play, and the parent's job is to follow her lead. The parent should be very animated, using hand gestures and lots of facial expressions as he encourages the infant or young child to choose an activity. With a young baby, for example, the parent can join in whatever the baby happens to be doing: clapping, making noises, playing with a rattle. The parent can mirror the baby's emotional gestures and entice the baby to exchange gestures with him. If an older child is painting or building with blocks, the parent can gently try to join her. If a verbal child insists that the parent merely watch her paint a picture, the parent can comply but also gesture to her and say something like, "Gee, I wonder if I could paint, too." If the child responds by listing five reasons why she is a better artist than mom or dad and insists that the parent just watch her paint, that creative interchange *is* a Floortime activity, one centered around the theme, "I'm better than you." By allowing himself to be drawn into this debate, the parent is helping his child string together long chains of two-way communication, use ideas creatively, and practice logical thinking.

Ideally, the parent should join in whatever activity the child chooses, even if it means playing dollhouse or superheroes for the umpteenth time. Any kind of playful sharing is valuable, however, as long as both parties find it enjoyable. If the parent winds up occasionally choosing the activity, she should still encourage the child to take the lead and play as creatively as possible. Letting the child make up new rules and suggest new ways of playing can be a way of building up his assertiveness.

In families with two parents, or two or more adults who play important roles in the child's life, each adult may prefer a different type of play with the child. One parent may be good at acting out stories, whereas the other may prefer art projects or active physical play. In such situations, the child has the opportunity to perceive what each adult enjoys and to initiate different types of interactions with each.

Note that Floortime is not a time for teaching rules; that should be done at other times. Floortime is one arena in which it is safe and appropriate to encourage a child to reign as benevolent dictator. Only two rules govern Floortime: the child cannot hurt people, and she cannot break toys. The adult must step in and enforce these rules if necessary. When limits do need to be set, they should be implemented gently, with lots of accompanying gesturing and verbal explanation, a process that will be explained later.

Opening and Closing Circles of Communication

When a parent follows the child's lead and builds on the child's interests and overtures, the child will usually be inspired, in turn, to build on what the parent does or says. If the child has arranged stuffed animals around a table, as participants in a festive party, the parent might pick up an animal from off to the side and have it say, "Gee, it looks like you guys are having so much fun! Can I join the party, too?" We call this "opening a circle of communication." The child will likely respond by including the new animal in the party or refusing an invitation; either way, the child has built on the parent's words and actions, thus closing that circle of communication. This ability to tune into a partner and build on his response is what makes communication truly interactive. Even when a child's response is a simple, "No!" or "Shhh!" he is closing the circle of communication that his partner opened.

Creating an Appropriate Play Environment

One way to facilitate a child's ability to open and close circles of communication is to stock her play environment with a sampling of age-appropriate play materials, such as dolls, action figures, cars, and blocks. Parent and child can use these materials together to explore the child's natural interests. The parent should try to become an extension of the child's props: when the parent picks up a toy frog, he can speak in a croak; as he pushes a toy car, he can make a "vroom!" sound. In this way, the parent will not be competing with the toys for the child's attention but instead will be using them to promote creative interaction with the child.

Some children do better with a few select toys, whereas others enjoy interacting with the parent while using a wide variety of toys. In addition to helping a child create new dramas, dolls and action figures make it easier for many children to imaginatively explore some of the real situations and real feelings that they experience in everyday life, including scary ones. Parents should avoid relying on board games and puzzles during Floortime. Though such toys definitely have their uses, they tend to create more structured interactions, rather than creative and spontaneous ones.

Extending the Circles of Communication

As parents and child participate in regular Floortime, the parents should help the child expand the scope and length of his playful interactions with them. In other words, they should help their child create longer and longer chains of communication circles. A parent has an opportunity to do this whenever the child is highly motivated to reach a goal. For example, suppose an 18-month-old is longingly looking and pointing at a toy train placed on a shelf too high for him to reach. Instead of simply handing him the train, a parent can say, while holding it out, "Want it?" When the toddler nods and reaches for the toy with a big smile, he is extending the interaction. If a 2-year-old is making loud noises with a hammer and bell, the parent could first acknowledge his activity by commenting, "What a terrific drummer you are!" Then, she could put a duck puppet on her hand, pick up a toy hammer to bang the bell, and exclaim, "Loud! Loud!" If the child shows an interest, or better yet, tries to take the duck puppet and imitate the parent, the parent could expand the activity still further by getting out a dog puppet and starting a simple dialogue between the dog and the duck.

At times, a parent will experience more success in expanding play or conversation with a child by interacting in a playfully obstructive manner. If the child is avoiding the parent during Floortime, the parent can try positioning himself between the child and whatever object or activity is absorbing the child's attention. For example, the parent can take on the role of a moving, talking fence that the child must climb over or under to reach her favorite truck. If the child still seems determined to tune out the parent's friendly overtures, the parent can try covering one of the trucks with his hand to create a tunnel. When the truck does not emerge from the tunnel on its own, the child may be motivated to search for it by picking up the parent's hand. By doing so, she will close a circle of communication, making the play truly interactive.

Broadening the Range of Emotions Expressed by the Child in Interactions

As child and parent play and interact, the parent should be looking for opportunities to add a new twist or plot line that builds on the child's interests. In this way, the parent can engage the child in all the marvelously varied themes of life: closeness and dependency; assertiveness, initiative, and curiosity; aggression, anger, and limit-setting; and pleasure and excitement. In addition, the parent will be introducing the child to themes involving right and wrong and to various thinking skills. The child will develop a growing understanding of new words and of spatial and mathematical concepts.

Despite the parent's best efforts to foster a supportive Floortime environment, there will be times when a child avoids or neglects certain emotional themes and types of interactions. At such times, the parent should gently challenge the child in the areas that the child seems to be bypassing. For example, consider a 3-year-old who is wonderfully easygoing but a little passive when it comes to asserting himself and claiming his own toys during playgroup. A parent could do something as simple as moving his favorite car away from his group of vehicles. The parent will want to appear impish, rather than malicious, and move the car away very slowly and deliberately. The child may well assert himself and come after his prized jeep.

When a child's pretend play seems to center disproportionately on themes of anger and aggression, the parent will need to steel himself not to interfere with the dramatic flow by asking questions like, "Why is [the character] so mad?" "Why doesn't he behave nicely?" Instead, the parent can comment, "Gee, he really wants to bop those bad guys. He's going to destroy them in a hundred different ways. I bet he must have a good reason for that!" By acknowledging both the depth of anger that the child is portraying and the fact that she must have good reason for it, the parent communicates empathy rather than appearing to have his own agenda. The parent's empathy is what eventually helps the child learn how to care about others herself.

All this is easier said than done, because a child's portrayals of anger and aggression tend to be very disturbing for parents. Parents must remember, however, that by supporting the child's verbal and imaginative exploration of such feelings, they are helping him understand and regulate them. Strong feelings, such as anger, that are not acknowledged tend to get acted out. The child who has not been helped to acknowledge and express angry feelings may act them out directly by behaving aggressively or indirectly by becoming overly inhibited or fearful. Recognizing the child's "pretend" agenda and helping him expand on it will help the child use ideas, rather than actions, to negotiate strong feelings. It will also strengthen the parent's ability to discuss and set relevant limits on aggressive behavior if it emerges at school or at home during nonpretend times.

Floortime does not replace discipline; it supplements it. When a child is misbehaving, pretend play can sometimes help reveal what is on her mind, why she is so angry and provocative. The parent's acknowledgment of the child's angry, negative feelings may eventually help the child to introduce positive themes into her dramatic play. Most children have a balance of feelings: if they receive empathic messages that it is okay to explore aggressive themes during play, themes like dependency, love, and concern for others will usually emerge, too. However, if the child senses that the parent does not understand or cannot tolerate her ideas, her frustration may cause her to polarize feelings.

Broadening the Child's Capacity to Use Muscles and Senses as He or She Processes Information

As parent and child interact using sounds, words, sights, touches, and movements, the parent should make a conscious effort to appeal to all the child's senses and to involve the muscles of his body at the same time. The players on the child's "mental team"—his emerging functional emotional capacities—learn to work together in an integrated manner as child and parent interact in an emotionally meaningful way. If the child is playing the conductor of a toy trolley and the parent is playing the trusty brake operator, the parent can do more than just make the screeching noise of the brakes, ring the bell, and call out the names of the stops. He can also introduce some visual and spatial elements into the scenario. Parent and child can spy some robbers hiding behind a nearby chair. The parent can wonder aloud if the thunderstorm that is raging around the trolley will put it behind schedule and ask if the conductor can smell the storm coming. What does it feel like to get drenched by the rain? How much does it cost to ride the trolley?

Similarly, spatial play, such as building towers and forts out of blocks, can promote a broadening of the child's range of sensory processing and motor capacities. Over time, the child may start to build entire cities. The parent can play the assistant architect or construction worker or step into countless other roles. After all, cities need people to deliver food, to provide security, and to keep monsters outside the gates. A child who is overly fond of sitting may be motivated to leap to his feet and play Batman as he tries to scare the monsters away.

Extending a child's capacities can combine fun with excellent learning. Parents, however, should be careful not to try to do too much too quickly. They can feel confident that they are helping their child extend his capacities if they simply keep the basic underlying principles of Floortime in mind as they play and have fun with the child.

Floortime Interactions and Games for Each Developmental Level

The following outline can serve as a guide for parents, daycare workers, and other caregivers to some of the many potentially useful and enjoyable Floortime interactions they can share with children. As the child progresses through each developmental level, the parent or caregiver can incorporate the capacities mastered at that stage and all the prior ones into Floortime interactions. For example, the parents of a 3-year-old can foster logical thinking, imaginative problem-solving interaction, gleeful gestures, love and trust, and concentrated attention all at the same time. This outline is not intended as a comprehensive checklist that caregivers must work through systematically. Instead, it is like a guidebook that a traveler might consult before visiting a foreign country: as intrigued as one might be by the descriptions of hundreds of interesting sights, one would not realistically expect or desire to visit all of them.

For vivid illustrations of the developmental stages and of Floortime approaches, parents and professionals may also want to view two videotapes, *Explor-*

ing First Feelings, produced by the Institute for Mental Health Initiatives, and *Floortime: Tuning in to Each Child*, published by Scholastic, Inc. (Greenspan 1985; Greenspan et al. 1990).

Level 1: Shared Attention and Regulation

Become aware of the baby's unique style of hearing, seeing, touching, smelling, and moving. Harness all her senses in enjoyable ways that simultaneously involve her hearing, vision, touch, smell, and movement. Entice her into the world.

- *The "Look and Listen" Game:* Enjoy face-to-face games with the baby in which you smile and talk to him about his beautiful lips, sparkly eyes, and button nose. As you slowly move your animated face to the right or left, try to capture the baby's attention for a few seconds. This game can be played while holding the baby in your arms, or you can hover near him when he is reclining in an infant seat or lying in another person's arms.
- *The "Soothe Me" Game:* Settle into a comfortable rocking chair and enjoy slow, rhythmic rocking with the baby when she's fussy or tired or during other times when you simply want to cuddle. As you soothingly touch the baby's arms, legs, tummy, back, feet and hands and relax into the lulling back-and-forth rocking rhythm, try to gently move her little fingers and toes in a "This Little Piggy" type of game. You can move her arms, legs, fingers and toes as you change her diaper as well.

Level 2: Engagement and Relating

Observe what kinds of interactions—silly sounds, kisses, tickles, or favorite games—bring the baby or child pleasure and joy. Peekaboo and hiding-the-toy-under-the-box are visual games that delight most babies, and rhythmic clapping games like pat-a-cake will especially intrigue babies with auditory strengths. Moving trucks will delight toddlers, and imaginative dramas will bring joy to most preschoolers.

Make the most of those "magic moments" of availability and relaxed alertness. Interact with the baby for 15- or 20-minute blocks of time at various points during the day. Tune in to the baby's or child's rhythms, to how he feels emotionally and uses his senses and movements. Follow his interests, even if this just involves making silly noises, and you will foster pleasure and closeness. Become a part of an object the child likes, instead of competing with it; for example, put a block he especially likes on your head, and make a funny face.

- *The Smiling Game:* Enjoy using words and funny faces to entice the baby into breaking into a big smile or producing other pleased facial expressions, such as sparkling or widened eyes. You can chatter about the spoon you have stuck in your mouth, or the rattle you have placed on your head, or simply about how "bee-you-ti-ful" his hair is.

- *The "Dance With Me" Sound and Movement Game:* Try to inspire the baby to make sounds and move her arms, legs, or torso in rhythm with your voice and head movements. You might say, "Are you going to dance with me, sweetheart? Oh, I bet you can—I know you can!" while looking for a gleam of delight in her eyes.

Level 3: Two-Way Intentional Affective Signaling and Communication

Be very animated as you exchange subtle facial expressions, sounds, and other gestures as well as words and pretend dramas with the child. Go for the gleam in the child's eye that lets you know he is alert and aware and enjoying this exchange. Help the child open and close circles of communication.

Treat all of a child's behaviors—even the seemingly random ones—as purposeful. For instance, if she flaps her hands in excitement, you could use this behavior as a basis for an interactive "flap your hands" dance step. If her play seems a little aimless as she idly pushes a car back and forth, you might announce that your doll has a special delivery letter that needs to be carried straightaway to one of her favorite television characters. See if she takes the bait!

Help the child go in the direction he wants to by first making his goal easier to achieve. For instance, you could move a bright new ball closer to him after he points his finger and indicates that he wants it. Then, encourage the child's initiative by avoiding doing things for him or to him. When it is time for him to go to bed, for example, see if he can put his favorite teddy bear to bed at the same time, rather than rely on you to do it for him.

Challenge the child to do things to you. For example, when the two of you are roughhousing, entice her to playfully jump on you or climb up onto your shoulders, rather than simply picking her up and swinging her yourself.

- *The Funny Sound, Face, and Feeling Game:* Notice the sounds and facial expressions the baby naturally uses when he's expressing joy, annoyance, surprise, or any other feeling, and mirror these sounds and facial expressions back to him in a playful way. See if you can get a back-and-forth going.
- *The Circle of Communication Game:* Try to see how many back-and-forths you can get going each time the baby touches a shiny red ball or pats your nose and you make a funny squeal or squawk in response. Or see how many times she will try to open your hand when you have hidden an intriguing object inside. Each time the baby follows her interests and takes your bait, she is closing a circle of communication.

Level 4: Long Chains of Coregulated Emotional Signaling and Shared Social Problem Solving

Create extra steps in Floortime plots. For example, try announcing, "This car won't move. What shall we do?" Create interesting barriers or obstacles to the child's goals. Work up to a continuous flow of circles of communication.

Many toddlers can string together 30, 40, and even 50 circles with your help. Be animated and show your feelings through your voice and facial expressions to help the child clarify his intentions. If the child vaguely points to a toy and grunts, you might sometimes feign confusion, put on a puzzled expression, and fetch the "wrong" toy. The child's gestures and vocalizations will become more elaborate and perhaps heated as he works harder to make his wishes understood.

Increase the child's ability to plan her movements and use her senses and imitative skills in different circumstances, such as hide-and-seek and treasure hunt games.

- *The Working Together Game:* Note the toddler's natural interest in various toys, such as dolls, stuffed animals, trucks, and balls, and create a problem that he needs your help to solve that involves that favorite toy.
- *The Copycat Game:* Copy the toddler's sounds and gestures and see if you can entice her to mirror all of your funny faces, sounds, movements, and dance steps. Eventually, add words to the game and then use the words in a purposeful manner to help her meet a need, for example by saying, "Juice" or "Open!"

Level 5: Creating Representations (or Ideas)

Support the child's use of ideas with meaning, intent, or affect, rather than by labeling objects or pictures. Challenge the preschooler to express his needs, desires, or interests. Encourage the child to use ideas both in imaginative play and in realistic verbal interactions. Help the toddler use ideas by fostering situations in which he wants to express his feelings or intentions.

Remember WAA (Words, Action, Affect): Always combine your words or ideas with your affect (expression of feelings) and actions. Encourage the use of all types of ideas; be open to all emotions or themes the child is inclined to explore. Do not forget to incorporate ideas in the form of pictures, signs, and complex spatial designs, as well as words.

- *Let's Chitchat.* Using the child's natural interests, see how many back-and-forth circles of communication you can get going using words, phrases, or short sentences. You can even turn a child's single-word response into a long chat. For instance, when she points to the door and says, "Open," you might reply, "Who should open it?" She's likely to say, ""Mommy do it," and you could shake your head from side to side and say, "Mommy can't now. Who else?" She'll probably turn to her father and ask, "Daddy do it?" Daddy might reply, "Do what?" When the child once again points to the door and says, "Open, open!" Daddy can walk toward her saying, "Okay, can you help me push the door open?" With her eager head nod, the child will be closing this long sequence of back-and-forth words and gestures.

- *Let's Pretend:* Initially, encourage the preschooler's imagination by helping him stage familiar interactions during pretend play. Then, entice him into introducing new plot twists. Become a dog or cat or superhero in a drama of the child's own choosing. Jump into the drama he has begun by assuming the role of a character, ham it up, and see how long you can keep it going. Challenge his dolls or teddy bears to feed each other, hug, kiss, cook, or go off to the park and play. From time to time, switch from becoming a character in one of the child's dramas to taking on the role of a narrator or sideline commentator. Your comments will thicken the plot. Periodically summarize the action and encourage the child to move the drama along.

Level 6: Building Bridges Between Ideas: Logical Thinking

Challenge the child to close all her circles of communication using ideas, both during pretend play and in reality-based dialogues. Challenge her to link different ideas or subplots in a drama. In this way, you will help her build bridges between various ideas. Pull her back on track by acting confused if her thinking becomes a little piecemeal or fragmented. For instance, if her conversation about a neighbor suddenly shifts to a discussion about peanut butter and jelly sandwiches, challenge her to fill in the missing pieces of her thoughts: "Hold on a minute—I thought you were talking about our neighbor, but now you're talking about sandwiches. I'm lost! Which thing do you want to talk about?" Challenge the child with open-ended questions, i.e., those beginning with who, what, where, when, why, and how. Your questions will help the child refocus in a logical way on her meandering thoughts.

Provide multiple-choice possible answers if the child ignores or avoids responding to your open-ended questions. Throw out some silly possibilities for him to consider: "Did the elephant or the iguana visit your classroom today?" Create unexpected situations to challenge the child into greater creativity and new solutions. Expand the child's theme by placing it in different contexts. Challenge the child to broaden the emotional range of his drama.

Encourage reflection on feelings in both pretend dramas and reality-based discussions. Try posing open-ended questions such as "Why do you want to go outside?" or "What's the reason for the space invaders' attack?" Gradually increase the complexity of the preschooler's reflective thinking by challenging her to suggest different motives or to consider different points of view on various subjects. Follow up later on themes that are expressed during pretend play. For instance, when the child returns home after preschool, you could inquire, "How is that new boy in school acting these days? Has he learned to share his blocks yet?" Challenge the child to give her opinion rather than recite facts.

Enjoy debating and negotiating with the child rather than simply stating rules (except when the rule is absolutely essential). Encourage and challenge the child's use of more and more ideas as part of logical, emotionally meaningful dialogues, instead of focusing on correct grammar. As the two of you get a rich exchange of ideas going, the child will be learning to express himself logically. His grammar will usually improve in a natural fashion as he becomes a better abstract thinker.

Foster motor planning and sequencing capacities in the child. You can even incorporate sketches and diagrams as well as search games, obstacle courses, and building projects into your pretend play together. Encourage the child's understanding and mastering of time concepts. Challenge her during real-life conversations and pretend play to incorporate concepts about the past, present, and future. For instance, you could pose questions such as, "What are the cowboys going to do tomorrow?"

Encourage the understanding and use of quantity concepts. Negotiate with the child when he asks you for an extra cookie or an extra slice of pizza. When you two of you play make-believe, speculate on how many cups of tea should be served to each doll at the tea party. Provide the child with an emotional, real-life understanding of basic concepts whenever you offer him any preacademic or early academic work. For example, you can negotiate using candies, cookies, or coins to learn the concepts of adding and subtracting. Keep the numbers small—under six—to avoid the child's having to rely on rote memory.

Keep challenging the child in both your pretend and reality-based conversations toward higher levels of abstraction by shifting back and forth between details and the big picture. Periodically ask her how all the things she's been talking about fit together to help her "see the forest for the trees." Press her for details if she has a harder time seeing individual branches and trees in the green blur of the forest. Gradually expand the child's range of experiences—inside and outside, socially, and physically—because emotionally based experiences are the seedbed for creative, logical, and abstract thought.

- *The Director Game:* See how many plot shifts or new story lines the child can initiate as the two of you play make-believe games together. After the tea party play becomes a little repetitive or lacks direction, you can subtly challenge the child to thicken the plot by announcing something like, "I'm so full of tea my tummy's sloshing! What can we do next?"
- *"Why Should I?" Game:* When the child wants you to do things for him, gently tease him with a response of "Why should I?" and see how many reasons he can give you. Then offer a compromise, such as "Let's do it together," when he

wants you to get his riding toy out of the garage or pick out a new outfit to wear, and so on.

Developmentally Based Prevention and Early Intervention for Children With Special Challenges

The kinds of experiences and interactions described in the previous sections will promote children's core developmental capacities and enable them to move "up the ladder" developmentally. Such experiences must be made available to every child. They will enable children without special challenges to build stronger social, intellectual, and emotional capacities. They can help children who have impairments or extreme differences in sensory processing and motor capacities overcome these challenges. They can be especially helpful to children with severe and pervasive developmental challenges such as autism. However, in applying developmentally based prevention and early intervention approaches to children with special needs, we must work much more intensively with each family and must spend much more effort tailoring Floortime exercises to each child's motor and sensory profile.

Children With Regulatory-Sensory Processing and Motor Challenges

Children come into the world with individual variations in physical makeup—that is, they differ in the ways in which they take in and experience sensations such as sights, sounds, touch, and smells and the ways in which they plan and execute motor actions. Children who have challenges in one or more of these areas have often been misunderstood; although parents, teachers, and others correctly sense something unusual about these children, they are described in global terms as "difficult babies" or as having "a difficult temperament." Because their specific processing and motor differences often go undiagnosed, parents and professionals alike have trouble figuring out how to interact with them in ways that help them attend and focus, calm down, and relate smoothly. The strategies that "work" with most children may not succeed, leaving parents and professionals discouraged.

Children with processing and motor challenges need the same Floortime strategies described earlier, but these strategies must be tailored to each child's regulatory profile. (For a full discussion of therapeutic approaches for children with regulatory-sensory processing differences or disorders, see Chapter 8, "Assessment and Treatment of Infants and Young Children With Regulatory-Sensory Processing Disorders.") As we have discussed elsewhere in this volume, children's regulatory capacities differ in the following areas:

- Sensory modulation, including hyper- or hyporeactivity in each sensory pathway
- Sensory processing, including the ability to register, decode, and comprehend sequences and abstract patterns in each sensory pathway

- Sensory-affective processing, or the ability to process and respond to affect
- Muscle tone
- Motor planning and sequencing, or the ability to purposefully organize a sequence of actions or symbols

In many cases, specialized clinical intervention with an occupational or physical therapist is needed to work directly with the child and/or help parents understand their child's unique processing and motor challenges and adjust their interactions accordingly, so that parent–child interactions promote rather than undermine the child's progress to higher developmental capacities. Many educators also need training and coaching to interact with and teach each child in ways that best fit her processing style and motor capacities and thus help her reach educational goals.

To understand how Floortime activities can be tailored to a particular child's regulatory pattern, consider the case of Jane, who from birth was extremely sensitive to sound, touch, and smell. Her mother's instinct was to cuddle and stroke her, approaches that had helped soothe her other children when they were infants. Jane, however, would squirm, cry, and be inconsolable. She experienced routine activities like having her hair brushed, getting her diaper changed, and being bathed as physically painful. Due to her sensitivity to sound, she found her parents' voices not soothing and comforting, but irritating and intrusive. Because she was easily upset by smells, clothes washed in certain detergents irritated her. In short, her sensory sensitivities made her experience of the physical world, and hence of daily human interactions, generally unpleasant for her.

As Jane got older, she was often inattentive and easily distracted, because she was unable to screen out sensory stimuli. When she found herself in a busy classroom for the first time, where kids bumped against her sensitive skin, startled her with yells and screams during recess, and sometimes intruded into the well-defined, protected space she had set out for herself, her reactions ranged from tantrums to fearful avoidance.

Parents and teachers of a child like Jane can learn to understand the child's sensitive makeup, read her signals, and interact in ways that help her avoid becoming overwhelmed. They can experiment to find just the right vocal tone and rhythm and the most soothing kind of touch. For example, children like Jane often calm down better with firm pressure on the back, arms, and legs, rather than a lighter touch, which tends to irritate and agitate them. Parents can be coached to introduce their child to new sensory experiences—a new shirt with an unfamiliar texture, a visit to a busy museum—very gradually, in small increments. As the child grows older, she can be helped to understand that she is very sensitive in certain ways, to predict which situations may trigger her sensitivities and upset her, and to practice and prepare for such situations. Eventually, her own emotional sensitivity may become a basis for developing a sense of empathy and compassion for others as well as leadership abilities. In many cases, as children learn to deal with their own physical tendencies and to become more flexible, assertive, and empathic, their physical tendencies may change. Certain types of touch or sound, for example, may become more comfortable.

Helping the Child Master His or Her Unique Way of Responding to Sensations: Floortime Interactions and Games for Various Regulatory Profiles

The following guide can be used to help parents and teachers tailor their interactions to children's unique processing and motor styles. The goal of Floortime remains the same as for any child: to help the child master all six critical learning experiences—attending, engagement, two-way communication, preverbal problem-solving, using ideas, and emotional and abstract thinking. Yet reaching this goal requires that the adult understand and adapt interactions to the child's regulatory profile. As adult and child play, the adult will begin to recognize whether soothing or vibrant, noisy or subdued, visual or aural, free-form or limit-setting approaches will work best for the individual child.

The overreactive infant and child.   Some children are sensitive to light touches, certain sounds, bright lights, or abrupt movements. As one interacts with them during play, they may be very cautious and may need lots of time to adjust to anything new. They may also have a special need to be the boss of all the action and to control others. Children with sensitivities naturally want to test the waters of life only one toe at a time and need to be wooed into pretend play gradually. It is vitally important to respect their need to be in charge and to let them use Floortime interactions as a way to experiment gradually with assertiveness.

The underreactive infant and child.   Underreactive children are very reluctant to assert their wills by gesturing, using words, or playing "Let's pretend." Instead of always doing *for* the child, however, one needs to woo or *entice* such a youngster into activity. Over time, the bits and pieces of opinions and assertiveness shown by the underwhelmed child will lead him to joyfully step into all sorts of make-believe roles. He will relish being one of the people who are in control, like teachers, kings, and superheroes, and will grandly order Mom and Dad around the room in an active, rather than passive, manner. Often a child may need to manifest assertiveness or aggression through gestures and pretend play before he can express it with words.

The infant and child who crave sensations.   Very active children provide a different challenge. Here the task is twofold: to "go with the flow" and build on their natural interests and to hold their attention and help them elaborate on their interests rather than flit from one topic to another. If such a child is not engaged in this flexible way, her craving for new sights, sounds, and touches may lead to frenzied, aimless behavior rather than to active and organized play. Once her energies are focused on a theme she has chosen herself, she may be able to sit down and concentrate for 15 minutes or more. Try to mix in "modulation" games, going from fast to slow, noisy to quiet, to help her learn to regulate her behavior. Provide extra soothing, warmth, and pretending to encourage empathy and the use of ideas as well as actions. Remember to be gentle but firm in providing the child with guidance and limits.

The infant and child who have a relative strength in comprehending what they see over what they hear. These children have a harder time figuring out certain sounds and often find it difficult to pay attention to others' words. Rather than simply naming objects, or pointing to pictures in a book, parents and teachers can use Floortime to give lots of extra opportunities to practice understanding words. Pretend play in which a child is naturally motivated to "talk" for his dolls or action figures is a far more natural and fun way to support verbalization. Chatting or debating with the child when he really wants something helps him pay attention to sounds as well.

The infant and child who have a relative strength in comprehending what they hear over what they see. Treasure hunts, building things, visualization, and the use of visually exciting props during pretend play are all useful in enticing children to pay attention to and figure out sights.

Children With Neurodevelopmental Disorders of Relating and Communicating

The developmental challenges in children with neurodevelopmental disorders of relating and communicating (NDRC) go beyond the differences in sensory modulation, sensory processing, and motor capacities described in the previous section. In autism spectrum disorders, regulatory-sensory processing challenges are not only present but also contribute to an overall derailment of the child's fundamental capacities to relate, communicate, and think. As described in Chapter 9 ("Assessment and Treatment of Infants and Young Children With Neurodevelopmental Disorders of Relating and Communicating"), early detection of such impairments is vital if intervention is to succeed in helping children reach their full potential. Because the early years of development are so important, every month of effective intervention can contribute to huge gains for the child, enabling her to begin mastering capacities that may be difficult or impossible to teach in the later years. Too often, parents and teachers have, with the best of intentions, lost precious time waiting for a child with evidence of an autism spectrum disorder to "grow out of it." By using the six functional-emotional developmental capacities as the basis for observing children, a parent, clinician, or educator can confidently detect the problem as soon as the child fails to master basic milestones, such as warm relatedness and communication with gestures. When problems are detected early, caregivers and children can, to varying degrees, learn to work around regulatory dysfunctions and their associated relationship and communication problems. They can, again to varying degrees, form warm, empathetic, and satisfying relationships. See Table 11–2 for an outline of early signs of autism spectrum disorders.

In addition to enabling early detection of problems, a comprehensive, developmentally based approach to assessment can offer families a picture of their child's unique challenges as well as his unique strengths. Traditionally, we have considered children with special needs in terms of syndromes, such as "autism," "pervasive developmental disorder," and "mental retardation," and assumed that the children who share each label have the same impairments, require the same treatment approaches, and have similar prognoses. Children labeled autistic, for example, have been expected to remain largely disengaged from other human beings and to lead limited lives. Most have not been expected to go to college or to live independently. When viewed in terms of their core developmental capacities, however, children who share this label turn out to be quite different from one another. Each child has a unique nervous system and requires unique types of interaction in order to reach his potential. In our clinical work, we have found that many children diagnosed as having autism spectrum disorders can indeed become warmly related and joyful.

As in DIR assessment of any child and family, the assessment process yields an individual developmental profile describing 1) which of the core developmental capacities the child has mastered fully, partially, or not at all; 2) how the child reacts to sensations, processes information, plans actions, and sequences behaviors and thoughts; 3) family dynamics and interaction patterns; and 4) the kinds of interactions—resulting from #2 and #3—that the child typically experiences and the kinds of interactions she needs in order to master missing or constricted core capacities. It is this profile, rather than the particular syndrome, that determines the appropriate intervention program. The traditional pessimistic prognosis for pervasive developmental disorder is based on experience with children whose treatment programs tend to be mechanical and structured rather than based on individual differences, relationships, affect, and emotional cuing. Approaches that do not pull the child into spontaneous, joyful relationship patterns may intensify rather than remediate the difficulty.

The goal of intervention is to get the child back into, or to establish, a continuous flow of natural, warm communication. To accomplish this goal, treatment must help the child master the six core development capacities (to attend, engage, interact purposefully, experience a range of feelings, and ultimately think and relate in an organized, logical manner). Caregivers must be helped to provide the kinds of interactive experiences necessary for the child to master these capacities. Because children with pervasive developmental delays do not provide the kind of interactive feedback that parents intuitively expect, engaging in Floortime with them presents a formidable challenge for parents. A smiling baby easily elicits smiles from most adults, but a child who gives only aimless, perseverative, or self-absorbed feedback will likely elicit confusion and perhaps frustration. The adult's natural response to these feelings may be to either become overly rigid and controlling or to withdraw. Most parents will need intensive, specialized intervention to help them understand their children's sensory and motor experience and tailor Floortime interactions accordingly. In addition, an educational setting must be selected or tailored to meet the child's need for both special teaching expertise and peer interaction that provides the kind of feedback the child needs to develop his capacity for intentional relating.

In helping parents learn to tailor Floortime interactions to each child, we have observed that a critical component of progress for children with NDRC resides in our ability to help these children use their own emotions, desires, and intentions to guide first their behavior and later their thoughts. This means harnessing their natural desires to give purpose to their gestures and meaning to their words—holding a cookie we know the child wants and challenging her to grasp it, and later challenging her to use the words "eat cookie" to get a cookie for herself or, during pretend play, for her favorite teddy bear. From the simplest gestures, such as smiling, frowning, and turning away, to more complex behaviors—imitating a sound, taking a parent by the hand to recruit help in finding a toy, using words and concepts—the child's behavior is driven by her emotions, wishes, and desires. The more we can help a child connect her emotions to her behavior and her thoughts, the more we can help her become a person with purpose, meaning, and the capacity to understand her world.

Parents, teachers, and clinicians can learn to build on even the most perseverative, repetitive, and withdrawn behavior in order to help children become more emotionally engaged and intentional. For example, suppose a child is sitting alone, endlessly spinning the wheel of a toy car. Instead of trying to get him to look up, switch to another activity, or play with the car differently, the adult can reach over, with a warm smile, and spin the wheel in the opposite direction. Chances are the child will feel motivated to respond in some way, perhaps by putting his hand over the adult's hand. If a child is mechanically opening and closing a door, the adult can playfully "get stuck" in the doorway, thus provoking a response. If the child tries to get the adult out of the way, he has closed a circle of communication. As these examples illustrate, by playing off the child's current interest, however perseverative it may be, the adult can get affective interaction going. (For additional case examples,

TABLE 11–2. Earliest signs of autism spectrum and related developmental disorders

What to encourage: healthy foundations for relating, communicating, and thinking	Early signs leading to autism spectrum disorders	Associated symptoms
Shared attention and regulation (begins at 0–3 months)		
Calm interest in and purposeful responses to sights, sound, touch, movement, and other sensory experiences (e.g., looking, turning to sounds)	Lack of sustained attention to different sights or sounds	Aimless or self-stimulatory behavior
Engagement and relating (begins at 2–5 months)		
Growing feelings of intimacy and relatedness (e.g., has a gleam in her eye and initiates and sustains joyful smiles)	No engagement or only fleeting expressions of joy rather than robust, sustained, engagement	Self-absorption or withdrawal
Two-way intentional affective signaling and communication (begins at 4–10 months)		
A range of back-and-forth interactions with emotional expressions, sounds, and hand gestures to convey intentions	No interactions or only brief back-and-forth interactions with little initiative-taking (i.e., mostly responding)	Unpredictable (random and/or impulsive) behavior

TABLE 11–2. Earliest signs of autism spectrum and related developmental disorders *(continued)*

What to encourage: healthy foundations for relating, communicating, and thinking	Early signs leading to autism spectrum disorders	Associated symptoms
Long chains of coregulated emotional signaling and shared social problem solving (e.g., joint attention; begins at 10–18 months)	Unable to initiate and sustain many back-and-forth social interactions in a row (showing dad a toy)	Repetitive or perseverative behaviors
Creating representations (or ideas; begins at 18–30 months)	No words or scripted use of words (e.g., mostly repeats what is heard)	Echolalia and other forms of repetition of what is heard or seen.
Building bridges between ideas: logical thinking (begins at 30–42 months) Creates logical connections between meaningful ideas ("Want to go outside *because* I want to play?")	No words or memorized scripts coupled with random, rather than logical, use of ideas	Illogical or unrealistic use of behaviors and/or ideas

Note. For more information, please visit http://www.icdl.com. In addition, see Greenspan SI, Wieder S: *The Child With Special Needs: Encouraging Intellectual and Emotional Growth.* Reading, MA, Perseus Books, 1998; and Greenspan SI: *Engaging Autism.* Reading, MA, DaCapo Press/Perseus Books, 2005.

see Chapter 9, "Assessment and Treatment of Infants and Young Children With Neurodevelopmental Disorders of Relating and Communicating.")

Many children with special needs have things done for them, rather than initiating activities in response to their own wishes. Because a child's own desires and interests are a critical part of who she is, caregivers, clinicians, and teachers seem to do best when they can entice a child to use her own initiative and desires to practice necessary skills. When we challenge a child to take initiative, she develops a little more sense of personhood, a little more understanding of who she is, what she wants, and what she is capable of doing. When parents and therapists work this way, the children often surprise them with unsuspected new skills.

Children With Other Types of Special Needs

The DIR approach to assessment and intervention can also help children with mental retardation, cerebral palsy, and other conditions to achieve their full potential. Traditionally, children with mental retardation were thought to lag equally in language, cognition, motor abilities, auditory processing, and visuospatial processing. We have assessed many such children, however, and found that their individual profiles included both strengths and weaknesses in auditory processing, visuospatial processing, muscle tone, and motor planning. In working with both mentally retarded children and children with cerebral palsy, we have also found that one deficit often keeps other capacities from developing properly. For example, a child who could move only her tongue was believed to have very severe cognitive delays and no communication ability at all. However, once we taught her to use movements of her tongue to indicate "yes" and "no," she revealed greater potential for deliberate two-way communication. In a fairly short time, she was using her tongue to indicate her wishes and intentions, abilities her clinicians had previously assumed were beyond her. Even much more subtle difficulties with motor planning or sequencing may undermine a child's ability to communicate (for example, to put together a sequence of gestures) and therefore cause her to miss out on the types of interactions likely to foster intellectual and emotional growth.

For a full discussion of therapeutic work with children who have a variety of special needs, see *The Child With Special Needs: Encouraging Emotional and Intellectual Growth* (Greenspan and Wieder 1998).

Developmentally Based Prevention and Early Intervention for Multirisk Families

In some families, as we saw in Chapter 10 ("Infants in Multirisk Families"), fostering healthy development in the children requires the social service system to intervene at all levels of the "service pyramid" (see Figure 11–1). Such families face multiple hardships that can compromise healthy development. These may include insufficient food, lack of affordable shelter, untreated psychiatric illnesses in one or both parents, maladaptive patterns of interaction among family members, and lack of connection to available social services. In "multirisk" families, we may see children who are developing in a healthy manner, children with regulatory disorders, or children with pervasive developmental disorders or other special needs. Once a family is discovered to be under severe stress from multiple hardships, it is critical that the service system reach out to offer comprehensive preventive intervention, even if the children are currently developing in a healthy way. By intervening early, we can prevent the family's dire situation from compromising the children's development. (For a full discussion of prevention and early intervention with multirisk families, see Chapter 10.)

Conclusion

A comprehensive approach to prevention and preventive intervention begins with understanding the infant's expected emotional, social, and cognitive progression and the types of caregiver and family patterns that support it. With this understanding, healthy development can be facilitated. In addition, risk factors can be identified and worked with, early signs of challenges or early expressions of disorders can be fully evaluated, and intervention begun as soon as possible. The DIR model provides a framework for pursuing these goals.

References

Greenspan SI: Exploring First Feelings (video). Washington, DC, Institute for Mental Health Initiatives, 1985

Greenspan SI: Greenspan Social-Emotional Growth Chart. Bulverde, TX, The Psychological Corporation, 2004

Greenspan SI, Wieder S: The Child With Special Needs: Encouraging Intellectual and Emotional Growth. Reading, MA, Perseus Books, 1998

Greenspan SI, Wilford S, Hanna S: Floortime: Tuning in to Each Child (video). New York, Scholastic, 1990

Greenspan SI, DeGangi GA, Wieder S: The Functional Emotional Assessment Scale (FEAS) for Infancy and Early Childhood: Clinical and Research Applications. Bethesda, MD, Interdisciplinary Council on Developmental and Learning Disorders, 2001

Index

Page numbers printed in **boldface** type refer to tables or figures.